Geriatric Dentistry

Caring for Our Aging Population

Geriatric Dentistry

Caring for Our Aging Population

EDITED BY

Paula K. Friedman DDS, CAGS, MSD, MPH

Past President, American Society of Geriatric Dentistry
Professor and Director
Geriatrics and Gerontology Section
Department of General Dentistry
Henry M. Goldman School of Dental Medicine
Boston University
Boston, MA
USA

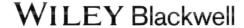

This edition first published 2014
© 2014 by John Wiley & Sons, Inc.

Editorial Offices

1606 Golden Aspen Drive, Suites 103 and 104, Ames, Iowa 50010, USA

The Atrium, Southern Gate, Chichester, West Sussex, PO19 8SQ, UK

9600 Garsington Road, Oxford, OX4 2DQ, UK

For details of our global editorial offices, for customer services and for information about how to apply for permission to reuse the copyright material in this book please see our website at www.wiley.com/wiley-blackwell.

Authorization to photocopy items for internal or personal use, or the internal or personal use of specific clients, is granted by Blackwell Publishing, provided that the base fee is paid directly to the Copyright Clearance Center, 222 Rosewood Drive, Danvers, MA 01923. For those organizations that have been granted a photocopy license by CCC, a separate system of payments has been arranged. The fee codes for users of the Transactional Reporting Service are ISBN-13: 978-1-1183-0016-9 / 2014.

A catalogue record for this book is available from the Library of Congress and British Library.

Wiley also publishes its books in a variety of electronic formats. Some content that appears in print may not be available in electronic books.

Cover image: iStock / © traffic_analyzer
Cover design by Meaden Creative

Set in 9/12 pt Meridien by SPi Publisher Services, Pondicherry, India

1   2014

Contents

List of Contributors

Douglas Berkey, DMD, MPH, MS
Professor (Emeritus)
University of Colorado School of Dental Medicine
Aurora, CO, USA

Mary Bertone, RDH, BScDH
Centre for Community Oral Health
Faculty of Dentistry
University of Manitoba
Winnipeg, MB, Canada

Jayne E. Cernohous, DDS
Associate Professor
Department of Dental Hygiene
Metropolitan State University
St. Paul, MN, USA

Elisa M. Chávez, DDS
Associate Professor
Department of Dental Practice
Director, Pacific Dental Program at Laguna Honda Hospital
University of the Pacific
Arthur A. Dugoni School of Dentistry
San Francisco, CA, USA

Jessica De Bord, DDS, MSD, MA
Pediatric Dentist
Children's Village
Yakima, WA, USA;
Affiliate Assistant Professor
Department of Pediatric Dentistry
University of Washington
Seattle, WA, USA

Teresa A. Dolan, DDS, MPH
Vice President and Chief Clinical Officer
DENTSPLY International
York, PA, USA;
Professor and Dean (Emeritus)
University of Florida College of Dentistry
Gainesville, FL, USA

Diane Ede-Nichols, DMD, MHL, MPH
Chairperson
Department of Community Dentistry
Nova Southeastern University College of Dental Medicine
Fort Lauderdale, FL, USA

Ronald L. Ettinger, BDS, MDS, DDSc, DABSCD
Professor
Department of Prosthodontics
Dows Institute for Dental Research
University of Iowa College of Dentistry
Iowa City, IA, USA

Ruth S. Goldblatt, DMD, FAGD, FASGD, DABSCD
Associate Clinical Professor
Department of Craniofacial Sciences
University of Connecticut, School of Dental Medicine
Farmington, CT, USA

Harold E. Goodis, DDS
Professor Emeritus
University of California School of Dentistry
San Francisco, CA, USA
Chief Executive Officer/Chief Academic Officer
Boston University Institute for Dental Research
and Education
Dubai, UEA

Dick Gregory, DDS
School of Dentistry
University of California
San Francisco, CA, USA

Saroj Gupta, DDS
Department of Periodontics
University of Maryland
Baltimore, MD, USA

Kelly A. Halligan, DDS, PC
Private Practitioner
Colorado Springs, CO, USA

Timothy J. Halligan, DMD, ABGD, DABSCD
Director, Advanced Education in General Dentistry (AEGD)
Consultant Surgeon General Hospital Dentistry
United States Air Force Dental Corps
Colorado Springs, CO, USA

Jadwiga Hjertstedt, DDS, MS
Clinical Associate Professor
Department of Clinical Services
Marquette University School of Dentistry
Milwaukee, WI, USA

Susan Hyde, DDS, MPH, PhD, FACD
Associate Professor of Preventive and
Restorative Dental Sciences
Chair, Division of Oral Epidemiology
and Dental Public Health
Interprofessional Education Faculty Lead, Dentistry
Director for Dentistry, Multidisciplinary Fellowship in Geriatrics
School of Dentistry
University of California
San Francisco, CA, USA

Deborah A. Jacobi, RDH, MA
Associate Director
Helping Services for Northeast Iowa
Decorah, IA, USA

Teresa E. Johnson, DDS, MS, MPH, FASGD, DABSCD
Education and Quality Assurance Director
Apple Tree Dental
Minneapolis, MN, USA

Peter Y. Kawamura, DDS, MS, FASGD, DABSCD, FACD
Staff Geriatric Dentist/Prosthodontist
Department of Veterans Affairs Medical Center
San Francisco, CA, USA

Bassam M. Kinaia, DDS, MS
Associate Professor
Department of Periodontology and Dental Hygiene
University of Detroit-Mercy School of Dentistry
Detroit, MI, USA

Harvey Levy, DMD, MAGD, DABSCD
Department Head
Frederick Memorial Hospital
Frederick, MD, USA

Paul Mulhausen, MD, MHS
Chief Medical Officer
Telligen
West Des Moines, IA, USA

Miriam R. Robbins, DDS, MS
Clinical Associate Professor
Director, Special Needs Clinic
Associate Chair
Department of Oral and Maxillofacial Pathology,
Radiology, and Medicine
New York University College of Dentistry
New York, NY, USA

Ralph H. Saunders, DDS, MS
Professor
Eastman Institute for Oral Health
University of Rochester
Rochester, NY, USA

Mary R. Truhlar, DDS, MS
Interim Dean
Professor and Chair
Department of General Dentistry
School of Dental Medicine
Stony Brook University
Stony Brook, NY, USA

Mickey Emmons Wener, RDH, BS(DH), MEd
School of Dental Hygiene
Faculty of Dentistry
University of Manitoba
Winnipeg, MB, Canada

Michael Wiseman,
DDS, M SND, RCS(Edin), FASGD
Assistant Professor
Faculty of Dentistry
McGill University
Montreal, QC, Canada;
Chief of Dentistry
Mount Sinai Hospital
Montreal, QC, Canada

Bei Wu, PhD
Professor
School of Nursing and Global Health Institute
Duke University
Durham, NC, USA

Carol-Ann Yakiwchuk, RDH, BScDH, MHS
Faculty of Dentistry
University of British Columbia
Vancouver, BC, Canada

Janet A. Yellowitz, DMD, MPH, FASGD, DABSCD
Director, Geriatric Dentistry
Director, Special Care Dentistry
Associate Professor
Department of Periodontics
University of Maryland Dental School
Baltimore, MD, USA

Dedication

This book is dedicated to a number of significant individuals in my life:

My mother, Beatrice Gibbs, who demonstrated every day of her life what it meant to age successfully. She was my inspiration, my supporter, and a role model of a woman achiever in a time when there were very few women pushing boundaries.

My husband Emanuel, who encouraged me throughout the extensive and demanding writing and editing process. He never complained about the amount of time I spent on this legacy project. He shares my passion for accomplishing goals, and I am grateful for his continual support.

My patient, committed, responsive, and receptive contributors. The book could not have happened without all of you.

Introduction

Caring for and about our aging population has been a priority for me since I was a child. I had a close relationship with my grandmother and grandfather. They were warm, wonderful people. When my grandmother was in her 60s, she developed Alzheimer's disease. It was painful to witness her slow, inexorable decline. My grandfather was a strong man in his youth – a wrestling champion, in fact, before he immigrated to the United States. But he too suffered the wounds and arrows of aging. Although he retained his mental sharpness, his physical status belied his mental acuity.

From the moment that each of us is born, we are aging. For some, the prospect of aging is a very serious matter. And there is no doubt that there may be serious issues associated with aging, including health issues, mental status, financial considerations, and housing and transportation challenges. However, there is humor associated with the aging process. Consider that aging is a very relative term. To a teenager, someone aged 25 is "old." Many of our patients, themselves senior citizens (often in their late 80s), refer to neighbors, friends, co-residents in assisted living facilities as "they are so old," when, in fact, the people to whom they refer are in their 90s and the person speaking may be aged 88 or 89. New phraseology has arisen to describe our aging phenomenon, such as "60 is the new 40," or professionally speaking, "Age is just a number; it is functional status that counts." Here is an important fact about the US population:

> The age cohort of 85 and older is the most rapidly growing age cohort in the country, and the subset of that population called the "centenarians" is the quickest growing segment percentage-wise.

The rapidly growing baby boomer cohort in the USA is turning 65 at the rate of approximately 10 000 people per day, and will continue to do so for approximately 15 more years by the time this book is published. The paradox that faces us is that although the aging population is increasing, to a large extent they are invisible – in a social sense, in a healthcare sense, and in a public policy sense.

The "demographic imperative," or the mandate of the numbers, makes clear that the training of all health professionals must include information about how to care for our aging population. This book was conceived on the premise that there were a number of very good books on geriatric dentistry that were robust reviews of the literature and full of evidence-based information and conclusions. There is far less resource information available on the practical aspects of treating and caring for elders, a "how to" guide, of sorts. This book is intended to address that void in the literature. The intended audiences are widely defined: dental students, dentists, hygiene students, hygienists, mid-level providers, allied (non-dental) health providers, and the lay public. Each of the author contributors was charged with providing the most practical information possible in their assigned/chosen area. We tried to include case studies, where appropriate, in each chapter to illustrate the content in a practical clinical application.

The reader will note a number of terms used throughout the book that are intended to be synonymous. They were not changed out of respect for the integrity of each contributor's work. Throughout the text, the terms "aged," "geriatric," "older adults," "senior citizens," and "elders" are all interchangeable. Terms like "cognitively impaired," "Alzheimer's disease," and "dementia" are similarly synonymous. We did not make all chapters read with the same terminology because all of those terms are commonly used in discussions by and with patients and families. Although the editor contributed to each and every chapter, the editor elected not to include her name as a co-author because the primary work of each chapter is that of the listed contributors.

A word about the process of writing and editing a book: I am confident that few of the contributors fully understood the magnitude of the time commitment that each was making in agreeing to participate in this endeavor. We are fortunate to have a combination of well-known, esteemed experts in the field and some newer authors whose contributions are equally valued. Our original timeline was extended a little bit due to a number of factors; the overarching theme for people not being able to meet original commitments is that "life happens." During the process of writing this book, we collectively experienced health, marriage, birth, death, illness, and recovery. Despite the powerful impact of life on the authors, people maintained their dedication and commitment to getting the job done. The motivation that drove everyone, I believe, was that we each want to leave a legacy of our knowledge and experience to pass on to dental providers of the future. There is no doubt that techniques, methodology, and materials may change over time, but the underlying tenet of the importance of caring for our aging population will always remain the same.

The book is organized into six sections: Underlying Principles of Aging, Clinical Practice, Decision Making and Treatment Planning, Common Geriatric Oral Conditions and their Clinical Implications, Care Delivery, and Future Vision. Each section contains a number of chapters and topics. In the section on Underlying Principles of Aging (**Part 1**), we will learn about implications for the oral cavity, racial and ethnic disparities in oral status and aging, death and dying, palliative care, and functional status. The next section (**Part 2**) is Clinical Practice. In this section, legal and financial considerations for the provider including living arrangements (assisted living and continuous care communities), informed consent, and advanced directives/living will, the Palmore's "Facts on Aging" attitudinal instrument, and practical tips and techniques for creating a senior-friendly dental office are discussed. **Part 3** covers Decision Making and Treatment Planning. In this section, assessing the elderly patient, treatment considerations, and evidence-based practice are covered. **Part 4** addresses common geriatric oral conditions and their clinical implication. In this section, we learn about root caries, periodontal disease, diseases of the pulp, diseases of the oral mucous membranes, xerostomia, prosthetic considerations, and medical complexities. **Part 5** focuses on care delivery, including delivery systems – nursing home dentistry, portable dentistry, home visits, and senior centers. Additionally, this section informs the reader about oral health care in long-term care facilities (including policies and practice); dental professionals as part of an interdisciplinary team and the expanding oral health team. The final part, **Part 6**, consists of a visionary and challenging chapter "Planning for the Future," which includes political implications and potential professional initiatives. Chapters may complement/supplement other chapters, but each is designed to provide information independent of other chapters.

Everyone who worked on this book is a champion. The contributors each gave of himself or herself to make this the best book possible. My liaison with Wiley Blackwell, Nancy Turner, gave regular guidance and support and was an additional invaluable interface with the authors. It is our collective hope and expectation that the many years of expertise reflected in the pages of these chapters will help to reinforce the importance of oral health to overall health in our aging population, and moreover will provide the tools, techniques, and resources for those committed to improving the oral health status of our aging population. We hope that you will use the valuable contents to benefit someone you care for, care about, or will care for in the future.

Paula K. Friedman, DDS, MSD, MPH
Editor

About the Companion Website

This book is accompanied by a companion website:

www.wiley.com/go/friedman/geriatricdentistry

The website includes:
- Powerpoints of all figures from the book for downloading
- Discussion questions and answers

Scan this QR code to visit the companion website:

PART 1

Underlying Principles of Aging

CHAPTER 1

Aging: Implications for the Oral Cavity

Bei Wu

School of Nursing and Global Health Institute, Duke University, Durham, NC, USA

Aging of the US population

The US aging population is increasing. The US older population, that is individuals aged 65 and older, reached 40.3 million in 2010. This is an increase of 5.3 million compared to the 2000 census. The percentage of the US population aged 65 and older also increased from 2000 to 2010. In 2010, the older population represented 13.0% of the total population, an increase from 12.4% in 2000 (Vincent & Velkoff, 2010). In the USA, by 2030 it is projected that there will be about 72.1 million older people, more than twice their number in 2000. Individuals aged 65 and older are expected to grow to become 19% of the US population by 2030 (Administration on Aging, 2012). By 2050, it is projected that there will be about 88.5 million older adults, 20.2% of the US population (US Census Bureau, 2008a).

Ethnic diversity

The US population is becoming increasingly diverse, and this is true for the aging population too. In the USA, among those aged 65 and older in 2050, 77% of the elder population are projected to be White-alone, down from 87% in 2010. Within the same age group, 12% are projected to be Black-alone and 9% are projected to be Asian-alone in 2050, up from 9% and 3%, respectively, in 2010. The Hispanic proportion of the older population is projected to quickly increase over the next four decades. By 2050, 20% of the US population aged 65 and over are projected to be Hispanic, up from 7% in 2010. The smallest race groups are projected to see the largest growth relative to their populations.

Among the population aged 65 and older, it is projected that in 2050, the American Indian and Alaska Native-alone population will be 918 000, up from 235 000 in 2010, and the Native Hawaiian and Other Pacific Islander-alone population will be 219 000, up from 39 000 in 2010 (Vincent & Velkoff, 2010). There is also a trend of increasing number of old-old (age 75 and older) and oldest-old (age 85 and older) populations in the USA. The old-old and oldest-old carry much of the chronic disease burden in the population.

In the USA, among those aged 65 and older in 2050, the White-alone population will comprise approximately 77% of the aging population, whereas in 2010 the racial composition of the elder population was 87% White-alone, 9% Black, 3% Asian-alone, 7% as Hispanics, and 0.6% American Indian and Alaska Native. Between 2010 and 2030, the percentage of minority elders will increase much faster than the White population. The White population aged 65 and older is projected to increase by 59% compared with an average increase of 160% for older minorities, including Hispanics (202%), African Americans (114%), American Indians, Eskimos and Aleuts (145%), and Asians and Pacific Islanders (145%) (Administration on Aging, 2012).

While an increasing number of studies have examined oral health disparities across race/ethnicity in the USA, a limited number of such studies have been conducted for older adults. Policy makers, public health officials, and other healthcare providers need to better understand how social factors, along with medical conditions, may contribute to racial/ethnic disparities in oral health with the demographic

Geriatric Dentistry: Caring for Our Aging Population, First Edition. Edited by Paula K. Friedman.
© 2014 John Wiley & Sons, Inc. Published 2014 by John Wiley & Sons, Inc.
Companion website: www.wiley.com/go/friedman/geriatricdentistry

transitioning to a more diverse older population in the USA (US Census Bureau, 2008b).

A report from the Surgeon General (US Department of Health and Human Services, 2000) noted ongoing racial/ethnic disparities in oral health across all ages, and it stressed the need for research to explain these differences. The first step towards explaining the disparities is to know how oral health differs between the groups.

Trends in oral health in older adults

There is substantial evidence that oral health in the USA has significantly improved in the past four decades. Dye *et al.*, using data from the National Health and Nutrition Examination Survey (NHANES, III, 1988–1994) and NHANES 1999–2004, found that the oral health of the USA has substantially improved during this period (Dye *et al.*, 2007). Specifically, Dye *et al.* show that the rates of periodontal disease and caries have decreased for most age groups.

Edentulism, or complete tooth loss, is one of the most important indicators of oral health. Edentulism reflects both the accumulated burden of oral diseases and conditions and the result of dental extraction treatment (Sanders *et al.*, 2004). Studies suggest that edentulism significantly affects quality of life, self-esteem, and nutritional status (Nowjack-Raymer & Sheiham, 2003; Slade & Spencer, 1994; Starr & Hall, 2010). In economically developed countries, the trend of edentulism has declined consistently. For example, in England and Wales, the prevalence of edentulism for the adult population declined from 37% in 1968 to 12% in 1998 (Kelly *et al.*, 2000). In Australia, the prevalence of edentulism for the adult population declined from 20.5% in 1979 to 8.0% in 2002. Among Australian older adults aged 65 and older, the reduction for males was from 59.7% to 26.5%, and for females was from 71.5% to 40.3% (Sanders *et al.*, 2004). Similarly in the USA, the few studies available on middle-aged and older adults have shown that edentulism in these age groups has been dropping for the past several decades. One study revealed that within the period of 1971 and 2001, for those in a low socioeconomic position (SEP), the prevalence of edentulism declined from 50% to 32% in adults

aged 55–64 and from 58% to 43% in adults aged 65–74; the comparable declines for these age groups for individuals in a high SEP were from 22% to 6% and from 30% to 9%, respectively (Cunha-Cruz *et al.*, 2007). A report conducted by the US National Centers for Health Statistics using the US National Health and Nutrition Surveys of 1988–1994 (NHANES III) and NHANES 1999–2004 found that the prevalence of edentulism declined in the USA over these two time periods from 34% to 27% among adults aged 65 and older (Dye *et al.*, 2007).

In the USA, minority elders have been identified as a key demographic group at greatest risk for edentulism (US Department of Health and Human Services, 2000). Black elders, in particular, have higher rates of edentulism than non-Hispanic Whites and Mexican Americans (Dye *et al.*, 2007; Schoenborn & Heyman, 2009; Wu *et al.*, 2011a). One study reported that the rates of edentulism among Blacks were declining, even though they were still higher than other ethnic groups (Dye *et al.*, 2007). This study reported that the rates of edentulism for Black elders declined from 38% in 1988–1994 to 33% in 1999–2004 (Dye *et al.*, 2007). For Whites, the percentages were much lower: 34% in 1988–1994 and 26% in 1999–2004. By comparison, Mexican American adults had even lower edentulism rates (27% and 24%, respectively).

Information regarding edentulism for Asian Americans and Native Americans is very limited. A recent report determined that 21% of Asian Americans aged 65 and older had lost all of their teeth compared to 25% of Whites. Asian Americans also had the lowest percentage of edentulism compared to other minority groups (Schoenborn & Heyman, 2009). The Third Oral Health Survey conducted by the Indian Health Service in 1999 found that 21% of Native American adults aged 55 and older were edentulous, representing a decrease of 5% over 15 years (Indian Health Services, 2001).

One recent study examined the trend of edentulism among adults aged 50 and older in five ethnic groups: Asians, Blacks, Hispanics, Native Americans, and non-Hispanic Whites (Wu *et al.*, 2012a). This study used the National Health Interview Survey (NHIS), which is a cross-sectional household interview survey conducted annually. Ten waves of NHIS data were aggregated from 1999 to 2008. Eligible

Table 1.1 Trend of edentulism by racial/ethnic groups (1999–2008) (%) (weighted)*

Year	White	Black	Hispanic	Asian American	Native American
1999	21.49	24.62	17.78	17.04	33.20
2000	21.18	23.74	17.60	13.54	34.02
2001	20.20	23.02	17.71	11.88	31.78
2002	19.77	22.42	16.68	13.55	29.72
2003	18.90	21.78	16.21	15.88	29.67
2004	18.80	20.60	15.44	14.09	28.12
2005	17.98	20.65	15.13	13.57	24.72
2006	17.58	20.62	15.20	15.26	30.18
2007	17.05	19.58	14.74	14.08	27.07
2008	16.90	19.39	14.18	14.22	23.98

*The predicted rates of edentulism were calculated adjusting for time, race/ethnicity, sociodemographic characteristics, and level of education.
From Wu *et al.* (2012a).

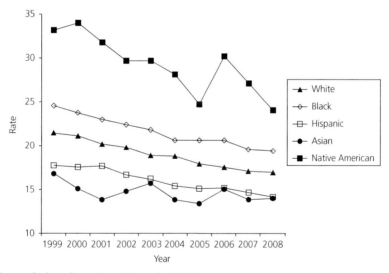

Figure 1.1 Predicted rate of edentulism. From Wu *et al.* (2012a).

respondents were those aged 50 and older who completed the question on tooth loss. The sample included 616 Native Americans, 2666 Asians, 15 295 Blacks, 13 068 Hispanics, and 86 755 non-Hispanic Whites. Self-reported responses to a question about whether the individual had lost all upper and lower natural teeth were used to determine edentulism. Results show that for the past 10 years, there was an overall declining trend of edentulism for all racial and ethnic groups, except for Native Americans (Table 1.1). Table 1.1 presents the predicted rate of edentulism adjusting for time, sociodemographic

characteristics and level of education. In 2008, Native Americans had the highest rate of edentulism (23.98%), followed by Blacks (19.39%), Whites (16.90%), Asians (14.22%), and Hispanics (14.18%). Figure 1.1 presents the trend of predicted rate of edentulism adjusting for time, sociodemographic characteristics and level of education.

This is the first study to provide national estimates for the rate of edentulism and associated trends over time for five major ethnic groups in the USA simultaneously: Native Americans, Asian Americans, Blacks, Hispanics, and non-Hispanic Whites. Significant disparities in edentulism exist across these ethnic groups. Relative to Whites, Blacks and Native Americans had a higher rate of edentulism, whereas the rate of edentulism was lower among Hispanics and Asians. After controlling for covariates (e.g., sociodemographic characteristics, smoking, and common chronic conditions), Blacks and Hispanics were less likely to be edentulous than White respondents, while Native Americans were still more likely to be edentulous. In contrast, when covariates were included in the models, no significant differences were found between Asian Americans and Whites in edentulous rates. Overall, there was a significant downward trend in edentulism rates between 1999 and 2008; however, oral health disparities, as measured by rates of edentulism, increased among Native Americans over time compared to Whites.

The improvement in tooth retention was not equally distributed across the five racial and ethnic groups examined in this study. Native Americans, in particular, were at a significant disadvantage. Compared to Whites, Native Americans were more likely to lose natural teeth over time, but the risk became smaller after controlling for individuals' socioeconomic status, health behaviors, and medical conditions. This study found that edentulism has continued to decline across the USA during the past decade. This comprehensive study supports previous reports about edentulism among adult populations collected in earlier time periods and across selected racial/ethnic groups (Dye et al., 2007; Indian Health Services, 2001; Schoenborn & Heyman, 2009).

One study found that current smoking and fewer years of education were two of the covariates most strongly associated with being edentulous (Wu et al., 2012a). Others have attributed the declining edentulous rate to the decrease in smoking and the increasing years of education among more recent cohorts (Cunha-Cruz et al., 2007). The authors also found that selected medical conditions were associated with edentulism; these were generally consistent with previous research (Holm-Pedersen et al., 2008). Self-reported memory problems and needing assistance with routine activities were also associated with increased risk of edentulism. Given the fact that the information on covariates was not collected prospectively, the authors cannot determine whether the factor preceded the edentulism. Many other factors could also contribute to the decrease of the edentulous rate, such as the introduction of fluoridation through community water treatment (Adair et al., 2001) and fluoridated toothpaste and mouth rinse (Featherstone, 1999; Marthaler, 2004). Health practices such as dietary supplements, and professionally applied or prescribed fluoride gel, foam, and varnish may also contribute to improved tooth retention (Adair et al., 2001; Marthaler, 2004; Weyant, 2004). Others point to advancements in dental technologies and treatment modalities, changes in patient and provider attitudes and treatment preferences (Starr & Hall, 2010), improved oral hygiene, and regular use of dental services (Eklund, 1999; Starr & Hall, 2010; Truman et al., 2002).

Oral health disparities in older adults

Some studies have reported that older Hispanic and Black Americans have more missing teeth, and decayed teeth than their White counterparts (Kiyak et al., 2002; Quandt et al., 2009; Randolph et al., 2001; Watson & Brown, 1995). Using the US National Health and Nutrition Examination Survey (NHANES 1999–2004), a Centers for Disease Control and Prevention (CDC) report found that both Blacks and Mexican Americans have a higher prevalence of untreated tooth decay and missing teeth than Whites (Dye et al., 2007). However, Mexican American adults were least likely to have lost all teeth compared to Whites and African Americans (Dye et al., 2007). In fact, a few studies have suggested that older Black adults have even worse oral health than Hispanics (Borrell et al., 2004; Craig et al., 2001; Kiyak et al., 2002). Many of the previous studies used small convenience samples or only individuals with low socioeconomic status; some were not able to compare the three racial/ethnic groups in the same sample, and some did not evaluate potential confounders that may help to explain differences among the racial/ethnic groups.

In order to address many of the methodologic issues noted earlier in this chapter, one study compared racial/ethnic differences in oral health among community dwelling non-Hispanic White, non-Hispanic Black, and Mexican American older adults aged 60 and older using NHANES (1999–2004) (Wu *et al.*, 2011a). The descriptive results of the study showed that in comparison with Whites and Mexican Americans, Blacks had a significantly higher number of missing teeth, with an average of 3.5 more than whites (12.7 missing teeth) ($P<0.05$) and 4.3 more than Mexican Americans (12.0 missing teeth) ($P<0.01$). Blacks also had significantly higher rates of edentulism (28.6%) than both Whites (24.5%) and Mexican Americans (18.1%). However, Mexican Americans had the lowest rate of edentulism (18.06%) among the three groups but the highest number of decayed teeth by comparison. Additionally, minorities had many fewer filled teeth than Whites, particularly Blacks who had 2.7 filled teeth compared with 7.3 for Whites and 4.7 for Mexican Americans. (Fig. 1.1)

The findings from this multivariate analysis (Wu *et al.*, 2011a) also showed that Blacks and Mexican Americans had significantly higher numbers of decayed teeth but fewer numbers of filled teeth than Whites, even controlling for many confounding variables. The results also found that Blacks were more likely to have a higher number of missing teeth than Whites; nonetheless, they were less likely to be edentulous. Compared with Whites, Mexican Americans were less likely to be edentulous, and dentate respondents were also less likely to lose their natural teeth. Further, the study reported that racial/ethnic differences were confounded by other health-related and social factors that often differ by race/ethnicity. Overall, oral health disparities across racial/ethnic groups persisted even after controlling for other covariates.

In this study (Wu *et al.*, 2011a), racial/ethnic differences remained even after controlling for all other covariates. The findings reflect a historic lack of access to dental care for racial/ethnic minorities (Davidson & Andersen, 1997; Manski & Magder, 1998). Minority elders often demonstrate a low use of dental services, particularly preventative services. Racial/ethnic disparities in dental care could be partially explained by differential treatment as a result of limited dental coverage and inadequate participation of dentists in the Medicaid program (Doty & Weech-Maldonado, 2003).

Oral health is associated with individual's socio-economic status (Borrell *et al.*, 2004). This association is often explained by the fact that individuals with higher income and a higher level of education are more likely than others to seek preventive dental care, have healthy behaviors, or to have access to dental services when they are needed. Another study confirmed the finding that individuals with higher level of education and income and education had better oral health outcomes, even controlling for the factors on health behaviors and preventive dental care (Wu *et al.*, 2011a). The authors suspect that the results may arise from unmeasured differences in the quality of dental care currently received. Another possibility is that the cross-sectional data do not capture the cumulative effects of access to dental care throughout the life course (Wu *et al.*, 2011a).

The observed disparities may also reflect current or lifetime dietary habits, and current or lifetime smoking habits and other negative health behaviors among minorities. Additionally, the results presented in this study could reflect unmeasured racial/ethnic differences in oral health beliefs and oral hygiene practice, and a lack of dental knowledge. Other researchers have suggested that clinicians should be aware that minorities may be less likely than Whites to believe in the benefits of preventative practices (Nakazono *et al.*, 1997).

Using the same NHANES data (1999–2004), one study also examined racial/ethnic differences in self-reported oral health (Wu *et al.*, 2011b). This study found that Blacks and Hispanics reported poorer self-rated oral health than Whites. In separate dentate and edentulous groups, socioeconomic status, social support, physical health, clinical oral health outcomes, and dental checkups accounted for much of the difference in self-rated oral health in Blacks, but significant differences remained for Hispanics. In addition to some potential reasons discussed earlier, other cultural factors could also contribute to the differences in self-rated oral health. Perception of health is socially constructed (Kaplan & Baron-Epel, 2003). Health beliefs and perceptions are rooted in social and cultural contexts and are influenced by prevailing social and medical ideologies. Responses to the self-rated oral health question may be the product of multiple present and past experiences. Factors such as differences in cultural perception and interpretation of overall health, and perceived needs of dental care, could contribute to the differences in self-rated oral health.

These cited studies suggest that reducing racial/ethnic oral health disparities requires multiple clinical approaches. First, it is important to improve access for dental care for minority elders. Second, it is critical to increase older adults' knowledge of the importance of oral health, including the linkage between oral health, referred to as "dental literacy", and systemic medical conditions, oral hygiene, and preventive dental care services. Third, programs are needed to improve individuals' overall health behaviors – perhaps through encouraging positive behaviors that can help older Americans retain their natural teeth and maintain good oral health later in life. Fourth, develop and improve culturally competent services for minority communities by recruiting more underrepresented minorities to the dental professions, and enrich dental education curriculum (Lopez, N. *et al.*, 2003; Wu *et al.*, 2011a).

Functional status and oral health

The aging population is at increased risk for physical disability. Among people aged 65 and older, 18.1 million people (51.8%) had a disability, defined as having at least one disability of Activities of Daily Living (ADL) or Instrumental Activities of Daily Living (IADL). About 12.9 million people aged 65 and older (36.9%) had a severe disability. The prevalence of disability increases as people get older. For those aged 65 and those aged 69, 37.4% had disability and 7% need personal assistance with ADL or IADL. For individuals aged 80 and older, the percentage increases to 71% and 29.2%, respectively (Brault, 2008). Disability leads to reduced quality of life for individuals and increased costs to society in the provision of services. It is likely that disabled older adults are at higher risk of oral diseases. One reason is that disability may affect individual's ability to maintain good oral hygiene and restrict their access to necessary dental care. Several cross-sectional studies have shown that elders with functional disability have more untreated caries, higher prevalence of edentulism, and use dental services less regularly than their counterparts (Gift & Newman, 1993; Jette *et al.*, 1993; Philip *et al.*, 2012; Wu *et al.*, 2007). One longitudinal study conducted among Swedish elders found that

individuals with recent decrease in functional status were associated with root caries while more severely disabled elders that needed personal assistance were more likely to have coronal caries (Avlund *et al.*, 2004). These findings suggest that those individuals with more severe functional impairment were more likely to have coronal caries while those with less severe level of functional impairment were associated with root caries. One possible explanation for the finding is that people who need help in daily activities (i.e., those with a more advanced stage of impairment) have had these problems over a longer period of time, and the development of coronal caries reflects a past caries burden that has been present over a period of time. A general decline in functional status may be regarded as an early sign of later deterioration, which is reflected in root caries, a condition that may reflect a caries burden in a period closer to the time of the examination. One factor that explains the association between functional impairment and poor oral health is that decline in functional performance could result in a decline in the quality and regularity of oral hygiene, which in turn, affects oral health. Using data from a randomized trial of community dwelling adults aged 75 and older, one study reported that functional status was positively correlated with frequency of dental visits over time (Dolan *et al.*, 1998). The findings suggest that functionally impaired older adults underutilize dental services. The authors' assumption is that these individuals' higher utilization of medical services due to health problems may cause them to use less dental care. Functionally disabled elders may see dental care as a lower priority for many reasons, including time availability, access to transportation, perceived importance of dental care, financial resources, and energy to seek dental care.

As indicated previously, functional disability may affect the individual's regular dental visits and ability to perform oral hygiene. Adherence to the American Dental Association's and the US Surgeon General's Oral Hygiene Self-care recommendations to brush twice and floss at least once a day and receive regular prophylactic dental hygiene visits have been associated with reducing the plaque-mediated conditions of periodontal disease and dental caries, as well as improving tooth retention (Kressin *et al.*, 2003; Sharma *et al.*, 2004; Sniehotta *et al.*, 2007). Biofilm is the aggregation of any cluster of microorganisms on a surface; in the oral cavity, removal of the biofilm that forms on teeth is associated with better oral health. Studies indicate that oral hygiene self-care can manage biofilm by mechanically removing the oral plaque biofilm mass, lowering the bacterial load, oxygenating the site, and changing the ecology of the biofilm (Schaudinn et al., 2009). The process can be achieved with good oral hygiene practice, such as brushing, rinsing, scraping, and flossing, or using other interdental cleaning (Schaudinn et al., 2009). One study conducted among community dwelling dentate individuals age 70 and older indicated a need for older adults to improve in their frequency of oral hygiene behavior, particularly for elderly men (Wiener et al., 2012). The study reported that a higher proportion of older adult women brushed their teeth more frequently than their male counterparts. Eighty-one percent of women reported brushing their teeth twice a day, while the percentage for males was 52%. Compared to brushing, all participants reported lower frequency of flossing and mouth rinsing. Forty-four percent of males and 32% females reported flossing intermittently, and the percentage for mouth rinsing was 41% and 37% respectively.

Xerostomia, medications, and oral health

Saliva provides a crucial role in oral health. It buffers acids, has antibodies, helps to prevent gingival mucosal erosions and ulcerations, and aids in remineralization of teeth. When salivary function is diminished, there is more risk for caries, denture discomfort, and diseases such as candidiasis (Guggenheimer & Moore, 2003; Turner et al., 2008).

Xerostomia is a person's *complaint* (subjective perception) of oral dryness/hyposalivation (Navazesh & Kumar, 2008). Hyposalivation is the condition of having a reduced *production* of saliva. Xerostomia is a common problem in older adults. One review article reported older adults to have rates between 17 and 29%, with more prevalence in women (Guggenheimer & Moore, 2003). Another study reported 46% of participants experienced xerostomia (Narhi, 1994). One recent study conducted among community dwelling elders aged 70 and older found that 20.5% of the participants reported having xerostomia (Wiener et al., 2010).

Medications with antisialogogic (inhibiting salivary flow) side-effects are the most frequent causes of xerostomia. These medications include anticholinergics, antidepressants, antipsychotics, diuretics, antihypertensives, sedative and anxiolytics, muscle relaxants, antihistamines, opioid analgesics, and nonsteroidal anti-inflammatories (Narhi, 1994; Navazesh & Kumar, 2008). Some biologic causes of xerostomia include a previous history of radiation to the head and neck, diseases of the salivary gland, diabetes, alcohol use, cystic fibrosis, hormonal imbalance, autoimmune diseases, and other diseases. Psychologic and social factors, such as depression, anxiety, and stress are also causes (Fox, 1996; Navazesh & Kumar, 2008).

As chronic conditions are more prevalent in later life, medication intake also increases. Based on a national survey, 81% of the adult population had taken at least one medication during the previous week (Kaufman et al., 2002). Rates of medication use increase with age and are greater in women. Among female individuals aged 65 and older, 94% had taken at least 1 medication during the previous week, 57% took 5 or more, and 12% took 10 or more; while for male counterparts, the percentage was 91%, 44%, and 12% respectively. The increasing number of prescribed and/or over the counter medications taken increases the risk of dry mouth, which in turn have potential negative impact on oral health.

Case study 1

Your patient is a 78-year-old woman who lives alone at her home in an urban community who comes to your office for routine check-up. She has multiple chronic conditions including hypertension, diabetes, and depression. She has been taking Exforge® to treat her hypertension and selective serotonin reuptake inhibitors (SSRIs) to treat her depressive symptoms. She tells you that she feels her eyes, mouth, and lips are dry. She has to sip liquids to aid in swallowing food or avoids certain food. She frequently feels thirsty at night and she has to get up to drink water. As a dental professional, what would you recommend to this patient to alleviate the symptoms? What would you do to communicate with the patient's primary care provider?

Cognitive function and oral health

Cognitive impairment is common among older adults. It is reported that between 2.6 million and 5.1 million Americans may suffer from the condition (National Institutes of Health, 2010), and the numbers are expected to more than double by 2050 (Hebert et al., 2003). In addition, an estimated 5.4 million people in the USA aged 71 and older (22.2%) have cognitive impairment without dementia (mild manifestations of impairment) (Plassman et al., 2008).

Evidence from clinical samples suggests that the elderly have an increased incidence of oral disease and that the frequency of oral health problems increases significantly in cognitively impaired older adults, primarily those with dementia. The few studies to examine the relationship between cognitive function and oral health have primarily focused on patients with Alzheimer's disease (AD) or other dementias. Results from three longitudinal studies have consistently shown higher rates of oral conditions such as salivary dysfunction (King, 1992; Ship & Puckett, 1994), coronal and root caries (Chalmers et al., 2002; Chalmers et al., 2004; Jones et al., 1993), and other oral diseases (Chalmers et al., 2002; Chalmers et al., 2004) in individuals with dementia compared to the nondemented controls. These findings involving individuals with diagnosed dementia may not apply to older individuals across the full range of cognitive function, including the large number of people with undiagnosed dementia (Callahan et al., 2002) or with cognitive impairment not severe enough to meet criteria for dementia (Lopez O.L. et al., 2003). To address this point, a few studies have investigated the association between cognitive status and oral health in later life. These studies provide preliminary support for an association between performance on brief cognitive status measures and poorer oral health based on the presence of more decayed teeth (Beck, 1990), greater dental functional impairment (Osterberg et al., 1990), and a trend toward more coronal and root caries (Avlund et al., 2004). However, interpretation of these studies has been limited by the use of cognitive measures insensitive to the full range of cognitive ability, inability to control for key variables associated with oral health, or a small sample size.

More recently, several epidemiologic studies have examined the relationship between cognitive function and oral health. Using data from NHANES III, Stewart et al. (2008) investigated the association between oral health and cognitive function in early, mid-, and late-adult life. A total of 5138 people aged 20–59 and 1555 people aged 70 participated in the study. The study included three measures of oral health: gingival bleeding, loss of periodontal attachment, and loss of teeth. Cognitive function was measured by the Symbol Digit Substitution Test (SDST), and the Serial Digit Learning Test (SDLT) (both in participants aged 20–59), and a Story Recall Test (in participants aged 70). The results show that worse scores on all three measures of oral health status were significantly associated with poorer performance on cognitive function. After adjustment for covariates (including individual's socioeconomic status and medical conditions), gingival bleeding (%), and loss of periodontal attachment (%) remained associated with relative impairment on SDST score, and gingival bleeding was associated with relative impairment on SDLT.

Almost all these previous epidemiologic studies used cross-sectional data. It is critical to conduct longitudinal studies to examine the linkages between cognitive function and oral health in older adults. Although the processes underlying this association remain unclear, there are some underline assumptions on the impact of cognitive impairment on oral health. Studies have shown that an individual's socioeconomic status (as represented by years of education) is strongly related to oral health. It is possible that the association between cognitive function and oral health, even after controlling for education, still may reflect unmeasured differences in life-course socioeconomic status. Cognitive function may reflect not only the level of educational attainment but also the quality of education and cumulative effect of socioeconomic status (e.g., previous or current occupational status, wealth, and cognition in childhood, etc.) across the life span (Froehlich et al., 2001; Moody-Ayers et al., 2005).

Dental care utilization likely serves as a mediating variable between cognitive function and oral health. Dental care utilization has a strong association with oral health outcomes such as number of decayed teeth, missing teeth, and filled teeth (Vargas et al., 2003). One study also found that cognitive function has a significant impact on dental care utilization

(Wu *et al.* 2007). Individuals with lower cognitive function may not view dental care as a high priority and may have limited self-awareness of dental care needs. In addition, a decline in cognition may be reflected as a decline in IADL performance, specifically a decline in the quality and regularity of oral hygiene. These changes may partially explain the association between cognition and oral health.

One study used longitudinal data from community dwelling elders to examine cognitive impairment's impact on oral hygiene (Wu *et al.*, 2012b). This study suggests that incident decline in oral hygiene practices, such as transitioning from brushing to not brushing teeth, is often associated with concurrent declines in cognition, which can be classified as incident cognitive impairment in many individuals. These findings add to the growing body of literature that indicates that decline in both oral hygiene and oral health may begin prior to the time an individual has advanced dementia and significant impaired function.

On the other hand, there are several potential reasons why poor oral health may itself be a risk factor for cognitive decline. Periodontal disease, at times resulting in tooth decay and loss, is a common source of chronic infection in humans and is associated with elevated levels of inflammatory markers (Li *et al.*, 2000). Even a low-grade infection in the oral cavity may be associated with a moderate, subclinical systemic inflammatory response, but appropriate treatment reduces the levels of inflammatory markers (D'Aiuto & Tonetti, 2004; Taylor *et al.*, 2006).

Chronic inflammation, as measured by serum interleukin-6 and C-reactive protein, is reportedly a risk factor for cardiovascular disease (D'Aiuto & Tonetti, 2004), cognitive decline (Weaver *et al.*, 2002; Yaffe *et al.*, 2003), and AD (Schmidt *et al.*, 2002). Current theories posit that inflammatory processes play a major role in the etiology of AD (Finch & Crimmins, 2004; McGeer & McGeer, 1995). Consistent with this, one study found that among monozygotic twin pairs, twins who reported the loss of all of their teeth prior to age 35 were more likely to develop dementia than their co-twins who retained half or more of their teeth (Gatz *et al.*, 2006). Furthermore, tooth loss is also associated with dietary changes (Nowjack-Raymer & Sheiham, 2003), which may cause cognitive impairment due

to potential nutritional deficiency. Finally, poor oral health is associated with systemic diseases such as cardiovascular disease and diabetes (Lamster *et al.*, 2008; Lockhart *et al.*, 2012) and smoking (Laxman & Annaji, 2008) that are risk factors for cognitive impairment.

Case study 2

A 74-year-old man was a regular visitor to your dental office for the past 20 years. Recently, he missed some dental appointments. In his most recent visit, his wife accompanied him to his dental visit. The dentist observed that the patient's oral hygiene had declined and that he had developed some new coronal and root caries. His wife told the dental hygienist that sometimes he forgets to brush his teeth. What advice would you give to the patient and his wife on how to improve the patient's oral health status?

Clinical and policy implications

Oral health problems (e.g., missing teeth, dental caries, and periodontal diseases) accumulate throughout the life span, but they occur with increasing frequency in later life. These differences may be partially due to cohort effects; younger cohorts may have higher levels of education and income, which are factors associated with better oral health status. However, many of these differences could be age-related. Genetic and biologic factors likely play a major role in deterioration of oral health in elders, but social, psychologic, and behavioral factors may also be important determinants. As discussed earlier, some major factors related to oral health deterioration in older adults include: (i) poor oral hygiene due to functional and cognitive impairment or other medical conditions; (ii) medications taken that may cause dry mouth; (iii) declining use of dental care services; and (iv) chronic illnesses. Given that increasing numbers of individuals are retaining their natural teeth, the issue of maintaining healthy teeth in later life is becoming more critical.

Maintaining oral health status in older adults needs multiple approaches which should focus on both prevention (use of professional dental care, use of preventive dental care products, oral health education, and improvement of self-care skills) and dental treatment. The use of professional dental care by US elders, which is critical to oral health, has increased steadily and rapidly during the past several decades. The proportion of Americans aged 65 and older who reported at least one dental visit during the preceding year rose from 15% in 1950 to 55% in 2003 (Brown, 2008). Despite this increase, rates of utilization remain lower in elders than in other age groups. Elders are more likely than the general population to have difficulty accessing dental care due to frailty, medical comorbidity, and functional and cognitive impairment.

Many elders report needing dental services and the needs are even higher for racial/ethnic minority elders. Cost is certainly a big concern with regard to dental use. Nonetheless, geriatric dental services also need to improve access and utilization by reducing barriers such as inadequate geriatric training, lack of culturally competent services, and a lack of portable dental equipment. While most elders with chronic diseases can get dental care from private dental offices, having dentists and dental hygienists provide mobile dental services at an individual's home, institutional care facility, or at a mobile unit would be very helpful to those who cannot easily access a dental clinic. In the meantime, increasing the number of dentists with geriatric training is an important step toward improving the quality of dental care for elders.

Despite the availability of a broad array of preventive measures for oral diseases, many elders are not aware of or do not use proven preventive procedures. Many do not realize that most oral diseases can be prevented or controlled by improved oral hygiene and the use of fluoride and other cost-effective measures. Thus, there is a clear need to provide education on the importance of oral health and prevention of oral health problems. It has been shown that generic oral health education has a consistent positive effect on knowledge level and a small positive (although temporary) effect on plaque accumulation and gingivitis (Boundouki et al., 2004; Renz et al., 2007). While such programs should be an integral part of interventions to improve oral health in older adults, the development of tailored

behavioral interventions deserves further attention. Given the heterogeneity of the elderly population, tailored educational messages may be more effective in prevention of oral diseases. Depending on individual needs, educational programs can cover topics such as evidence-based recommendations on oral hygiene behaviors; signs of oral diseases and conditions that require immediate attention (e.g., cancer and abscess); strategies for reducing symptoms of minor oral conditions; cueing techniques for daily oral hygiene; diet and nutrition; and information about adverse effects of tobacco and certain medications.

Given that many older adults do not or cannot afford to use the oral healthcare system, interventions to improve oral health in older adults need to be readily accessible, easily incorporated into daily routines, and economical. Innovative interventions need to be implemented to empower elders and their family members with knowledge of oral health, and improve dental self-care skills. A recent US Department of Health and Human Services report (US Department of Health and Human Services, 2010) emphasized the importance of using proven self-care management approaches that include informing and motivating patients and treating them as partners in their own care. The report stressed that even the highest quality care for individuals with chronic conditions cannot guarantee improved health outcomes, and also pointed to the important role played by families and other caregivers in providing assistance with self-care tasks to individuals with significant declines in physical and cognitive function. Its conclusions support the importance of involving family members or informal caregivers to help implement oral health interventions for older adults with functional/cognitive impairment or chronic disease. The list of daily activities for which spouses, adult children, or friends provide assistance and regular reminders should include oral hygiene tasks, which are all too often neglected. Well-established practices from the field of occupational therapy show that with sufficient repetition, hygiene tasks (e.g., tooth brushing) can become automatic when triggered by cues, events, or other environmental factors (Levy & Burns, 2005), and can be maintained even with advancing cognitive decline.

DISCUSSION QUESTIONS

1 If you are the director of the dental office in your statue, what would you do to increase the use of dental care services for older adults in various settings (residential homes, senior centers, public housing, nursing homes)?

2 An increasing number of elders are from minority groups and/or are first-generation immigrants; many of them do not seek dental care on a regular basis. What systems would you establish to increase the use of dental care for these elders?

3 For older adults that reside at home with functional and cognitive impairment, what suggestions you would like to make to improve, or at least maintain their oral health status?

4 Many of the homebound elders have difficulty visiting dentists regularly due to physical constraints.

   A What can nondental professionals do to improve oral health care for these homebound elders? How would you establish networking structures for dental referrals by nondental professionals?

   B How can a trained nondentist perform an initial assessment of dental care needs? How can they provide preventive needs? Can you design a checklist to assist nondental providers in these functions?

   C What can dental professionals do to train family members to assist in helping these frail elders to improve or at least maintain oral health status?

References

Adair, S.M., Bowen, W.H., Burt, B.A., *et al.* (2001) Recommendations for using fluoride to prevent and control dental caries in the United States. Centers for Disease Control and Prevention. *MMWR. Recommendations and Reports*, **50**(RR–14), 1–42.

Administration on Aging (2012) *A Profile of Older Americans: 2011.* From http://www.aoa.gov/aoaroot/aging_statistics/Profile/2011/4.aspx. Accessed April 16, 2014.

Avlund, K., Holm-Pedersen, P., Morse, D.E., *et al.* (2004) Tooth loss and caries prevalence in very old Swedish people: the relationship to cognitive function and functional ability. *Gerodontology*, **21**(1), 17–26.

Beck, J. (1990) The epidemiology of root surface caries. *Journal of Dental Research*, **69**(5), 1216–21.

Borrell, L.N., Burt, B.A., Neighbors, H.W. & Taylor, G.W. (2004) Social factors and periodontitis in an older population. *American Journal of Public Health*, **94**(5), 748–54.

Boundouki, G., Humphris, G. & Field, A. (2004) Knowledge of oral cancer, distress and screening intentions: longer term effects of a patient information leaflet. *Patient Education and Counseling*, **53**(1), 71–7.

Brault, M. (2008) *Americans with Disabilities: 2005.* Current Population Reports. US Census Bureau, Washington, DC.

Brown, L.J. (2008) Dental services among elderly Americans: utilization, expenditures, and their determinants. In: *Improving Oral Health for the Elderly* (eds. I.B. Lamster & M.E. Northridge), pp. 439–80. Springer, New York.

Callahan, C.M., Unverzagt, F.W., Hui, S.L., *et al.* (2002) Six-item screener to identify cognitive impairment among potential subjects for clinical research. *Medical Care*, **40**(9), 771–81.

Chalmers, J.M., Carter, K.D. & Spencer, A.J. (2002) Caries incidence and increments in community-living older adults with and without dementia. *Gerodontology*, **19**(2), 80–94.

Chalmers, J.M., Carter, K.D. & Spencer, A. J. (2004) Oral health of Adelaide nursing home residents – a longitudinal study. *Australasian Journal on Ageing*, **23**, 63–70.

Craig, R.G., Boylan, R., Yip, J., *et al.* (2001) Prevalence and risk indicators for destructive periodontal diseases in three urban American minority populations. *Journal of Clinical Periodontology*, **28**(6), 524–35.

Cunha-Cruz, J., Hujoel, P.P. & Nadanovsky, P. (2007) Secular trends in socio-economic disparities in edentulism: USA, 1972–2001. *Journal of Dental Research*, **86**(2), 131–6.

D'Aiuto, F. & Tonetti, D. (2004) Periodontal disease and C-reactive protein associated cardiovascular risk. *Journal of Periodontal Research*, **39**, 236–41.

Davidson, P.L. & Andersen, R.M. (1997) Determinants of dental care utilization for diverse ethnic and age groups. *Advances in Dental Research*, **11**(2), 254–62.

Dolan, T.A., Peek, C.W., Stuck, A.E. & Beck, J.C. (1998) Functional health and dental service use among older adults. *Journals of Gerontology. Series A, Biological Sciences and Medical Sciences*, **53**(6), M413–18.

Doty, H.E. & Weech-Maldonado, R. (2003) Racial/ethnic disparities in adult preventive dental care use. *Journal of Health Care for the Poor and Underserved*, **14**(4), 516–34.

Dye, B.A., Tan, S., Smith, V., *et al.* (2007) Trends in oral health status: United States, 1988–1994 and 1999–2004. *Vital and Health Statistics, Series 11*, **248**, 1–92.

Eklund, S.A. (1999) Changing treatment patterns. *Journal of the American Dental Association*, **130**(12), 1707–12.

Featherstone, J.D. (1999) Prevention and reversal of dental caries: role of low level fluoride. *Community Dentistry and Oral Epidemiology*, **27**(1), 31–40.

Finch, C.E. & Crimmins, E.M. (2004) Inflammatory exposure and historical changes in human life-spans. *Science*, **305**(5691), 1736–9.

Fox, P.C. (1996) Differentiation of dry mouth etiology. *Advances in Dental Research*, **10**(1), 13–16.

Froehlich, T.E., Bogardus, S.T., Jr. & Inouye, S.K. (2001) Dementia and race: are there differences between African Americans and Caucasians? *Journal of the American Geriatrics Society*, **49**, 477–84.

Gatz, M., Mortimer, J.A., Fratiglioni, L., *et al.* (2006) Potentially modifiable risk factors for dementia in identical twins. *Alzheimer's & Dementia*, **2**(2), 110–17.

Gift, H.C. & Newman, J.F. (1993) How older adults use oral health care services: results of a National Health Interview Survey. *Journal of the American Dental Association*, **124**(1), 89–93.

Guggenheimer, J. & Moore, P.A. (2003) Xerostomia: etiology, recognition and treatment. *Journal of the American Dental Association*, **134**(1), 61–9; quiz 118–19.

Hebert, L.E., Scherr, P.A., Bienias, J.L., *et al.* (2003) Alzheimer disease in the US population: prevalence estimates using the 2000 census. *Archives of Neurology*, **60**(8), 1119–22.

Holm-Pedersen, P., Schultz-Larsen, K., Christiansen, N. & Avlund, K. (2008) Tooth loss and subsequent disability and mortality in old age. *Journal of the American Geriatrics Society*, **56**(3), 429–35.

Indian Health Services (2001) *An Oral Health Survey of American Indian and Alaska Native Dental Patients: Findings, Regional Differences & National Comparisons*. US Department of Health and Human Services, Rockville, MD.

Jette, A M., Feldman, H.A. & Douglass, C. (1993) Oral disease and physical disability in community-dwelling older persons. *Journal of the American Geriatrics Society*, **41**(10), 1102–8.

Jones, J.A., Lavallee, N., Alman, J., *et al.* (1993) Caries incidence in patients with dementia. *Gerodontology*, **10**, 76–82.

Kaplan, G. & Baron-Epel, O. (2003) What lies behind the subjective evaluation of health status? *Social Science and Medicine*, **56**(8), 1669–76.

Kaufman, D.W., Kelly, J.P., Rosenberg, L., *et al.* (2002) Recent patterns of medication use in the ambulatory adult population of the United States: the Slone survey. *JAMA*, **287**(3), 337–44.

Kelly, M., Steele, J., Nuttall, N., *et al.* (2000) *Adult Dental Health Survey Oral Health in the United Kingdom 1998*. UK Office for National Statistics, The Stationery Office, London.

King, P.L. (1992) *A dental health education program for caregivers of elderly people in nursing homes*. Masters thesis, University of Sydney, Sydney, Australia. From http://hdl.handle.net/2123/4745. Accessed March 13, 2014.

Kiyak, H.A., Kamoh, A., Persson, R.E. & Persson, G.R. (2002) Ethnicity and oral health in community-dwelling older adults. *General Dentistry*, **50**(6), 513–18.

Kressin, N.R., Boehmer, U., Nunn, M.E. & Spiro, A., 3rd. (2003) Increased preventive practices lead to greater tooth retention. *Journal of Dental Research*, **82**(3), 223–7.

Lamster, I.B., Lalla, E., Borgnakke, W.S. & Taylor, G.W. (2008) The relationship between oral health and diabetes mellitus. *Journal of the American Dental Association*, **139**(Suppl), 19S–24S.

Laxman, V.K. & Annaji, S. (2008) Tobacco use and its effects on the periodontium and periodontal therapy. *Journal of Contemporary Dental Practice*, **9**(7), 97–107.

Levy, L.L. & Burns, T. (2005) Cognitive disabilities reconsidered: rehabilitation of older adults with dementia. In: *Cognition and Occupation Across the Life Span* (ed. N. Katz), 2nd edn, pp. 347–88. American Occupational Therapy Association, Bethesda, MD.

Li, X., Kolltveit, K.M., Tronstad, L. & Olsen, I. (2000) Systemic diseases caused by oral infection. *Clinical Microbiology Reviews*, **13**, 547–58.

Lockhart, P.B., Bolger, A.F., Papapanou, P.N., *et al.* (2012) Periodontal disease and atherosclerotic vascular disease: does the evidence support an independent association? A scientific statement from the American Heart Association. *Circulation*, **125**(20), 2520–44.

Lopez, N., Wadenya, R. & Berthold, P. (2003a) Effective recruitment and retention strategies for underrepresented minority students: perspectives from dental students. *Journal of Dental Education*, **67**(10), 1107–12.

Lopez, O.L., Jagust, W.J., DeKosky, S.T., *et al.* (2003b) Prevalence and classification of mild cognitive impairment in the Cardiovascular Health Study Cognition Study: part 1. *Archives of Neurology*, **60**(10), 1385–9.

Manski, R.J., & Magder, L.S. (1998) Demographic and socioeconomic predictors of dental care utilization. *Journal of the American Dental Association*, **129**(2), 195–200.

Marthaler, T.M. (2004) Changes in dental caries 1953–2003. *Caries Research*, **38**(3), 173–81.

McGeer, P.L. & McGeer, E.G. (1995) The inflammatory response system of brain: implications for therapy of Alzheimer and other neurodegenerative diseases. *Brain Research. Brain Research Reviews*, **21**(2), 195–218.

Moody-Ayers, S.Y., Mehta, K.M., Lindquist, K., *et al.* (2005) Black–white disparities in functional decline in older persons: the role of cognitive function. *Journal of Gerontology: Medical Sciences*, **60A**, 933–9.

Nakazono, T.T., Davidson, P.L. & Andersen, R.M. (1997) Oral health beliefs in diverse populations. *Advances in Dental Research*, **11**(2), 235–44.

Narhi, T.O. (1994) Prevalence of subjective feelings of dry mouth in the elderly. *Journal of Dental Research*, **73**(1), 20–5.

National Institutes of Health (2010) *Alzheimer's Disease*. National Institutes of Health, Bethesda, MD. From http://report.nih.gov/NIHfactsheets/Pdfs/Alzheimers-Disease(NIA).pdf. Accessed March 13, 2014.

Navazesh, M. & Kumar, S.K. (2008) Measuring salivary flow: challenges and opportunities. *Journal of the American Dental Association*, **139**(Suppl), 35S–40S.

Nowjack-Raymer, R.E. & Sheiham, A. (2003) Association of edentulism and diet and nutrition in US adults. *Journal of Dental Research*, **82**(2), 123–6.

Osterberg, T., Mellstrom, D. & Sundh, V. (1990) Dental health and functional ageing. A study of 70-year-old people. *Community Dentistry and Oral Epidemiology*, **18**(6), 313–18.

Philip, P., Rogers, C., Kruger, E. & Tennant, M. (2012) Caries experience of institutionalized elderly and its association with dementia and functional status. *International Journal of Dental Hygiene*, **10**(2), 122–7.

Plassman, B.L., Langa, K.M., Fisher, G.G., *et al.* (2008) Prevalence of cognitive impairment without dementia in the United States. *Annals of Internal Medicine*, **148**(6), 427–34.

Quandt, S.A., Chen, H., Bell, R.A., *et al.* (2009) Disparities in oral health status between older adults in a multiethnic rural community: the rural nutrition and oral health study. *Journal of the American Geriatrics Society*, **57**(8), 1369–75.

Randolph, W.M., Ostir, G.V. & Markides, K.S. (2001) Prevalence of tooth loss and dental service use in older Mexican Americans. *Journal of the American Geriatrics Society*, **49**(5), 585–9.

Renz, A., Ide, M., Newton, T., *et al.* (2007) Psychological interventions to improve adherence to oral hygiene instructions in adults with periodontal diseases. *Cochrane Database of Systematic Reviews* **2**, CD005097.

Sanders, A.E., Slade, G.D., Carter, K.D. & Stewart, J.F. (2004) Trends in prevalence of complete tooth loss among Australians, 1979–2002. *Australian and New Zealand Journal of Public Health*, **28**(6), 549–54.

Schaudinn, C., Gorur, A., Keller, D., *et al.* (2009) Periodontitis: an archetypical biofilm disease. *Journal of the American Dental Association*, **140**(8), 978–86.

Schmidt, R., Schmidt, H., Curb, J.D., *et al.* (2002) Early inflammation and dementia: a 25-year follow-up of the Honolulu–Asia Aging Study. *Annals of Neurology*, **52**(2), 168–74.

Schoenborn, C.A. & Heyman, K.M. (2009) Health characteristics of adults aged 55 years and over: United States, 2004–2007. *National Health Statistics Reports*, **16**, 1–31.

Sharma, N., Charles, C.H., Lynch, M.C., *et al.* (2004) Adjunctive benefit of an essential oil-containing mouthrinse in reducing plaque and gingivitis in patients who brush and floss regularly: a six-month study. *Journal of the American Dental Association*, **135**(4), 496–504.

Ship, J.A. & Puckett, S.A. (1994) Longitudinal study on oral health in subjects with Alzheimer's disease. *Journal of the American Geriatrics Society*, **42**(1), 57–63.

Slade, G.D. & Spencer, A.J. (1994) Social impact of oral conditions among older adults. *Australian Dental Journal*, **39**(6), 358–64.

Sniehotta, F.F., Araujo Soares, V. & Dombrowski, S.U. (2007) Randomized controlled trial of a one-minute intervention changing oral self-care behavior. *Journal of Dental Research*, **86**(7), 641–5.

Starr, J.M. & Hall, R. (2010) Predictors and correlates of edentulism in healthy older people. *Current Opinion in Clinical Nutrition and Metabolic Care*, **13**(1), 19–23.

Stewart, R., Sabbah, W., Tsakos, G., *et al.* (2008) Oral health and cognitive function in the Third National Health and Nutrition Examination Survey (NHANES III). *Psychosomatic Medicine*, **70**(8), 936–41.

Taylor, B.A., Tofler, G.H., Carey, H.M., *et al.* (2006) Full mouth tooth extraction lowers systemic inflammatory and thrombotic markers of cardiovascular risk. *Journal of Dental Research*, **85**, 74–8.

Truman, B.I., Gooch, B.F., Sulemana, I., *et al.* (2002) Reviews of evidence on interventions to prevent dental caries, oral and pharyngeal cancers, and sports-related craniofacial injuries. *American Journal of Preventive Medicine*, **23**(1 Suppl), 21–54.

Turner, M., Jahangiri, L. & Ship, J.A. (2008) Hyposalivation, xerostomia and the complete denture: a systematic review. *Journal of the American Dental Association*, **139**(2), 146–50.

US Census Bureau (2008a) *2008 National Population Projections*. From http://www.census.gov/population/projections/data/national/2008/downloadablefiles.html. Accessed January 27, 2013.

US Census Bureau (2008b) *Population Projections of the United States by Age, Sex, Race and Hispanic Origin: 1995 to 2050*. From http://www.census.gov/prod/1/pop/p25-1130.pdf. Accessed March 17, 2013.

US Department of Health and Human Services (2000) *Oral Health in America: A Report of the Surgeon General*. National Institutes of Health, Rockville, MD. From http://purl.access.gpo.gov/GPO/LPS13826. Accessed March 13, 2014.

US Department of Health and Human Services (2010) *Multiple Chronic Conditions: A Strategic Framework. Optimum Health and Quality of Life for Individuals with Multiple Chronic Conditions*. US Department of Health and Human Services, Washington, DC.

Vargas, C.M., Dye, B.A. & Hayes, K. (2003) Oral health care utilization by US rural residents, National Health Interview Survey 1999. *Journal of Public Health Dentistry*, **63**(3), 150–7.

Vincent, G.K. & Velkoff, V.A. (2010) The next four decades: the older population in the United States: 2010 to 2050. US Census Bureau, Washington, DC.

Watson, M.R. & Brown, L.J. (1995) The oral health of US Hispanics: evaluating their needs and their use of dental services. *Journal of the American Dental Association*, **126**(6), 789–95.

Weaver, J.D., Huang, M.H., Albert, M., *et al.* (2002) Interleukin-6 and risk of cognitive decline: MacArthur studies of successful aging. *Neurology*, **59**(3), 371–8.

Weyant, R.J. (2004) Seven systematic reviews confirm topical fluoride therapy is effective in preventing dental caries. *Journal of Evidence-Based Dental Practice*, **4**(2), 129–35.

Wiener, R.C., Wu, B., Crout, R., *et al.* (2010) Hyposalivation and xerostomia in dentate older adults. *Journal of the American Dental Association*, **141**(3), 279–84.

Wiener, R.C., Wu, B., Crout, R., *et al.* (2012) Oral hygiene self-care of older adults in West Virginia: effects of gender. *Journal of Dental Hygiene*, **86**(3), 231–8.

Wu, B., Plassman, B.L., Liang, J. & Wei, L. (2007) Cognitive function and dental care utilization among community-dwelling older adults. *American Journal of Public Health*, **97**(12), 2216–21.

Wu, B., Liang, J., Plassman, B.L., *et al.* (2011a) Oral health among white, black, and Mexican-American elders: an examination of edentulism and dental caries. *Journal of Public Health Dentistry 2011;* **71**(4): 308–17.

Wu, B., Plassman, B.L., Liang, J., *et al.* (2011b) Differences in self-reported oral health among community-dwelling black, Hispanic, and white elders. *Journal of Aging and Health*, **23**(2), 267–88.

Wu, B., Liang, J., Plassman, B.L., *et al.* (2012a) Edentulism trends among middle-aged and older adults in the United States: comparison of five racial/ethnic groups. *Community Dentistry and Oral Epidemiology*, **40**(2), 145–53.

Wu, B., Plassman, B.L., Liang, J., *et al.* (2012b) *Cognitive Function and Oral Hygiene Behavior In Later Life*. Alzheimer's Association International Conference, Vancouver, BC, Canada.

Yaffe, K., Lindquist, K., Penninx, B.W., *et al.* (2003) Inflammatory markers and cognition in well-functioning African-American and white elders. *Neurology*, **61**(1), 76–80.

CHAPTER 2

Palliative Care Dentistry

Michael Wiseman

Faculty of Dentistry, McGill University, Montreal, QC, Canada; Mount Sinai Hospital, Montreal, QC, Canada

Introduction

Palliative care dentistry focuses on the treatment of terminally ill patients in which the oral cavity is affected directly or indirectly by the illness and the principle is symptom relief (Wiseman, 2000). Palliative care involves more than simply treating the patient. Care is directed both to the patient and to their loved ones (Fig. 2.1). It must be noted that the interdisciplinary palliative care team should include a dentist, as patients often suffer from oral problems that other members of the team may not realize or know how to manage.

The palliative care team must be careful not to become prognostic as to life expectancy, as this could influence the treatment choices for the patient, the family, and the dentist. When physicians were asked to predict life expectancy, physicians were only correct 20% of the time (Christakis & Lamont, 2000); this is important as an incorrect prognosis may lead the dentist to change from comfort-providing care to more advanced dental care. The dentist must always remember that the prime goal is comfort/pain control ("comfort care"). Although studies have indicated that palliative care patients have frequent oral problems, the inclusion of a dentist on the treating team is often overlooked. The oral cavity is vastly important to the palliative care patient. It provides an important route for nutrition, medications, speech, and affection by kissing (Table 2.1).

The oral cascade of problems associated with palliative care is found in Fig. 2.2. As can be seen in this schematic, palliative care patients may have an array of problems, which will be discussed in the following sections.

Mucositis and stomatitis

As part of their treatments, patients may receive chemotherapy and/or radiotherapy. These treatments may be extended during their palliative care period in order to decrease pain or improve function. The oral cavity is affected by chemotherapy and radiotherapy at different rates. Chemotherapy affects mitotically active cells. Tissues of the oral cavity with high mitotic turnover are affected by such treatments, leading to atrophy of the tissues. Younger patients are of greater risk of atrophy of the tissues than older patients as they have a higher mitotic rate (Sonis *et al.*, 1978). Radiotherapy affects the oral cavity by sclerosing the small vessels which vascularise the oral tissues. An index to grade the severity of mucositis exists as outlined in Box 2.1.

A key element in mucositis/stomatitis prevention is to keep the mouth moist and clean. Oral care can actually decrease the rate of mucositis/stomatitis within cancer patients, probably by preventing or minimizing secondary infections (Sonis & Kunz, 1988).

Treatments for stomatitis/mucositis are primarily aimed at pain management. Failure to alleviate patient discomfort may lead to poor nutrition and hydration. This will further decrease the ability of the patient to recover. Topical anaesthetic agents are used to reduce pain. These include 2% viscous xylocaine, 10% xylocaine spray, 0.5–1.0% dyclonine hydrochloride, and 2% morphine. These agents except

Geriatric Dentistry: Caring for Our Aging Population, First Edition. Edited by Paula K. Friedman.
© 2014 John Wiley & Sons, Inc. Published 2014 by John Wiley & Sons, Inc.
Companion website: www.wiley.com/go/friedman/geriatricdentistry

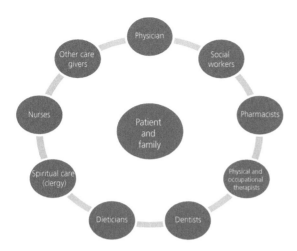

Figure 2.1 Palliative care team treating the patient and family.

Table 2.1 Impact of oral problems in palliative care

Physical impact	Social impact	Emotional impact
Difficulty in eating/drinking	Difficult to speak	Emotional pain
Taste disorders	Self-conscious of cancer	Fear of dying
Denture instability	Embarrassed	Fear for family
Xerostomia	Difficult to socialize	Depressed
Fungal infections	Halitosis	Depression
Viral infections ⎫ Mouth ulcers ⎬ Pain ⎭	Physically unable to display emotions; e.g., kiss	

Box 2.1 Index for mucositis

National Cancer Institute common terminology criteria for mucositis severity*

1 Asymptomatic or mild symptoms; intervention not indicated
2 Moderate pain, not interfering with oral intake; modified diet indicated
3 Severe pain, interfering with oral intake
4 Life-threatening consequences. The health professional must alleviate the pain to increase comfort and ameliorate the mastication process
5 Death

*National Cancer Institute (2012).

for morphine can be swished and swallowed. Patients must be instructed to expectorate the morphine. This can be modified by initially giving the patient saline to practice expectoration (Cerchietti, 2007).

Additional agents include sucralfate suspension, honey, benzydamine, and magic mouthwash. Sucralfate suspension as an agent in mucositis has had mixed results (Cengiz *et al.*, 1999; Dodd *et al.*, 2003). Its efficacy has to be evaluated on a case by case basis. Honey was found to effective in reducing mucositis; this may be due its natural bacteriostatic action (Biswal *et al.*, 2003). Magic mouthwash is a generic term that describes a number of formulations of a palliative solution used to allay the pain and discomfort of mucositis. One study surveyed 40 institutions and found that most of the prescribed formulations included diphenhydramine, lidocaine, Maalox®/Mylanta®, nystatin, and corticosteroids (dexamethasone, hydrocortisone and prednisone). Some of the other formulations included the ingredients tetracycline, chlorhexidine, sucralfate, and Orabase®/Ulcerase® (Chan & Jenoffo, 2005). The author's opinion is that treatment should be directed to the specific patient's chief complaint and the patient should not be treated with ingredients not required to alleviate the oral problem. The formulation selected must be prepared specifically for the patient by a pharmacist according to the dentist's prescription.

Nutrition

Oral problems can significantly affect a patient's ability to eat. Furthermore as the patient functionally declines, he or she becomes more prone to an anorexia–cachexia syndrome (Yavuzsen *et al.*, 2005). This syndrome involves the emaciation of the body of the patient. It is important that the dentist evaluates the patient's oral cavity for any interference with mastication. Anorexia may be a result of some of the medications prescribed to the terminally ill patient; these include psychostimulents, antidepressants, and chemotherapy. Additional factors include depression, pain, stomatitis, dysphagia, nausea, and depression. It is estimated that 70% of terminally ill patients will have anorexia (Yavuzsen *et al.*, 2005).

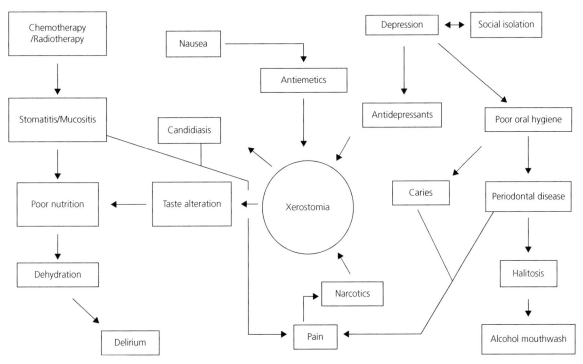

Figure 2.2 Oral problems in palliative care. From Bruera & Neumann (1998).

Suggestions that are nonpharmacologic include the provision of more frequent, small high-energy meals, attempting to make the presentation of food on the plate as appetizing as possible (use colorful foods, arrange in a visually pleasing way, accent with a piece of parsley/mint/flower), and simply asking the patient if there is anything that he or she may want to eat or drink. Pharmacologic agents to stimulate the appetite include megestrol and corticosteroids. These should be prescribed by the physician. Additionally as the patient's mouth can be xerostomic, meals should be moist and soft so that it is easier for the patient to swallow. Using high-calorie shakes can promote nutrition, be gentle on the mucosa, and be appetizing for the patient. Some are available commercially (e.g., Ensure®) or they can be easily be prepared in a blender by family members or caregivers. The careful use of seasonings may enhance flavors and promote nutrition; some may have the potential to irritate the mucosa so use of seasonings should be monitored for patient tolerance.

Dysphagia

Dysphagia can be divided into two different phases; one being the oropharyngeal phase and the other the esophageal phase. Causes of dysphagia may involve one or both of these phases.

The oropharyngeal phase begins in the mouth. If the patient's dentition is poor, mastication of the food bolus may not be adequate. The other components for the bolus preparation include adequate saliva production, sufficient muscular function, clear oral pathway, and freedom from pain such as ulcers, herpes, or fungi.

Inability to masticate foods can be the result of fewer teeth, poor fitting dentures, caries, or advanced periodontal disease. The palliative-care dentist should evaluate all patients for pain and function. Caries and periodontal disease should be treated. The choice of method to restore oral function should be based on prognostic longevity of the patient. For example, the patient may not be a good candidate for crowns or implants but may benefit from partial dentures.

Patients frequently do not have sufficient saliva production. This can be due to radiotherapy to the head and neck region leading to sclerosis of the salivary glands. Patients are often taking medications that cause xerostomia such as pain medications, antidepressants, and antihypertensives. (See Chapter 14 for further discussion of xerostomia.)

Muscular causes of dysphagia range from poorly functioning muscles of mastication, to poor tongue control. Causes for this include neurologic conditions such as Parkinson's disease, cerebral vascular accident, or amyotrophic lateral sclerosis; or nerve damage (cranial nerves V, VII, or XII) due to surgical or radiation treatment of intraoral tumors. Patients with poor tongue control will lack the ability to propel the food posteriorly to the oral pharynx.

Pain from fungal, herpes, or mucositis can lead to oral pain which will affect the patient's ability to swallow food. (See Stomatitis and mucositis section, earlier in this chapter.)

The esophageal component of swallowing can be inhibited by a physical obstruction from a tumor, or esophageal constrictions caused by radio/surgical therapy of a tumor. Additionally neurologic damage can lead to the lack of function.

Nausea and vomiting

Nausea and vomiting are common side effects of chemotherapy. Additionally, vomiting may be associated with bowel obstruction, constipation, electrolyte imbalance, autonomic failure, peptic ulcer disease, malignancy-associated gastroparesis, metabolic abnormalities, brain metastasis-associated increased intracranial pressure, and drug use such as opioids. Most patients will have at least two of these contributing factors as a causative factor. Chronic vomiting can have oral sequelae, and is discussed in greater detail later in the chapter. The acid content of vomit can erode tooth enamel and cause sensitivity. It is important to recommend the use of fluoride rinses and to prescribe fluoride varnish applications to counteract the erosive effect of the dentition's chronic exposure to vomit in the oral cavity. Anticholinergic agents such as scopolamine are used to alleviate vomiting and nausea. It is administered transdermally (1.5 mg every 72 h), and its primary side effects are drowsiness, xerostomia, and visual disturbances (Clissold & Heel, 1985). Dexamethasone, a glucocorticoid, is a good antiemetic (0.5–9.0 mg/day in divided doses every 6–12 h). Its side effects include insomnia, mood swings, and increased energy (Basch et al., 2011). Serotonin receptor antagonists, also called 5-HT3 (type three 5-hydroxytryptamine) receptor antagonists, are excellent antiemmetics with few side effects. Agents of this class include ondansetron (Zofran®) given at a dose of 8 mg twice daily.

Nonpharmacologic agents/methods used to control nausea and vomiting include ginger and acupuncture. In a study of 576 patients undergoing chemotherapy for breast cancer, ginger reduced nausea during the first day of chemotherapy (Ryan et al., 2012). Some studies indicate that acupressure/acupuncture may be of benefit to patients (Ezzo et al., 2005). This study did not involve an appropriate control, and the authors concluded that more studies would have to be done to verify its clinical relevance.

Prolonged vomiting may also lead to dehydration. The palliative team may suggest to replace fluids by parenteral routes such as intravenous or subcutaneous routes. Once the patient is able to tolerate oral fluids, they should be encouraged to drink. It is important for the palliative team to recognize that possible causes are hypercalcemia due to bone metastasis and the use of bisphosphonates may alleviate this cause.

The major oral problem associated with vomiting and nausea is that vomiting erodes teeth and increases the severity of mucositis and stomatitis. Vomiting robs the body of vital nutrients needed for repair. Nausea can prevent patients from wearing dentures, which are important for mastication and, perhaps of greater importance, their quality of life by affecting their social interactions due to vanity with loved ones. The use of antiemetics helps prevent this pathology but has a major side effect of xerostomia and possible tardive dyskinesia. Tardive dyskinesia is the repetitive muscular movements often seen as either frequent tongue, lip, or jaw movements. The use of a fluoride varnish or rinse will help protect the teeth. Oral care must be instituted as a strict regimen even though the patient may be nauseous. The use of a smaller toothbrush (child size) may help prevent triggering the nausea as its smaller size may not illicit a gagging reflex.

Delirium

Delirium is defined as a quick-onset change in cognitive condition and is very common in palliative care patients. They will exhibit cognitive difficulties, varying levels of consciousness, and changes in their sleep/wake cycle, and have varying degrees of agitation (Pereira et al., 1997). Delirium can be caused by the accumulation of opioid metabolites and other drugs. Patients that are dehydrated due to problems in swallowing, nausea and vomiting, or inability to eat/drink from stomatitis/mucositis will experience decreased urine output and, thus, decreased drug clearance. This can lead to certain drugs to have extended half-lives and increased toxicity. Patients do not require large volumes of fluids to maintain urine output, volumes of ≤1 L/day should be sufficient to maintain urine flow and electrolyte balance (Bruera et al., 1996).

Xerostomia and salivary gland hypofunction

Xerostomia and salivary gland hypofunction are terms that are easily confused. Xerostomia is the subjective sense of oral dryness. The oral cavity may appear to be moist; however, if the patient subjectively states that his or her mouth is dry, then he or she is xerostomic. Salivary gland hypofunction is defined by a quantitative flow rate of saliva less than 0.7 ml/min (Navazesh, 2003). It is more practical in dealing with palliative care patients to utilize the xerostomia definition as the aim of care is comfort measures. Xerostomia is one of the most frequent symptoms associated with terminally ill patients (Jobbins et al., 1992). Medication usage is the most common cause of xerostomia. One study indicated that in patients taking 4–5 medications daily, the incidence of xerostomia was 50% (Sreebny et al., 1989). Medications for pain management, antidepressants, diuretics, and antiemetics frequently prescribed to palliative care patients are among the major contributors to xerostomia. Additionally, the use of alcohol mouthwashes,and caffeinated beverages can lead to further drying of the mouth. The impairment generated by xerostomia affects the quality of life of the patient as it affects their ability to eat, communicate, and interact with loved ones (Gerdin et al., 2005).

Saliva is important as it lubricates the oral cavity, preventing trauma to the oral tissues; it contains ions responsible for remineralization of teeth; has buffers to maintain the pH of the oral cavity; and has antimicrobial components (Mandel, 1989). Caries rate is significantly higher in xerostomic mouths (Hopcraft & Tan, 2010). Additionally those patients with dry mouths are more prone to eat foods that are softer and cariogenic (Guggenheimer & Moore, 2003). The palliative care dentist should strive to keep the mouth moist. A dry mouth impacts the patient's ability to speak, chew, swallow, taste food, wear dentures, and kiss (Kleinegger, 2007).

Measures to ensure sufficient saliva levels include hydration, and having the patient's room humidified. The use of artificial saliva agents may help the patient. The ideal formulation for an artificial saliva agent would be one that is long lasting, a good lubricant, antimicrobial, neutral pH, has remineralization abilities, and is pleasant tasting. Most salivary substitutes are carboxymethylcellulose or mucin-based. Mucin-based products are usually preferred over carboxymethylcellulose products (Duxbury et al., 1989; Visch et al., 1986). Mucin products are not available in the USA, carboxymethylcellulose products include Mouth Kote® (Parnell Pharmaceuticals), Xerolube® (Colgate Pamolive), and Salivart® (Gebauer). Saliva substitutes must be evaluated for their pH. The pH of these products is important to prevent demineralization of dentin/enamel in the xerostomic mouth (Table 2.2) (Kielbassa et al., 2000; Smith et al., 2001).

Table 2.2 The pH of artificial saliva agents

Agent	pH
A S Saliva Orthana Spray®*	5.45
Salivace Spray®*	5.86
Glandosane Spray® natural flavor*	5.15
Glandosane Spray® lemon flavor*	5.12
Glandosane Spray® peppermint flavor*	5.12
Luborant*	5.99
Saliveze® spray*	6.88
Artisial®[†]	6.66
Oralube®[†]	6.89
Biotène®[†]	5.15
Meridol®[†]	3.88

*Smith et al. (2001).
[†]Kielbassa et al. (2000).

Saliva can be stimulated by proprioceptive agents, such as sugarless chewing gums and mints, and organic acids (Grovenko *et al.*, 2009; Jensdottir *et al.*, 2006; Turner & Ship, 2008). Flavoring agents, such as cinnamon, should be avoided in gums and mints as they may irritate fragile tissues (Kleinegger, 2007). Organic acids, such as ascorbic acid, citric acid, or malic acid, should be used cautiously as they may cause rapid demineralization of natural teeth in the xerostomic patient (Anneroth *et al.*, 1980). Sugarless products that contain xylitol may be advantageous due to their bactericidal effect of cariogenic bacteria (Van Loveren, 2004). One study indicated that patients' preferred sugarless chewing gum over mucin-based saliva agents in the management of their xerostomia (Davies, 2000). There are reports that acupuncture and electrostimulation may increase salivary flow, but these studies are few in number (Cho *et al.*, 2008; Strietzel *et al.*, 2007). Caffeine-based products should be avoided if possible to decrease their diuretic properties. Use of mouthwash that does not contain alcohol is recommended for xerostomic patients, as alcohol desiccates tissues,

A major problem for xerostomic patients is the dryness during sleep or when semi-comatose. The use of water-soluble lubricants, such as Biotene Oral Balance® gel, K-Y® jelly, Muko® jelly, or Taro® gel, can be helpful. These agents are spread over surfaces thinly using a foam brush, like a Toothette® (Sage Dental Products). The use of an adhesive mucocutaneous disk (OraMoist®) by Quantum Research has been suggested to provide short-term relief (Kerr *et al.*, 2010). Patients that are xerostomic are prone to caries. They may decide to use a variety of mouth rinses, caution should be noted with alcohol-based rinses as they will desiccate tissues.

Systemic agents include the use of agents such as pilocarpine (Salagen®) 5–10 mg three times daily, or cevimeline (Evoxac®) 30 mg three times daily. These drugs are cholinergic mimetic agents and may have a variety of side effects, including sweating and increased pulmonary secretions. These may not be tolerable for the palliative care patient; physician and pharmacist consultations are suggested.

Xerostomia can affect the ability of the patient to retain their dentures (Turner & Ship, 2008). In patients with normal salivary flow, there exists an layer of saliva between the acrylic and the soft tissues

of the mouth. This layer promotes the generation of a vacuum to improve retention. Additionally it acts as a lubricant to reduce denture trauma-associated sores. Palliative care patients may benefit from rinsing the mouth and wetting the denture prior to placement. The use of adhesives can also aid in denture retention. Toward the end-of-life, patients may decide not to wear their dentures for a variety of reasons. There may be poor denture adhesion due to xerostomia and poor muscle tone, and/or the patient may be anorexic and is no longer eating. This may become a source of concern to family members.

Patients that are xerostomic or patients that are on oxygen may experience dry lips. Using a petroleum distillate such as Vaseline® is dangerous as it can catch fire, as well it "protects" microorganisms from the body's defense mechanisms. It is probably best to use lanolin. This product is available as a protectant to nursing mothers' nipples.

Candidiasis

The most frequent pathogen causing candidiasis is *Candida albicans.* This organism is present in healthy moist mouths but is kept at subclinical levels by the competition of normal microbial biota. Fungal infections are frequently seen in cancer patients, ranging from 7.2% to 57% (Schlenz *et al.*, 2011). Oral candidiasis is frequently found in patients using inhaled steroids, undergoing chemotherapy, or suffering from xerostomia. Immunosuppression and/or xerostomia explain the high incidence of candidiasis, as the natural microbial environment alters from non-pathogenic organisms to opportunistic pathogenic organisms (Hopcraft & Tan, 2010).

There are two different types of *Candida* infections; one being pseudomembranous and characterized by white plaques, and the second being an atrophic form without white plaques just erythemic, seen frequently as denture stomatitis (Butz-Jorgensen, 1981). Fungal infections in the mouth may cause a painful burning sensation (Turner & Ship, 2007). Fungal infections are exacerbated by xerostomia.

Treatment of candidiasis can be either topical or systemic. Topical treatments include nystatin products, clotrimazole, and miconazole treatments. Systemic agents include fluconazole and ketoconazole. These agents should be reserved for cases in which topical measures fail. Using these products can create opioid toxicity by displacing albumin-bound opioids to dangerous levels. These medications must be used carefully with close cooperation between the treating physician and pharmacist.

Nystatin should be given at a dose of 400 000–600 000 IU, swished in the mouth for about 20–30 seconds, and then swallowed. Two major problems exist with nystatin suspension: firstly, this agent works best topically and, although patients are urged to swish this product for as long as possible, it is often swallowed quickly. The second problem is that nystatin suspension contains 33% sucrose. This is primarily used to mask the taste of nystatin. The high sugar content feeds the fungus as it attempts to kill it, and also increases the risk for caries. A sugarless formulation for nystatin suspension is found in Fig. 2.3.

Other topical measures to treat the candidiasis include the use of clotrimacazole lozenges, the use of vaginal antifungals such as the sucking of nystatin suppositories, and the use of creams such as miconazole (Monistat® cream), clotrimazole (Canestan® cream), or nystatin (Mycostatin® cream) to line the tissue-bearing side of dentures. As stated earlier, the xerostomic patient is more prone to fungal infections and may experience a burning sensation. The author has used "nystatin popsicles" (5 ml nystatin suspension : 5 ml sugarless fruit juice [see Fig. 2.4]) for these patients. The benefits of the nystatin popsicles are that the antifungal stays topically for extended periods of time, the patient is being hydrated, and the cryotherapy aids decrease the burning pain. The semi-comatose patient presents a different clinical problem as these patients cannot use rinses or pills due to the risk of aspiration. The author has used a mixture of a water-soluble lubricant (e.g., K-Y® jelly, Muko® jelly, or Taro® gel) and nystatin suspension (50 : 50 v/v) and painted it upon oral tissues (Fig. 2.5) to provide relief.

Cancer and quality of life

Cancer in any form will affect the quality of life for the patient and family. It must be noted that cancer of the head and neck area may be more psychologically disturbing to the patient, family, and care staff (Dropkin *et al.*, 1983). Head and neck cancer patients

**Nystatin 100,000 IU
Sugar-Free Oral Suspension**

Directions:
1. Triturate nystatin, stevioside 90% powder, potassium acesulfame, sodium saccharin, xanthan gum, and sodium benzoate in glass mortar and pestle.
2. Add enough glycerin to make a smooth paste to eliminate all of the brown bumps from the xantham gum.
3. Add the flavour and peppermint oil if needed.
4. Add purified water. Keep refrigerated. Shelf life 30 days.

**Nystatin 100,000 IU
Sugar-Free Oral Suspension**

Ingredients:
- Nystatin   6,000,000 IU
- Stevioside 90% powder   120 mg
- Potassium Acesulfame   100 mg
- Sodium saccharin   45 mg
- Sodium Benzoate   120 mg
- Xanthan gum   120 mg
- Glycerin to make paste
- Raspberry/Tutti Frutti   2 ml
- Peppermint oil (if needed)   0.1–0.2 ml
- Purified water   60 ml

Figure 2.3 Formulation for sugar-free nystatin solution.

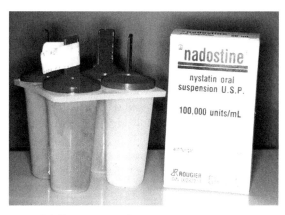

Figure 2.4 Nystatin popsicles.

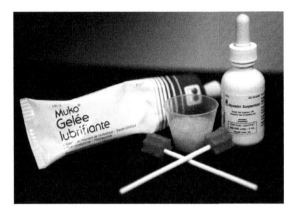

Figure 2.5 Nystatin suspension plus lubricant.

may develop impairments in their physical or functional ability, affect patient's social interactions, and cause psychologic distress. This will affect the patient's quality of life. Many instruments have been developed to assess quality of life in cancer patients (Kirkova *et al.*, 2006).

Herpes and palliative care

Palliative care patients may have reactivation of herpetic lesions in the mouth. This can lead to a painful herpetic stomatitis. A palliative measure is the use of a mixture of Benadryl® suspension with Kaopectate® at a 50 : 50 dilution painted onto oral lesions. The use of antivirals such as acyclovir (400 mg three times daily for 5 days) is given to treat herpetic infections. Herpetic zoster may result in neuropathic pain. A nonopioid approach to pain relief is the use of peppermint oil applied to the lesions (Davies *et al.*, 2002).

Depression and the oral cavity

Within the dying process, patients will frequently exhibit depression, grief, sadness, and feelings of loss. The extent of depression is associated with the form of cancer. Patients with head and neck cancer exhibited greater depression than patients with pancreatic, breast, or lung cancer (Massie, 2004). This is probably related to the loss of self-image associated with head and neck lesions. Depression can be treated with antidepressants. These include the tricyclic antidepressants, selective serotonin reuptake inhibitors (SSRIs), and monamine oxidase inhibitors (MAOs). Unfortunately, a major side effect of these medications is varying degrees of xerostomia.

Depressed palliative care patients may neglect their oral care. The probable resulting caries and periodontal disease may cause pain and, thus, increased pain medications are required. On a social level, neglect of oral care leads to increased social isolation as loved ones may not want to be near them due to halitosis. Patients may decide to treat the halitosis by using alcohol-based mouth rinses, which in turn further increase xerostomia, caries, and periodontal disease. Patients should be instructed to use a saline rinse or an alcohol-free mouth rinse.

An important asset to every member of the palliative care team is the ability to converse with the patient. This not only improves the level of social interactions for the patient but may help alleviate their fears by talking about death and the process of dying.

Caries prevention

The palliative care patient is at high risk for dental caries because of the many xerogenic medications prescribed, radiotherapy to the head and neck, dehydration, and a lack of will to perform oral care. Dental care for these patients should be divided into either prevention or treatments. Prevention should be aimed to reduce new decay if possible. Patients can receive fluoride varnishes and use high-level fluoride toothpastes. Examples include Duraphat® (Colgate Pamolive) and PreviDent® 5000 (Colgate Pamolive). Treatment of carious lesions includes the smoothing of rough edges and using restorative agents, such as glass ionomers or amalgam. Glass ionomers are anticariogenic due to their fluoride release but are limited in a dry mouth (De Gee *et al.*, 1996). The patient should be given a mouthwash with fluoride to protect the oral cavity. Agents include ACT® fluoride rinse (Chattem) or Crest Pro-Health® (Proctor and Gamble).

Taste disorders

Taste disorders can be seen in 25–50% of palliative care patients, with xerostomia being of prime etiology (Tanaka, 2002; Twycross & Lack, 1986). Taste disorders can be differentiated into dysgeusia (distorted taste), hypogeusia (reduced taste), or ageusia (total loss of taste). Altered taste disorders seem to affect women at a higher rate than men (Ripamonti & Fulfaro, 2004). Some patients will increase the sugar content of their diet to improve taste. As taste mediators must be dissolved to be sensed by the tongue, rinsing the mouth with artificial saliva and having moist foods, such as those with gravy, will increase taste. Zinc deficiency has been linked to taste disorders; zinc supplementation (220 mg) may improve taste (Tanaka, 2002).

Treatment planning

The dentist must strive to ensure that the patient is free of pain from the oral cavity, and has sufficient dental function. The dentist should listen to both the patient and family members to determine the chief complaint and desired outcomes. The dentist must provide an oral hygiene plan to nursing staff in order to provide the best quality of life for the patient. Treatment suggestions must be tailored to the patient's health status. It must be based on reality, taking into account the patient's and/or family member's ability to aid in their oral care. The author has suggested that dental teams use the CARE anagram to guide comprehensive treatment assessment for the palliative care patient (Box 2.2):

Box 2.2 CARE anagram

> **C**omfort measures
> **A**ssessment of changing health and dental status
> **RE**ality dictating treatment options

Communication

Every health professional should maintain an honest, direct approach when talking with both the patient and his/her family. It is also important that everyone on the palliative care team share the same treatment vision and approach. This can be best attained by having team meetings at which the members of the palliative care team discusses the patient and reach a consensus on treatment.

Case study 1

Mrs. S. is a 75-year-old woman with incurable breast cancer with metastasis to bone and lungs. She is presently on a fentanyl patch (Duragesic®) 75 mg/h for pain. Her chief complaints are nausea, constipation, and a dry mouth. Upon the dentist's arrival to her room, she is bare-breasted with a fulminating mass over her left breast. This is a mass that has punctured the skin and is odorous. She has discomfort from the bed sheets resting upon her breast. A request for a dental consultation was issued because of her dry mouth.

Dental appraisal and approach

The first approach for the treating dentist is to gain the patient's trust. The dentist should introduce him or herself; and explain his or her role in helping to alleviate some of the patient's discomfort. The dentist must not use any body language that may cause embarrassment to the patient. The dentist should ask Mrs. S. if her mouth is dry or if she has any pain or discomfort in her mouth. Mrs. S. states that her mouth is indeed dry. You can discuss the decision to give her an artificial saliva agent and water-soluble lubricant to ease her dryness. It is important to explain the reasons why you are prescribing these agents. You should ask if you may look into her mouth. Upon oral examination, you notice that her tongue and oral cavity are very dry. You ask her if she is having pain elsewhere in her body. She states that her left breast and chest are very painful and that she is scared. It is important for the palliative care dentist to provide care with a humanistic approach. You hold her hand and state that you will discuss her pain with her physician.

The following week she begins to complain of a burning sore mouth. Upon inspection you notice that she has white plaques over the mucosal tissues of her cheeks. These are easily removed leaving an erythemic area. You diagnose this as being a fungal infection (*Candida*). You conduct a further review of her medication list and note the use of systemic antifungals may affect her midazolam and morphine (pain medication) blood levels. You decide to treat her with a nystatin rinse (5 ml of 100 000 IU four times daily for 10 days). It is important to provide encouragement and emotional support.

After 7 days, her fungal infection has resolved. You continue to visit her, making sure that her mouth is as moist as possible. After a couple of weeks Mrs. S. becomes semi-comatose and unresponsive; you use a Toothette® to spread the water-soluble agents over her mouth. Mrs. S. dies shortly thereafter. You provide emotional support to her family.

Case study 2

Mr. M. is an 83-year-old patient presenting to the dental clinic with pain in the lower right angle of the jaw. A radiograph reveals a large radiopaque lesion, which is confirmed by excisional biopsy to be squamous cell carcinoma (Fig. 2.6).

Dental management

A family meeting was held and instead of opting for a surgical resection of the patient's mandible, palliative care radiotherapy was used to shrink the lesion and decrease his pain. Unfortunately radiotherapy led to the destruction of healthy tissue which resulted in an oral fistula through the patient's cheek (Fig. 2.7). Although the resulting treatment minimized his discomfort, the resulting lesion allowed food and medications to exit his mouth through this fistula. His mouth was continuously lubricated and cleaned. He died a natural death after 10 months.

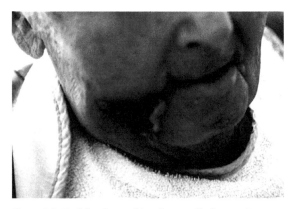

Figure 2.7 Oral fistula resulting from radiotherapy (see Case study 2).

DISCUSSION QUESTIONS

1 Oral care is often overlooked in patients receiving palliative care. What protocol would you recommend to the healthcare staff for patients for routine oral care in a palliative care setting?
2 You are asked to provide a dental consultation to a patient in hospice who is complaining of a burning mouth after several rounds of radiation therapy. How would you approach the situation? What would you discuss with the patient? What would you discuss with the healthcare staff?

References

Anneroth, G., Nordenram, G. & Bengtsson, S. (1980) Effect of saliva stimulants [Hybrin and malic acid] on cervical root surfaces in vitro. *Scandinavian Journal of Dental Research*, **88**, 214–18.

Basch, E., Prestrud, A.A., Hesketh, P.J., *et al.* (2011) Antiemetics: American Society of Clinical Oncology clinical practice guideline update. *Journal of Clinical Oncology*, **29**(31), 4189–98.

Biswal, B.M., Zakaria, A. & Ahmad, N.M. (2003) Topical application of honey in the management of radiation mucositis. A preliminary study. *Supportive Care in Cancer*, **11**, 242–8.

Bruera, E. & Neumann, C.M. (1998) Management of specific symptom complexes in patients receiving palliative care. *Canadian Medical Association Journal*, **158**(13):1717–26.

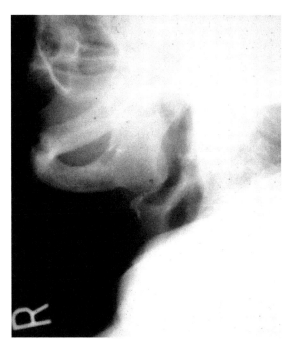

Figure 2.6 Radiograph of jaw (see Case study 2).

Bruera, E., Belzile, M., Watanabe, S. & Fainsinger, R.L. (1996) Volume of hydration in terminal cancer patients. *Supportive Care in Cancer*, **4**(2), 147–50.

Butz-Jorgensen, E. (1981) Oral mucosal lesions associated with the wearing of removable dentures. *Journal of Oral Pathology*, **10**, 65–80.

Cengiz, M., Ozyar, E., Ozturk, D., *et al.* (1999) Sucralfate in the prevention of radiation-induced oral mucositis. *Journal of Clinical Gastroenterology*, **28**, 40–3.

Cerchietti, L. (2007) Morphine mouthwashes for painful mucositis. *Supportive Care in Cancer*, **15**, 115–16.

Chan, A. & Jenoffo, R.J. (2005) Survey of topical oral solutions for the treatment of chemo-induced oral mucositis. *Journal of Oncology Pharmacy Practice*, **11**, 139–43.

Cho, J.H., Chung, W.K., Kang, W., et al. (2008) Manual acupuncture improved quality of life in cancer patients with radiation-induced xerostomia. *Journal of Alternative and Complementary Medicine (New York, NY)*, **14**, 523–6.

Christakis, N.A. & Lamont, E.B. (2000) Extent and determination of error in doctors' prognoses in terminally ill patients: prospective cohort study. *BMJ (Clinical Research Ed.)*, **320**, 469–73.

Clissold, S.P. & Heel, R.C. (1985) Transdermal hyoscine (Scopolamine). A preliminary review of its pharmacodynamic properties and therapeutic efficacy. *Drugs*, **29**(3), 189–207.

Davies, A.N. (2000) A comparison of artificial saliva and chewing gum in the management of xerostomia in patients with advanced cancer. *Palliative Medicine*, **12**, 197–203.

Davies, S.J., Harding, L.M. & Baranowski, A.P. (2002) A novel treatment of postherpetic neuralgia using peppermint oil. *Clinical Journal of Pain*, **18**, 200–2.

De Gee, A.J., van Duinen, R.N., Werner, A. & Davidson, C.L. (1996) Early and long-term wear of conventional and resin-modified glass ionomers. *Journal of Dental Research*, **75**, 1613–19.

Dodd, M.J., Miaskowski, C., Greenspan, D., *et al.* (2003) Radiation-induced mucositis: a randomized clinical trial of micronized sucralfate versus salt and soda mouthwashes. *Cancer Investigation*, **21**, 21–33.

Dropkin, M.J., Malgady, R.G., Scott, D.W., *et al.* (1983) Scaling of disfigurement and dysfunction in postoperative head and neck patients. *Head & Neck Surgery*, **6**, 559–70.

Duxbury, A.J., Thakker, N.S. & Wastell, D.G. (1989) A double-blind cross-over trial of mucin-containing artificial saliva. *British Dental Journal*, **166**, 115–20.

Ezzo, J., Vickers, A., Richardson, M.A., *et al.* (2005) Acupuncture-point stimulation for chemotherapy-induced nausea and vomiting. *Journal of Clinical Oncology*, **23**(28), 7188–98.

Gerdin EW, Einarson S, Jonsson M, *et al.* (2005) Impact of dry mouth conditions on oral health-related quality of life in older people. *Gerondontology*, **22**, 219–26.

Grovenko, M., Clark, D.C. & Aleksejuniene, J. (2009) Over the counter xerostomia remedies currently available in Canada. *Canadian Journal of Dental Hygiene*, **43**, 71–7.

Guggenheimer, J. & Moore, P.A. (2003) Xerostomia etiology, recognition and treatment. *Journal of the American Dental Association*, **134**, 61–9.

Hopcraft, M.S. & Tan, C. (2010) Xerostomia an update for clinicians. *Australian Dental Journal*, **55**, 238–44.

Jensdottir, T., Nauntofte, B., Buchwald, C., *et al.* (2006) Effects of sucking acidic candies on saliva in unilaterally irradiated pharyngeal cancer patients. *Oral Oncology*, **42**, 317–22.

Jobbins, J., Bagg, J., Finlay, I.G., *et al.* (1992) Oral and dental disease in terminally ill cancer patients. *BMJ*, **304**, 1612.

Kerr, A.R., Corby, P.M., Shah, S.S., *et al.* (2010) Use of a mucoadhesive disk for relief of dry mouth: a randomized, double-masked, controlled crossover study. *Journal of the American Dental Association*, **141**, 1250–6.

Kielbassa, A.M., Shohadai, S.P. & Schulte-Monting, J. (2000) Effect of saliva substitutes on mineral content of demineralized and sound dental enamel. *Supportive Care in Cancer*, **9**, 40–7.

Kirkova, J., Davis, M.P., Walsh, D., *et al.* (2006) Cancer symptom assessment instruments: a systematic review. *Journal of Clinical Oncology*, **24**(9), 1459–73.

Kleinegger, C.L. (2007) Dental management of xerostomia: opportunity, expertise, obligation. *Journal of the California Dental Association*, **35**, 417–24.

Mandel, I.D. (1989) The role of saliva in maintaining oral homeostasis. *Journal of the American Dental Association*, **119**, 298–304.

Massie, M.J. (2004) Prevalence of depression in patients with cancer. *Journal of the National Cancer Institute. Monographs*, **32**, 57–71.

National Cancer Institute (2012) *Common Terminology Criteria for Adverse Events v.3.0.* From http://ctep.cancer.gov/protocolDevelopment/electronic_applications/docs/ctcaev3.pdf. Accessed August 24, 2012.

Navazesh, M. (2003) How can oral health care providers determine if patients have dry mouth? *Journal of the American Dental Association*, **134**(5):613–18.

Pereira, J., Hanson, J. & Bruera, E. (1997) The frequency and clinical course of cognitive impairment in patients with terminal cancer. *Cancer*, **79**(4):835–42.

Ripamonti, C. & Fulfaro, F. (2004) Taste disturbance. In: *Oral Care in Advanced Disease* (eds A. Davies & I. Finlay), pp. 115–24. Oxford University Press, Oxford.

Ryan, J.L., Heckler, C.E., Roscoe, J.A., *et al.* (2012) Ginger (*Zingiber officinale*) reduces acute chemotherapy-induced nausea: a URCC CCOP study of 576 patients. *Supportive Care in Cancer*, **20**(7), 1479–89.

Schlenz, S., Abdallah, S., Gray, G., *et al.* (2011) Epidemiology of oral yeast colonization and infection in patients with hematological malignancies, head neck and solid tumors. *Journal of Oral Pathology & Medicine*, **40**, 83–9.

Smith, G., Smith, A.J., Shaw, L. & Shaw, M.J. (2001) Artificial saliva substitutes and mineral dissolution. *Journal of Oral Rehabilitation*, **28**, 728–31.

Sonis, S. & Kunz, A. (1988) Impact of improved dental services on the frequency of oral complications of cancer therapy for patients with non-head-and-neck malignancies. *Oral Surgery, Oral Medicine, and Oral Pathology*, **65**(1), 19–22.

Sonis, S.T., Sonis, A.L. & Lieberman, A. (1978) Oral complications in patients receiving treatment for malignancies other than of the head and neck. *Journal of the American Dental Association*, **97**(3), 468–72.

Sreebny, L.M., Valdini, A. & Yu, A. (1989) Xerostomia part II: relationship to nonoral symptoms, drugs, and diseases. *Oral Surgery, Oral Medicine, and Oral Pathology*, **68**, 419–27.

Strietzel, F.P., Martin-Granizo, R., Fedele, S. *et al.* (2007) Electrostimulating device in the management of xerostomia. *Oral Diseases*, **13**(2), 206–13.

Tanaka, M. (2002) Secretory function of the salivary gland in patients with taste disorders or xerostomia: correlation with zinc deficiency. *Acta Oto-laryngologica. Supplementum*, **546**, 134–41.

Turner, M. & Ship, J.A. (2007) Dry mouth and its effects on the oral health of elderly people. *Journal of the American Dental Association*, **138**, 15S–20S.

Turner, M. & Ship, J.A. (2008) Hyposalivation, xerostomia and the complete denture: a systematic review. *Journal of the American Dental Association*, **139**, 146–50.

Twycross, R.G. & Lack, S.A. (1986) *Control of Alimentary Symptoms in Far-Advanced Cancer*. Churchill Livingstone, Edinburgh.

Van Loveren, C. (2004) Sugar alcohols: what is the evidence for caries-prevention and caries-therapeutic effects? *Caries Research*, **38**, 286–93.

Visch, L.L., Gravenmade, E.J., Schaub, R.M., *et al.* (1986) A double-blind crossover trial of CMC- and mucin-containing saliva substitutes. *International Journal of Oral and Maxillofacial Surgery*, **15**, 395–400.

Wiseman, M.A. (2000) Palliative care dentistry. *Gerodontology*, **17**(1), 49–51.

Yavuzsen, T., Davis, M.P., Walsh, D., *et al.* (2005) Systemic review of the treatment of cancer-associated anorexia and weight loss. *Journal of Clinical Oncology*, **23**, 8500–11.

PART 2
Clinical Practice

CHAPTER 3

Living Arrangements for the Elderly: Independent Living, Shared Housing, Board and Care Facilities, Assisted Living, Continuous Care Communities, and Nursing Homes

Timothy J. Halligan[1] and Kelly A. Halligan[2]

[1] United States Air Force Dental Corps, Colorado Springs, CO, USA
[2] Private Practitioner, Colorado Springs, CO, USA

Introduction

In 2010, Americans aged 65 and older numbered over 40 million (approximately 13% of the US population). Since 2000, this age group has increased almost twice as fast as those aged under 65. By 2030, 20% of the US population is expected to be over the age of 65. The fastest growing age groups of Americans are those over the age of 85. From 2010 to 2020, this population will increase 19%, more than any other age group. This growth of the older adult population has been spurred by the aging of the baby boomers and the increased longevity of the elderly due to improved medical care, more availability of community services, and improved quality of care in long-term living facilities (US Department of Health and Human Services, 2011).

As mentioned in previous chapters, growth in the elderly population is growing at an astounding rate. This growth impacts present and future housing markets through development of more living communities that cater to seniors' lifestyles and values. Housing options for the elderly include: (a) independent living/age in place (including unassisted elderly communities); (b) shared housing; (c) assisted living facilities; (d) board and care

facilities; (e) continuous care communities; and (f) nursing homes. This chapter will highlight the various options for living facilities for the elderly, describe factors to consider when choosing a particular arrangement, and explain why people prefer certain arrangements over others. Understanding these available options prior to time of immediate need will help seniors and their family members make informed decisions for future living arrangements.

According to the 2010 US Census Bureau Report, 22% of Americans aged 65 and over currently live alone, 63% live with a spouse, 13% live with other relatives, and 2% live with nonrelative caregivers, in self-owned, single-family, detached houses in mixed-age, higher-income neighborhoods. Three-fourths of the elderly live in metropolitan areas, with a majority living in the suburbs (US Census Bureau, 2010). Living arrangement choices are affected by multiple factors, including preference, proximity to family, cost, need for medical care, desire for more social interaction, etc. However, fragility, or the need for assistance to perform Activities of Daily Living (ADLs), usually determines which living situation is the best option. The six ADLs assessed when determining level of independence are: (a) walking;

Geriatric Dentistry: Caring for Our Aging Population, First Edition. Edited by Paula K. Friedman.
© 2014 John Wiley & Sons, Inc. Published 2014 by John Wiley & Sons, Inc.
Companion website: www.wiley.com/go/friedman/geriatricdentistry

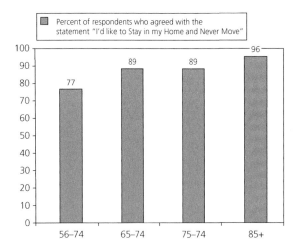

Figure 3.1 Summary of the results of an American Association of Retired Persons' survey on seniors' choices for living arrangements. From Hobbs and Damon (1996).

(b) dressing; (c) bathing, personal hygiene; (e) eating; (f) getting in and out of bed; and (g) toileting. Failure to independently perform any of these ADLs increases fragility (McDowell & Newell, 1996). Additionally, Instrumental Activities of Daily Living (IADLs), including, but not limited to, ability to independently perform housework, prepare meals, shop for groceries, use the telephone or other technology, take medications, manage finances, or use transportation within the community, are not necessary for fundamental functions that can be supplemented with assistance from family, friends, or outside agencies to enable the individual to live independently in a community (Bookman *et al.*, 2007; McDowell & Newell, 1996; Schafer, 1999). IADLs can also be helpful in deciding which living arrangement option is best, and failures in ability to independently perform IADLs could potentially be overcome with in-home services.

Most people believe seniors' living arrangements of choice are assisted living communities. However, almost 90% of people aged 65–74, and over 95% of people aged 85 and older would rather stay in their homes. Figure 3.1 summarizes the results of a 1996 American Association of Retired Persons' (AARP) survey on seniors' choices for living arrangements (AARP, 1996).

Knowing these statistics, seniors and their family members must consider home design, level of needed care, the seniors' desires, and cost when choosing the appropriate living arrangement for themselves or loved ones. Below, are descriptions of living arrangement options for seniors to consider.

Independent living/age in place

Building or designing a home that is modifiable as ADLs levels deteriorate is an ideal choice for those seniors who plan to age in place. This design requires preplanning a single-story building to include minimal outside grade and stairs for access, wider door openings for wheelchair passage, and/or creating a bedroom with a full bath off the main living area. If the home was not selected or designed for future needs, simple alterations in an existing home may allow the senior to stay at home for many more years. As the senior's ADLs and IADLs levels deteriorate, they can implement various home care options. These options include: (a) home management assistance (assistance with household chores and shopping); (b) home meal delivery (e.g. Meals on Wheels); (c) personal nonmedical assistance (assistance with ADLs); (d) personal medical assistance (home health aide); and (e) licensed home health care (registered nurse, physical therapists, and occupational therapists). A rapidly growing profession, geriatric care managers, specializes in assessing living arrangements for the elderly and can give objective recommendations. Services provided include conducting home care assessments (recommendations to meet resident's needs), conducting interviews to hire and manage home health care, providing counsel on legal issues, determining fragility, recommending best housing options; and transition support for seniors and their family members.

Geriatric care manager agencies are often expensive for seniors not enrolled in a senior managed care organization (SCO). The monthly cost of retaining a geriatric care manager agency is in addition to the cost of the required service personnel. SCOs are managed care groups for Medicaid recipients who receive a capitated payment per individual per month to manage all the enrollees healthcare needs – acute, chronic, inpatient, and outpatient.

Congregate housing/retirement communities

Ambulatory seniors who can perform most of their ADLs but desire more social interaction should consider congregate housing or retirement communities. Often, these communities provide a variety of social and recreational activities for their residents. Seniors live in their own apartment units, share some meals in a central dining room, and are eligible to receive some housekeeping services (Fig. 3.2). Typically, these communities do not require entrance fees. Some of them, however, receive public subsidies that help keep rental fees down. Therefore, rental fees vary widely, and meals and other services may cost extra. Unfortunately, many of these facilities have years long waiting lists and stringent income requirements, catering to lower income individuals.

The option to stay at home may become unreasonable due to a medical complexity, physical fragility, or the development of a disability. In 2010, 37% of older persons reported some type of disability (i.e., loss of function in the following areas: hearing, vision, cognition, ambulation, self-care, or independent living). Although some of these disabilities may be relatively insignificant, others could force seniors into some form of assisted living (US Department of Health and Human Services, 2011). Typically, a spouse, family member, physician, or other trusted source determines the need for changing the living arrangement from independent to assisted living. Sometimes the other party (spouse, family member, clergy, etc.) may realize the need for a change in living arrangements before the senior does. This can often lead to discussions between and among the parties over an extended period of time before a transition can be made. As shown in Fig. 3.1, almost all older adults would like to stay in their homes forever and never move.

Assisted living

Assisted living residences are aimed at helping residents remain as self-sufficient as possible with the assurance of assistance with ADLs when needed. Typically, residents are provided board (either as a single room or an apartment with a small kitchen), meals, personal care and support, social activities (Table 3.1), 24-hour supervision and, in some facilities, health services. Residents in these facilities pay regular monthly rent for room and board plus additional fees for the services they receive. Assisted living facilities offer residents an advantage over other living arrangements, as they offer different levels of care as needs change. Because each state decides how they are licensed, assisted living facilities vary from state to state and may also vary in size, appearance, cost, and services offered or regulated by the federal government. Board and care homes could also be placed under this category (AARP, 1996).

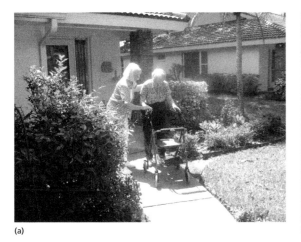

(a)

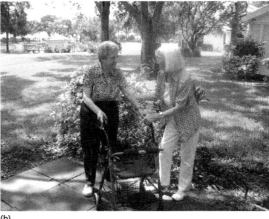

(b)

Figure 3.2 (a,b) Theresa Dewar, aged 83, leaving her unassisted living facility to move to a nursing home with the help of Lois Halligan.

Table 3.1 Sample of week's activities in an assisted living facility

Sunday	Monday	Tuesday	Wednesday	Thursday	Friday	Saturday
	9:30 AM Chair fitness	9:30 AM Chair fitness	9:30 AM Chair fitness	9:30 AM Chair fitness	9:30 AM Chair fitness	9:30 AM Chair fitness
11:00 AM Church: Meadow Creek First Baptist Church		10:00 AM Bible study	1:00 PM Crazy Eights	11:00 AM Special music	11:00 AM Coffee, tea, and party	11:00 AM Trivial Pursuit
3:30 PM Super Bowl party	3:30 PM Blackout bingo	2:30 PM Bingo	3:00 PM Bingo	3:30 PM Bingo	3:30 PM Bingo	
				6:00 PM Movie night		

Board and care home

Board and care homes are considered a smaller version of an assisted living arrangement, and are an attractive option for seniors who need some assistance. Residents are provided nonmedical custodial care in various facilities, including a single family residence, a retirement residence, or in any appropriate care facility. These residences provide a private or shared room, meals, and help seniors with daily activities. They are not always licensed, however, and are, therefore, not always monitored by local authorities. In some states, board and care homes can provide nursing services, but they are not medical facilities. More than 90% of board and care homes are licensed for six or fewer residents housed in a private residential home setting (AARP, 1996).

Continuing care retirement communities

These facilities are designed to meet the changing needs of older people by providing a variety of housing options and services on the same campus (Fig. 3.3). Residents might initially live independently in an apartment and then move to an assisted living unit as assistance with daily activities are needed. A nursing unit is also available on-site for when skilled nursing care is needed. The average entrance fee for each unit ranges from $160 000 to $600 000, based on size and amenities, and is used to pay for resident care, facility maintenance, and operations. Charges can range from $2500 to $5400, but

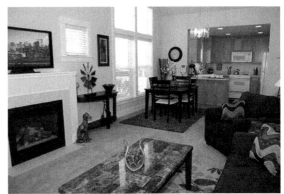
(a)

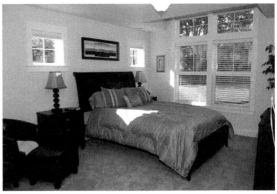
(b)

Figure 3.3 (a,b) Photographs from McMinnville, Oregon Continuing Care Retirement Community.

may increase as needs change (US Government Accountability Office, 2010). Some contacts allow for some or all entrance fees to be returned to beneficiaries when resident dies.

This option is most often used by higher-income individuals who afford the entrance fee by selling their home and using the proceeds to pay this expensive fee. Some continuing care retirement communities have dementia units so residents can transition through all potential phases of need in one location.

Typically, residents are offered three contract options:

1 **Life care or extended contract:** Most expensive, but offers unlimited care without additional charges.
2 **Modified contract:** Offers defined set of services for a limited length of time. When time is expired, services can be obtained for higher monthly fees.
3 **Fee-for-service contract:** Enrollment fee is reduced, nursing care is paid on as needed basis.

Nursing homes

Nursing home residents are among the frailest Americans. In 2005, nearly half of all residents had dementia, and more than half were confined to a bed or wheelchair (AARP, 2007; Harrington *et al.*, 2006) These residences offer room, board, assistance with daily living activities, and skilled nursing care for both short- and long-term care (Fig. 3.4).

In 2013, the median cost for a private room in a nursing home was $230 per day ($83 950 per year) (Table 3.2). For a semi-private room, usually a room shared with a curtain or other partition between the beds, the average cost was $207 per day ($75 555 per year) (Genworth, 2013). The number of nursing home stays has increased since 2000. This growth is because of increasing use for short-term respite care and post-acute care. Because of reimbursement provisions and limitations under Medicare, patients are discharged from hospitals "quicker and sicker" than in the past. They need an intermediate level of care and supervision before they are able to return home. In 2005, total nursing home stays in Medicare- and Medicaid-certified facilities reached 3.2 million, up from 3.0 million in 2000 (CMS, 2006).

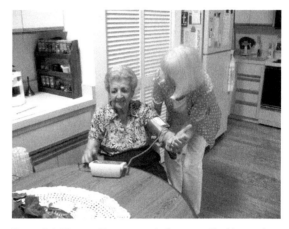

Figure 3.4 Theresa Dewar now in her new Florida nursing home.

Table 3.2 Comparison and cost of different living options*

Care type	Median daily cost ($)	Median monthly cost ($)	Payment options	Advanced fee?	Respite care?
Home care	65	1950	Private/Medicare/ Medicaid via home health aid	No	No
Assisted living	115	3450	Mostly private, some Medicaid	Some can be high	Yes
Board and care homes	Variable based on service	1500–3000	Private. Some Medicaid	No	Some
Nursing home (double occupancy)	207	6210	Private, Medicare, Medicaid	No	Yes
Nursing home (single occupancy)	230	6900	Private, Medicare, Medicaid	No	Yes
Continuous care communities	Variable based on service	2500–5400	Private	Yes, very expensive	No

*From Genworth (2013).

Projecting future trends is difficult, since nursing home use is driven by care preferences, as well as life expectancy and disability trends. Current estimates suggest that 35% of Americans who turned 65 by 2005 will need some nursing home care in their lifetime, 18% will live in a nursing home for at least 1 year, and 5% for at least 5 years (AARP, 2007; Kemper *et al.*, 2005). Women, with longer life expectancy and higher rates of disability and widowhood, are more likely than men to need nursing home care, and their stays will be lengthy (CMS, 2006).

Long-term care insurance

Most adults buy all types of insurance (home, car, health, and now we even have even pet insurance). But when it comes to long-term health care, which potentially could be most devastating, relatively few sign up. Low participation in long-term care insurance (LTC or LTCI) is due to its high cost. It's an insurance product that provides for the cost of long-term care long beyond what standard health insurance covers. Generally it covers the full spectrum of care from home assistance to nursing home and Alzheimer's facilities, and everything in-between. Premium costs can be pricy, especially if the person waits until retirement age to purchase. Rates are determined by six main factors: age, benefit, how long the benefits pay, elimination period, inflation protection, and the health rating.

Conclusion

The ultimate decision for elderly living arrangements will remain a very personal one based on multiple factors, including: ability to perform ADLs, presence of a surviving spouse, location preference, support systems, social requirements, and economic realities. Understanding the services that each living arrangement option provides, as well as consideration of the above factors, help seniors and their family members choose the home that best suits their needs.

Case study 1

Mrs. Winslow was a 70-year-old very independent widow who lived in a 3500-square foot home in Sarasota, Florida. The master bedroom was on the second floor and the home and surrounding landscaping had become difficult to live in, maintain, or modify. At that time she was very healthy with no issues with ADLs. Knowing that this home would eventually become impossible to stay in, she elected to move into a single-story unassisted senior living facility that could have minor modifications to increase her personal safety. Thirteen years later, her health and ambulation deteriorated to a point where something needed to be done. Consideration was made to sell the home and use the proceeds to move into an assisted living facility or continuing care retirement community. Realizing, because of personal (her independent nature) and financially realities, neither of these options were viable, the decision was made to purchase a home-health monitor that she could use in an emergency. Presently, she is 83-years-old and lives a very independent lifestyle. The family continues to monitor the situation and hope to allow her to age in place. If required, they will provide delivered meals and home health care.

Case study 2

Mrs. Sanchez was a 75-year-old widow who had lived in a 3000 square foot home in Texas. Her adult daughter and son-in-law lived three miles away in the same community and visited her once a day to check on her regarding safety and nutrition, as well as provide companionship, and make sure her needs were being met. Over a period of 2 years, the family noticed a deterioration in her memory and cognition. Then, while on a visit, her daughter realized the stove had been left on all day, with a pot of boiling water over the burner, and her mother was placing deodorant on her face instead of face cream. The daughter discussed the situation with her sister, who was located in another state, and other family members. The sisters decided to have their mother tested for Alzheimer's disease. After positive results and their concerns of safety for their mother, the daughters decided to move their mother into an assisted living community with an Alzheimer's unit and sell her house. She lived a very fulfilling life in the facility and passed away five years later secondary due to complications of a orthopedic injury.

References

AARP (American Association of Retired Persons) (1996) *Understanding Senior Housing into the Next Century: Survey of Consumer Preferences, Concerns, and Needs.* AARP, Washington, DC.

AARP (American Association of Retired Persons) (2007) *Nursing Homes.* From http://www.aarp.org/home-garden/livable-communities/info-2007/fs10r_homes.html. Accessed March 17, 2014.

Bookman, A., Harrington, M., Pass, L. & Reisner, E. (2007). *Family Caregiver Handbook.*: Massachusetts Institute of Technology, Cambridge, MA.

CMS (Centers for Medicare and Medicaid Services) (2006) *Nursing Home Data Compendium, 2006 Edition.* From http://www.cms.gov/Research-Statistics-Data-and-Systems/Statistics-Trends-and-Reports/DataCompendium/18_2006DataCompendium.html. Accessed March 17, 2014.

Genworth (2013) *Compare Cost of Care Across the United States, 10th Edition.* https://www.genworth.com/cost-of-care/landing.html. Accessed March 17, 2014.

Harrington, C., Carrillo, H. & LaCava, C. (2006) *Nursing Facilities, Staffing, Residents, and Facility Deficiencies, 1999 through 2005.* University of California, San Francisco, CA. From http://www.pascenter.org/documents/OSCAR2005.pdf. Accessed March 17, 2014.

Hobbs, F.B. & Damon, B.L. (1996). *65+ in the United States* (Current Population Reports Special Studies P23–190). US Bureau of the Census, Washington, DC. From https://www.census.gov/prod/1/pop/p23-190/p23-190.pdf. Accessed March 17, 2014.

Kemper, P., Komisar, H.L. & Alecixh, L. (2005) Long-term care over an uncertain future: what can current retirees expect? *Inquiry,* **42**(4), 335–50.

McDowell, I. & Newell, C. (1996) *Measuring Health: A Guide to Rating Scales and Questionnaires,* 2nd edn. Oxford University Press, New York, NY.

Schafer, R. (1999) *Determinants of the Living Arrangements of the Elderly, W99-6.* Joint Center for Housing Studies, Harvard University, Cambridge, MA, p. 5.

US Census Bureau (2010) *America's Families and Living Arrangements; Table A2. Family Status and Household Relationship of People 15 Years and Over, by Marital Status, Age, Sex, Race, and Hispanic Origin: 2010.* From http://www.census.gov/population/www/socdemo/hh-fam/cps2010.html. Accessed March 17, 2014.

US Department of Health and Human Services (2011) *A Profile of Older Americans: 2011.* From http://www.aoa.gov/Aging_Statistics/Profile/2011/docs/2011profile.pdf. Accessed March 17, 2011.

US Government Accountability Office (2010) *Older Americans: Continuing Care Retirement Communities Can Provide Benefits, but Not Without Some Risk. GAO-10-611. June 21, 2010.* From http://www.gao.gov/products/GAO-10-611. Accessed March 17, 2014.

CHAPTER 4

Palmore's Facts on Aging Quiz: Healthcare Providers' Perceptions of Facts and Myths of Aging

Ralph H. Saunders

Eastman Institute for Oral Health, University of Rochester, Rochester, NY, USA

Introduction

Conclusions from psychology literature form the basis for today's general awareness of a continuum of relationships beginning with knowledge and extending to attitudes and then to behavior (Ajzen & Fishbein, 1977; Allport, 1954). It is plausible, therefore, that a certain level of knowledge about older adults is important for generating attitudes which can lead to the provision of optimal care for this population. It is also important that a relatively simple tool help to distinguish fact from fiction, and truth from myth about aging and older adults. In this chapter the methods by which the level of knowledge about geriatrics has been assessed and interpreted will be examined. Also, the extent to which the level of knowledge about older adults relates to the level of care for this population will be discussed.

Tests of knowledge about older adults

Several tests have been developed to assess the knowledge of healthcare professionals about older adults (International Academic Nursing Alliance, 2010; Ming *et al.*, 2004; Palmore, 1977; Towner, 2006). Palmore's Facts on Aging Quiz (FAQ) has been used widely in surveys of dental professionals as well as other health professionals and it is discussed here in some detail (Table 4.1).

After several early efforts to assess knowledge about geriatrics (Golde & Kogan, 1959; Kogan, 1961; Tuckerman & Lorge, 1952), Palmore's FAQ became the first attempt to incorporate elements that were evidence-based and which sought to avoid responses based on attitudes and suppositions. It is likely the most widely used assessment instrument currently; a literature search by the author utilizing PubMed® and Medline® revealed 207 citations.

In 1980, Palmore himself reviewed findings of 25 studies using the FAQ and reported that training in gerontology usually resulted in higher scores (Palmore, 1980). However, also in 1980, Miller and Dodder suggested, in a critical review, that unintended bias was inherent in the wording of several of the FAQ items used in the instrument that Palmore developed (Miller & Dodder, 1980).

In 1981 Palmore published a revision of the first FAQ (FAQ1), termed FAQ2, which included more content on social aspects of behaviors of the population (Palmore, 1981). Lusk and others, in a detailed analysis of content of both studies, reported that the correlation between the two was low ($r=0.04$) and Cronbach's alpha, which reflects the internal validity of the quiz items, was just 0.45 for FAQ1 and 0.32 for FAQ2 (Lusk *et al.*, 1995) [A good score on the scale for Cronbach's alpha would be >0.70 (George & Mallory, 2003).]

Although other modifications of FAQ1 have followed, it appears that most applications since have utilized the original. In 2008, Unwin and colleagues

Geriatric Dentistry: Caring for Our Aging Population, First Edition. Edited by Paula K. Friedman.
© 2014 John Wiley & Sons, Inc. Published 2014 by John Wiley & Sons, Inc.
Companion website: www.wiley.com/go/friedman/geriatricdentistry

Table 4.1 Palmore's Facts on Aging Quiz*

Directions: Circle "T" for true or "F" for false

(NOTE: For odd numbered questions, the answers are FALSE; for even questions, the answers are TRUE)

T	F	Question
		1 The majority of old people (past age 65) are senile (i.e., defective memory, disoriented, or demented)
		2 All five senses tend to decline in old age
		3 Most old people have no interest in, or capacity for, sexual relations
		4 Lung capacity tends to decline in old age
		5 The majority of old people feel miserable most of the time
		6 Physical strength tends to decline in old age
		7 At least one-tenth of the aged are living in long-stay institutions (i.e., nursing homes, mental hospitals, homes for the aged, etc.)
		8 Aged drivers have fewer accidents per person than drivers under age 65
		9 Most older workers cannot work as effectively as younger workers
		10 About 80% of the aged are healthy enough to carry out their normal activities
		11 Most old people are set in their ways and unable to change
		12 Old people usually take longer to learn something new
		13 It is almost impossible for most old people to learn something new
		14 The reaction time of most old people tends to be slower than reaction time of younger people
		15 In general, most old people are pretty much alike
		16 The majority of old people are seldom bored
		17 The majority of old people are socially isolated and lonely
		18 Older workers have fewer accidents than younger workers
		19 Over 15% of the US population are now age 65 or over
		20 Most medical practitioners tend to give low priority to the aged
		21 The majority of older people have incomes below the poverty level (as defined by the federal government)
		22 The majority of old people are working or would like to have some kind of work to do (including housework and volunteer work)
		23 Older people tend to become more religious as they age
		24 The majority of old people are seldom irritated or angry
		25 The health and socioeconomic status of older people (compared to younger people) in the year 2000 (or 2020) will probably be about the same as now

From Palmore (1977).

reported the FAQ1 results of 428 medical students at the Uniformed Services University (Unwin *et al.*, 2008). The average score on the FAQ1 in this study was 15.0 ± 2.0 out of 25; this is very similar to the proportion of correct answers in the original report (60%). Results overall indicate that some of the inaccurate negative perceptions about older adults have persisted and even worsened over the past 30 years.

The level of knowledge, using FAQ1, about geriatrics and aging among dental health students and providers has been assessed and reported previously (Friedman & Brecknock, 2003; Kiyak & Brudvik, 1982; Wood & Mulligan, 2000). The following new data adds to these reports.

Scores of recent dental graduates on the FAQ1

From 1986 through 2010, FAQ1 was administered to all of the 413 incoming dental residents who were matriculating in the Advanced Education in General

Dentistry (AEGD) program in the Division of General Dentistry at the Eastman Institute for Oral Health in Rochester, New York from 1986 to 2010. Of these, 222 were graduates of North American dental schools and 191 were graduates of schools in Asia, Europe, or South America. Sixty-one countries were represented among the residents.

Most residents were recent dental school graduates but a few had other postdoctoral education or had been engaged in clinical practice. Throughout the period of the study (1986–2010) the quiz was administered, during a class of the Orientation Summer Lecture Series, by the same instructor. Residents were instructed to answer each question to the best of their knowledge and regardless of the country of their training, and at a relaxed pace. Mean time to complete the quiz was approximately 12 minutes.

Overall mean scores for the entire study period by country of training and gender are displayed in Tables 4.2 and 4.3.

Graduates of dental schools in North America had slightly higher scores than graduates from other countries. Among all graduates, males scored slightly higher.

During the study period (1986–2010) the number and variety of opportunities for education in geriatrics and gerontology for dental health professionals have increased significantly internationally (Bullock et al., 2010; Ettinger, 2010; Hebling et al., 2007;

Table 4.2 Mean Facts on Aging Quiz scores by country of training

Country of training	Overall mean scores (SD)
North America (N=222)	16.74 (2.69)[*]
Asia, Europe, South America (N=191)	15.83 (2.62)

[*]P<0.005

Table 4.3 Mean Facts on Aging Quiz scores by gender

Gender of graduates	Overall mean scores (SD)
Males (N=256)	16.52 (2.70)[*]
Females (N=157)	15.44 (2.62)

[*]P<0.001

Table 4.4 Changes in Facts on Aging Quiz scores with time by selected variables

Selected variable	P value
Greater percent of population ≥ age 65	0.001
Higher life expectancy	0.110
Higher literacy rate	0.001
Higher % GDP for education	0.001

GDP, gross domestic product

Kossioni et al., 2009; Mohammad et al., 2003; Shah, 2005). However, analysis of variance (ANOVA) of mean scores across the entire period of 25 years revealed no significant change. ANOVA was also used to explore the possible roles of four demographic and socioeconomic variables with time in students' country of training. The FAQ scores with time. Results are displayed in Table 4.4.

What is the relationship between results of tests of knowledge about older adults and good care?

The face validity of a positive relationship between results of tests of knowledge about older adults and good geriatric care seems logical. However, although scores on the FAQ have not improved with time, correlating evidence that the performance of geriatric oral health professionals has not improved is lacking. Rather, available studies suggest that it is properly designed clinical experiences rather than general knowledge about the population that has led to the greatest changes in attitudes and improvements in the effectiveness of oral healthcare providers (Devlin et al., 1994; Kiyak & Brudvik, 1992; MacEntee et al., 2005; Nochajski et al., 2011).

Planning for the future of education in dental geriatrics may benefit from considering the data presented in this chapter.

Summary

As the older adult population continues to grow, the knowledge, attitudes, and behaviors of all health professionals towards the aging population becomes increasingly important. The Palmore FAQ is a simple instrument to help educators and practicing health professionals assess their knowledge and attitudes towards elders. Evidence shows that creating positive learning experiences and environments in learning about and treating senior citizens is critically important in developing healthcare professionals who treat elders with the respect and understanding that they deserve.

DISCUSSION QUESTIONS

1 What is the test most widely used for assessing knowledge about geriatrics among health professionals?

2 Why is general knowledge about the population of older adults thought to be important for health professionals?

3 According to results from the FAQ over time, has knowledge about geriatrics among dental health professionals increased, stayed about the same, or decreased?

4 According to results from the FAQ over time, has knowledge about geriatrics among "nondental" health professionals increased, stayed about the same, or decreased?

5 Among dental professional trainees which type of educational content appears to be most positively related to later caring for more older adults:
   A clinical
   B didactic
   C research

References

Ajzen, I. & Fishbein, M. (1977) Attitude-behavior relations: a theoretical analysis and review of empirical research. *Psychological Bulletin*, **84**, 888–918.

Allport, G. (1954) *The Nature of Prejudice*. Addison-Wesley, Reading, MA.

Bullock, A., Berkey, D. & Smith, B. (2010) International education research issues in meeting the oral health needs of geriatric populations: an introduction. *Journal of Dental Education*, **74**, 5–6.

Devlin, H., Mellor, A. & Worthington, H. (1994) Attitudes of dental students toward elderly people. *Journal of Dentistry*, **22**, 45–8.

Ettinger, R. (2010) The development of geriatric dental education programs in Canada: an update. *Journal of the Canadian Dental Association* **76**, a1.

Friedman, P. & Brecknock, S. (2003) A comparison of dental and dental hygiene students' performance on the Facts-on-Aging quiz. *Journal of the Massachusetts Dental Society* **52**, 36–9.

Golde, P. & Kogan, N. (1959) A sentence-completion procedure for assessing attitudes toward old people. *Journal of Gerontology* **14**, 355–63.

George, D. & Mallory, P. (2002) *SPSS for Windows Step by Step: A Simple Guide and Reference. 11.0 Update*, 4th edn. Allyn & Bacon, Boston, MA.

Hebling, E., Mugayar, L. & Dias, P. (2007) Geriatric dentistry: a new specialty in Brazil. *Gerodontology* **24**, 177–80.

International Academic Nursing Alliance (2010) *Geriatric Nursing Knowledge Assessment*. From http://www.nursingknowledge.org/geriatric-nursing-knowledge-assessment-4599.html. Accessed March 17, 2014.

Kiyak, H. & Brudvik, J. (1992) Dental students' self-assessed competency in geriatric dentistry. *Journal of Dental Education*, **56**, 728–34.

Kogan, N. (1961) Attitudes toward old people. *Journal of Abnormal Psychology*, **62**, 44–54.

Kossioni, A., Vanobbergen, J., Newton, J., et al. (2009) European College of Gerodontology: undergraduate curriculum guidelines in gerodontology. *Gerodontology*, **26**, 165–71.

Lusk, S., Williams, R. & Hsuing, S. (1995) Evaluation of the Facts on Aging Quizzes I and II. *Journal of Nursing Education*, **34**, 317–24.

MacEntee, M., Pruksapong, M. & Wyatt, C. (2005) Insights from students following an educational rotation through dental geriatrics. *Journal of Dental Education*, **69**, 1368–75.

Miller, R. & Dodder, R. (1980) A revision of the Palmore's Facts on Aging Quiz. *The Gerontologist*, **20**, 73–9.

Ming, L., Wilkerson, L., Reuben, D. & Ferrell, B. (2004) Development and validation of a geriatric knowledge test for medical students. *Journal of the American Geriatrics Society*, **52**, 532–41.

Mohammad, A., Preshaw, P. & Ettinger, R. (2003) Current status of predoctoral geriatric education in US dental schools. *Journal of Dental Education*, **67**, 509–14.

Nochajski, T., Davis, E., Waldrop, D., et al. (2011) Dental students' attitudes about older adults: do type and amount of contact make a difference? *Journal of Dental Education*, **75**, 1329–32.

Palmore, E. (1977) Facts on Aging: a short quiz. *The Gerontologist*, **17**, 315–20.

Palmore, E. (1980) The Facts on Aging Quiz: a review of findings. *The Gerontologist*, **20**, 669–72.

Palmore, E. (1981) The Facts on Aging Quiz: Part two. *The Gerontologist*, **21**, 431–37.

Shah, N. (2005) Need for gerodontology education in India. *Gerodontology*, **22**, 104–5.

Towner, E. (2006) Assessment of geriatric knowledge: an online tool for appraising entering APN students. *Journal of Professional Nursing,* **22,** 112–15.

Tuckman, J. & Lorge, I. (1952) The effect of institutionalization on attitudes toward old people. *Journal of Abnormal Psychology,* **47,** 337–44.

Unwin, B., Unwin, C., Olsen, C. & Wilson, C. (2008) A new look at an old quiz: Palmore's Facts on Aging Quiz turns 30. *Journal of the American Geriatric Society,* **56,** 2162–4.

Wood, G. & Mulligan, R. (2000) Cross-sectional comparison of dental students' knowledge and attitudes before geriatric training: 1984-1999. *Journal of Dental Education,* **64,** 763–71.

CHAPTER 5

The Senior-Friendly Office

Ruth S. Goldblatt[1] and Janet A. Yellowitz[2]

[1]*Department of Craniofacial Sciences, University of Connecticut, School of Dental Medicine, Farmington, CT, USA*
[2]*Department of Periodontics, University of Maryland Dental School, Baltimore, MD, USA*

Helen Keller is credited with noting that blindness cuts us off from things, but deafness cuts us off from people.

Case study

Mrs. Gonzalez

Today is Mrs. Gonzalez's first visit to your dental practice, and she is hoping to establish her care with you. She heard about you from her daughter-in-law. She is 78 years old, newly widowed, and has recently moved to a 55+ community. Mrs. Gonzalez was dropped off at the dental office by the community van that services senior citizens and takes her to appointments. She uses a walker and struggles a bit walking up the small set of stairs at the front door of the office building. She climbs the stairs slowly, using the one railing for support. At the top of the stairs, she has a hard time opening the large glass door, as it is too heavy for her to open. She knocks on the glass as there is no doorbell, and is eventually able to get into the building.

From the entry door, she walks down a short, carpeted, brightly lit hallway to your practice. As she enters, she attracts the attention of others in the waiting area as she needs assistance opening the door to the practice. The newly renovated, dimly lighted waiting area is designed to be inviting and calming, with soft, subtle colors used throughout the space. At the receptionist desk, Mrs. Gonzalez is handed a clipboard and pen and told to fill out three pages of forms and to return them when she is done. The top form is a light photocopy, written with small typeface.

Mrs. Gonzalez goes to a padded chair with arms, and completes the forms as best she can, leaving many questions unanswered. She returns the forms to the receptionist who glances at them and tells her you are running late and will see her as soon as possible. Mrs. Gonzalez is concerned about the time because her pre-arranged community van return ride is coming in 90 minutes to pick her up, and she doesn't know how to contact the driver.

When it is her turn to be seen, the dental assistant calls her name in the waiting area but Mrs. Gonzalez did not initially hear her as the television was playing in the waiting area. When she hears her name, she has a difficult time getting out of the chair, and the dental assistant tells her to go to the blue room down the hall.

The clinical areas are brightly lighted, compared to the waiting area. Mrs. Gonzalez walks down the hall toward the operatories, but is unsure which room to enter. She is directed to sit in the dental chair, and the assistant places her walker in the hallway so it is out of the way.

As you enter the operatory, the assistant whispers to you that the patient has some problems because she seems: (a) slow, (b) didn't complete the medical history, and (c) ignored her when she was called in the waiting room.

You enter the operatory, introduce yourself to the patient and begin to review her medical history forms. The patient wants to know when you will be finished. What do you do?

(Continued)

Geriatric Dentistry: Caring for Our Aging Population, First Edition. Edited by Paula K. Friedman.
© 2014 John Wiley & Sons, Inc. Published 2014 by John Wiley & Sons, Inc.
Companion website: www.wiley.com/go/friedman/geriatricdentistry

Case study questions

1 Does the scenario seem familiar? Does this resemble your practice?
2 Can you identify any areas of concern in the scenario?
    a) If so, which conditions are concerns?
3 How could this scenario be designed to better accommodate older patients?
4 How might this have played out if the office were more appropriate for an older adult population?

Introduction

As the population of older adults increases, dental practitioners will be challenged by having more older adults with impairments in their practice. A senior-friendly dental practice makes good business sense. Healthcare offices that accommodate the physical and emotional needs of a wide range of individuals demonstrate an awareness of patient concerns and safety issues. Having a good office design, utilizing appropriate lighting, and having appropriate seating help patients and staff negotiate the space with ease and confidence. Understanding that the "office" extends beyond the walls to include the lighting, the patient forms, and the building entrance, hallways, walkways, stairwells, and parking lot are important concepts when considering the patient's comfort and overall experience.

The atmosphere that an office projects originates from its physical design and can affect the interactions of patients with staff and doctors. In this chapter we will provide design recommendations to aid in your interactions with and care of older adults. From the first telephone contact to the time when they pay their bill, there are multiple opportunities to enhance the communication and quality of experiences of everyone involved. Positive interactions lead to valued patient experiences and positive clinical outcomes.

From today to 2030, older adults will continue to dominate the growth of the population as 10 000 people turn 65 every day (Pew Research Center, 2010). With this ever-increasing population of older adults, ensuring that healthcare offices are accessible and user friendly to all ages makes sense from a business and safety perspective. A senior-friendly office can reduce patient and provider stress as well as ensuring an appropriate environment for all. Environments designed for older adults can be achieved with ease and without much fuss or expenditure, and perhaps most importantly, they are welcomed by all age groups.

As a result of age-related changes and the probability of having one or more chronic diseases, older adults are often challenged by their environment. The American with Disabilities Act (ADA) of 1990 requires healthcare facilities meet specific construction standards (Department of Justice, 2014). The 2010 ADA Standards set a minimum scope and technical requirements for newly designed and constructed or altered state and local government facilities, public accommodations, and commercial facilities. These facilities must be readily accessible to, and usable by, individuals with disabilities. The newly revised standards address all aspects of design, from restrooms to parking lot spaces (Department of Justice, 2010). Adoption of the 2010 Standards establishes a revised reference point for any planned construction or renovations. The referenced web site highlights the changes between the 1990 and 2010 standard (Department of Justice, 2011). The 2010 rule became effective on March 15, 2011 and by March 15, 2012, compliance with this Standards is required for new construction and alterations (Department of Justice, 2011). When planning major renovations to an office space consider using an architect familiar with designing healthcare spaces and the law to ensure the office is compliant, comfortable, and efficient for all.

Sensory impairments

Hearing loss and vision changes are frequent occurrences for older adults and can affect almost every interaction they have with professionals. Between 1999 and 2006, sensory impairments were identified as a significant issue for older adults, with one out of six Americans having impaired vision, and one out of four having impaired hearing (Dillon *et al.*, 2010). Vision and hearing impairments increase with age, often doubling in those aged 80+ compared with persons aged 70–79. Addressing these issues through practice strategies and design modifications will enable your office to provide a user friendly and safe environment that allows patients to maintain their independence and self-esteem. Satisfied patients are return customers and are more likely to refer others to your practice.

By taking a closer look at some of these common issues it will be easier to understand the design suggestions.

Vision in older adults

Vision is defined as a combination of visual acuity, color sense, the ability to distinguish contrasts and the ability to evaluate the location of objects in the environment (Orr, 1998). Age-related eye diseases and vision loss are very common in older adults and often overlooked by individuals, caregivers, and healthcare providers. After age 40, age-related visual changes are almost universal, with a decline in the normal functions of the eyes and an increase in eye disorders. In 2008, 15% of males and 19.4% of females aged 65+ years, and 28% of those aged 85+ reported having trouble seeing (Federal Interagency Forum on Aging Related Statistics, 2010). The most common age-related eye diseases or conditions are presbyopia, cataracts, age-related macular degeneration (AMD), glaucoma, and diabetic retinopathy (National Eye Health Education, 2007). These and other conditions will be described and discussed later in this chapter. Visual impairments can be the result of a combination of diseases, that is a patient may have a combination of several conditions causing total vision loss. Visual impairments interfere with an individual's ability to live independently – including, but not limited to, completing their daily activities such as dressing, effective oral care, and traveling to the dental office.

Since the incidence of vision loss increases with age, visual impairments are an increasing concern for those providing care to older adults. Due to age-related changes, attention to environmental conditions – such as having adequate lighting, eliminating glare from a shiny floor, and using color contrast – are significant issues that need to be addressed for

improved visual functioning and comfort of older adults (Orr, 1998).

Although many age-related eye changes are correctable, visual acuity (sharpness of vision) often declines in older adults. The **pupils** of a 60 year old are about one third the size of a 20 year old, and react slower in response to rapid changes in light. With age, the **lens** becomes yellowed, less flexible, and slightly cloudy; the cornea flattens, becoming less sensitive to letting light into the eye. Additionally, there is decreased transparency of the **lens**, which reduces the ability of the eye to receive short wavelength colors such as blue and violet. The aged lens filters the blue out of the color spectrum, making it harder to differentiate between shades of blue, unique colors, and between colors with similar tone or value. As these changes occur slowly, most older adults are unaware that this is happening. Blues are usually the first colors to appear different to older adults, often looking greener, while warmer colors like reds and oranges appear stronger as compared to blues and greens. This change in vision may be the reason the clothes of some older adults do not match as they did when they were younger, or when patients present with stained or soiled clothing. Patients may not be aware that the clothes don't match, are stained, or soiled.

As the result of having a decreased blood supply in the eye of older adults, the **retina** becomes less functional resulting in decreased spatial discrimination, black and white contrast challenges, and reduced flicker sensitivity. These changes impair one's ability to tolerate glare and to adapt to sharp changes of light. A decline in accommodation also results as the lens hardens and there is a decrease in muscle tone. In general, older adults need more light to see than younger adults, and those aged 80+ require 10 times more light to read than the average 25 year old. One example of this change can be observed when older diners use small flashlights to read the menu in dimly lighted restaurants.

Presbyopia

Presbyopia, a common age-related eye change, is the result of a progressive change in the optic compartment, where the lens becomes less elastic. Presbyopia is the result of the eye's decreasing capacity to focus at close range, or loss of accommodation. Presbyopia also affects one's ability to read small print,

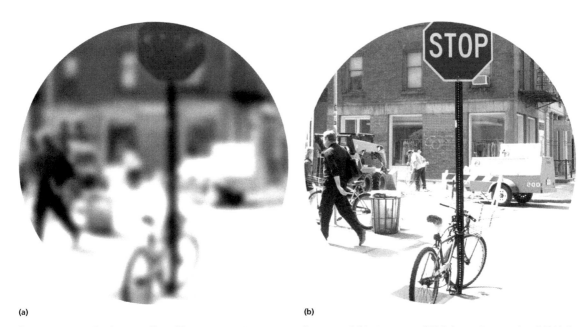

(a)   (b)

Figure 5.1 Example of vision affected by cataracts (a) as compared to normal (b). Courtesy of Lighthouse International (2014).

see well in dim lighting, and to differentiate colors. Often times, individuals with presbyopia compensate for this visual loss by holding reading materials at a longer distance than usual; however, eventually, reading glasses or multifocal contact lenses or corrective surgery is needed. Because it occurs gradually over time, most individuals do not notice a visual loss until after age 40. By age 55, most people require corrective lenses or "readers" that magnify the visual field for reading or up-close work.

Reading is a joy of many older adults, but due to print size, lack of contrast, and the availability of adequate lighting, many have difficulty reading newspapers, magazines, and books. From a health-care provider's perspective, this challenge can impact the health of patients due to a decreased ability to read medication labels, follow home-care instructions, read the small print on your business card, or visualize oral hygiene. Even reading food labels and preparation instructions on packages can be challenging. This decrease or loss of vision can affect quality of life for the older adults in many ways.

Cataracts

Cataracts are a clouding or opacity of the lens of the eye, and can range from a small to a diffuse area. Cataracts develop slowly over time in all older adults.

Like most age-related changes, cataracts are usually not treated until a severe decline has occurred. As cataracts develop, the opacity of the lens causes light to scatter resulting in decreased visual acuity . Colors appear faded, night vision is poor, and glare is often experienced from sunlight, streetlights, and headlights. Individuals with cataracts have difficulty seeing in low light levels. Because cataract changes are insidious (slow-onset), many people do not realize their visual loss until late in the cataracts' development. There is no preventive strategy for cataracts, though once treated, individuals realize the level of loss they had experienced prior to the surgery. An example of vision affected by cataracts as compared to normal is shown in Fig. 5.1.

Glaucoma

Glaucoma is a group of diseases wherein the optic nerve is damaged as a result of increased pressure resulting in a visual field loss (Fig. 5.2). It is a chronic, progressive, degenerative disease that is generally asymptomatic in its early stages. There are two main types of glaucoma, with 90% being open-angle or chronic glaucoma. Other causes of glaucoma include tumors, advanced cataracts, and inflammation. Glaucoma can occur rapidly; it can cause acute pain

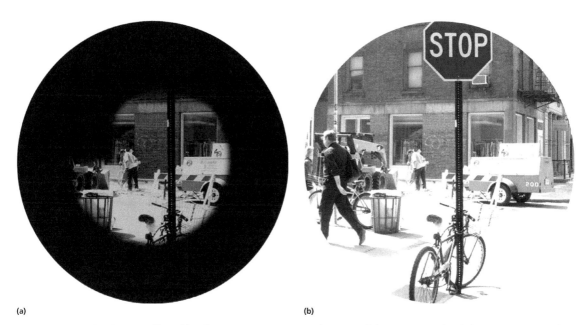

(a)

(b)

Figure 5.2 Example of vision affected by glaucoma (a) as compared to normal (b). Courtesy of Lighthouse International (2014).

or it can be silent, and if not treated, glaucoma can cause permanent vision loss or even blindness (National Eye Institute, 2014c).

Diabetic retinopathy

Diabetic retinopathy is a common, vascular complication of diabetes, the result of damage to the blood vessels in the retina, often caused by poor blood glucose control (Fig. 5.3). Diabetic retinopathy damage can take several forms including proliferation of the blood vessels on the retina surface or can be due to a swelling and leaking of fluid from blood vessels. Although early treatment can prevent blindness, diabetic retinopathy often results in vision loss (National Eye Institute, 2014b).

Age-related macular degeneration

Age-related macular degeneration (AMD) is an incurable and progressive retinal disease that can occur in one or both eyes. It is associated with increasing age and is the leading cause of low vision, severe vision loss, and legal blindness for people aged 60+ in the USA (Vision Aware, 2012). As age increases, the prevalence of AMD increases, ranging from 10% for those aged 66–74 to 30% for those aged 75–85 (Maylahn *et al.*, 2012).

Ninety percent of AMD is considered atrophic or dry, with the remainder identified as neovascular or wet. Individuals with AMD have a loss of clarity in the center of the visual field, lose contrast sensitivity and color perception. People with AMD attempt to compensate by using their peripheral vision, so that it appears that they are not looking at the person with whom they are speaking. AMD interferes with one's ability to recognize faces, watch television, navigate stairs safely, read, drive, and perform daily tasks (Fig. 5.4) (National Eye Institute, 2014a). Like other age-related conditions, individuals with AMD can lose their independence and are challenged in all settings. Since AMD can progress rapidly, whenever you are suspicious that a patient is having AMD symptoms, a prompt referral to an ophthalmologist is highly recommended.

Hemianopia or hemianopsia

Hemianopia or hemianopsia develops as the result of trauma, tumor, or stroke. As a result of damage to the optic nerve pathway, a partial blindness results leading to what is termed a visual-field cut (Fig. 5.5). Individuals with hemianopsia may ignore the side of the mouth with the brain damage as they do not perceive its presence. This condition can lead to the pocketing of

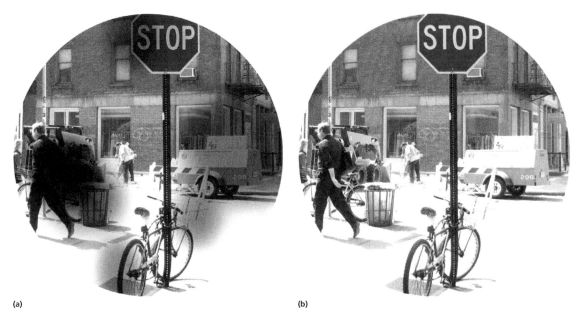

(a)   (b)

Figure 5.3 Example of vision affected by diabetic retinopathy (a) as compared to normal (b). Courtesy of Lighthouse International (2014).

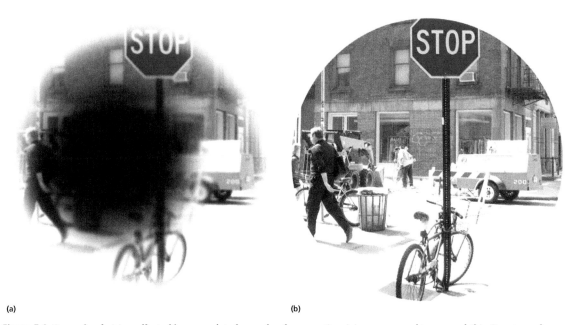

(a)   (b)

Figure 5.4 Example of vision affected by age-related macular degeneration (a) as compared to normal (b). Courtesy of Lighthouse International (2014).

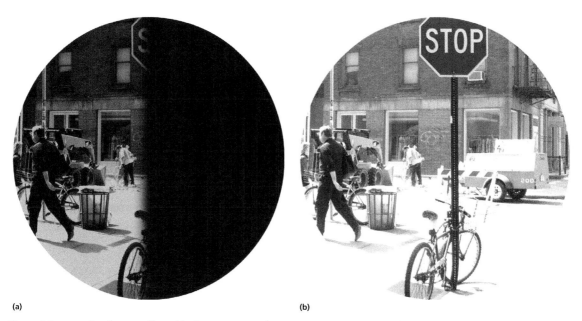

(a)   (b)

Figure 5.5 Example of vision affected by hemianopia or hemianopsia (a) as compared to normal (b). Courtesy of Lighthouse International (2014).

food on the effected side and the oral/dental sequelae that ensue. Similarly, people who pocket food are at greater risk of aspiration pneumonia.

Creating a functional senior-friendly office for patients with vision impairments

Modifying a dental practice to accommodate patients with vision impairments can have a great effect on the patients' overall experience. Changes in vision can be minimized by using proper lighting throughout the office and being aware of the needs of the patients. The accommodations used for those with low vision or vision impairments can provide a welcoming environment for all.

Managing and caring for patients with vision impairments can be challenging. Each approach must be individualized to accommodate to the patient's visual impairment. Understanding the patient's medical history and knowing his or her specific challenge(s) will assist in the development of a customized treatment and care plan. Utilizing the guidelines shown in Box 5.1, below, will optimize your practice, provide meaningful care, and result in appreciative patients.

Hearing loss

Humans can hear sounds at frequencies from about 20 Hz to 20 000 Hz, though most people hear sounds best at 3000–4000 Hz, where human speech is centered. With advancing years, sensitivity to high-frequency sounds usually declines, and can later involve all sound frequencies. Hearing loss is reported to be inevitable with advancing years, although the etiology is unknown.

Older adults often have difficulty in following the meaning of what is being said in ordinary conversation. Some older adults with hearing impairments are often unaware of the frequency with which they misunderstand words. Older adults with good low frequency hearing can perceive vowels but are likely to have difficulty with consonant sounds. As a result, they often conclude that other people are not speaking clearly when in reality the problem is faulty consonant perception resulting from hearing loss in the high frequency range (Jerger *et al.*, 1995).

In 2008, 42% of males and 30% of females aged 65+ reported having trouble hearing. For those aged 85+, 60% reported having difficulty hearing (Federal Interagency Forum on Aging Related Statistics,

Box 5.1 Recommended strategies for patients with vision impairments

1 Ask how an individual prefers to be assisted. Some patients appreciate learning about the procedures that are to occur during the appointment
2 Use a verbal approach to those with severe vision loss. Advise the patient when you are leaving and returning to the room
3 Document strategies used to inform team members and to facilitate future appointments
4 In reading and writing areas, use task lighting with full-spectrum or fluorescent light bulbs
   a) Full-spectrum light bulbs provide light that is very close to natural sunlight and help to increase black and white contrast and shows other colors in their true hues
5 Task or spot lighting assists with acuity issues and minimizes perceptual confusion that heightened shadows produce when overall light is increased (Cooper, 1986)
6 Keep clinical areas, restrooms, and hallways well lit:
   a) Maintain uniform lighting throughout to avoid shadows
   b) Reduce glare by eliminating lighting that reflects off of mirrors or floors
7 Keep magnifying glasses or over-the-counter nonprescription readers available for patients to use so they can independently complete health history forms, sign treatment plans, write checks, and enjoy reading materials in your waiting area
8 Remove obstacles that may be in their walkway, such as scatter rugs, high-pile rugs, electrical cords, or furniture
9 Use adjustable window coverings to adjust natural light and reduce glare
10 Within the operatory reduce sharp contrast between bright and dark areas
11 Use flat paint to reduce the potential glare from semi-gloss paint
12 Use contrast to help patients identify specific objects and switches (e.g., a dark table next to a white wall or a black switch plate on a white wall).
13 Use contrasting colors to identify:
   • door numbers/signs
   • doorways to walls
   • floors to baseboard
   • knobs to doors
   • edges of steps and ramps, stairwells, landing ,and railings
14 Consider signage in Braille for those who use Braille in their daily activities
15 **Typeface:** The choice of typeface is less important than contrast, type size, weight, and the spacing of the characters:
   a) Quirky, unusual, script, and titling typefaces (fonts) are inappropriate in continuous text
   b) Although there is no valid research to support the preference for a sans-serif typeface (such as Arial or Helvetica) over a serif one (such as Times or Century), serif typefaces are regarded as more "readable" in continuous text while sans-serif fonts are recommended for questionnaires:

Sans-serif typeface	**Serif typeface**
Arial font	Times New Roman font
Calibri font	Century font
Helvetica font	Book Antigua font

   c) Have the medical history forms, appointment cards, and business cards available in large print, such as 14 bold san-serif fonts
   d) Use matt paper when designing any brochures or informational handouts, such as postoperative instructions
   e) Use distinct contrast print color to paper color to ease reading. It is the difference between colors that enables people to discern the colors, not the individual color itself. Figure 5.6 provides examples of good contrast versus poor contrast

2010). With increasing age, people both lose their ability to hear high frequencies and experience a decline in the speed of processing speech information. Although volume is often perceived to be the problem of older adults with hearing loss, the hallmark of age-related hearing loss is that speech is perceived not to be clear, involving problems with sound and word discrimination.

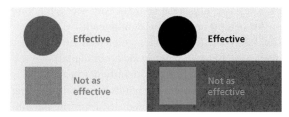

Figure 5.6 Examples of good contrast (left) versus not so good contrast (right). Courtesy of Lighthouse International. From Arditi (2014).

Presbycusis

Presbycusis or age-related hearing loss is typically sensorineural, involving the structures in the inner ear or cochlea and/or the auditory pathways in the brain. Presbycusis is one of the most common chronic conditions among older adults, predisposing victims to a diminished quality of life, increased risk for social isolation, depression, and a decline in physical functioning. (Pratt *et al.*, 2009). Presbycusis is progressive, more common in men than women and usually develops slowly over time (Jerger *et al.*, 1995). It involves decreased hearing sensitivity due to a peripheral cochlear defect and a defect in central auditory processing. The peripheral component results in the loss of hearing sensitivity or decreased signal audibility. Peripheral hearing loss increases hearing thresholds and distorts sounds. Presbycusis usually occurs in both ears, though there may be a significant variation between ears.

Age-related hearing loss is related to genetic factors and exposure to loud noises. Hearing loss reduces the range of frequencies a person can hear with ordinary conversation (ranging between 250 and 3000 Hz). The enunciation of many consonants is in the range of 2000–8000 Hz. Many people with hearing impairment mishear the consonants of "s, sh, f, v, t, p, and b," which are important to understanding speech (Jerger *et al.*, 1995). For many older adults, hearing aids and/or assistive devices can alleviate many of the handicaps of hearing impairment. For those with peripheral sensory loss, **hearing aids** are helpful as they improve the auditability of sounds often too faint to hear. They function best in one-to-one conversational situations or in listening to the radio or television; that is, where there is only one target sound source and little competing background noise. Studies have shown that between 10 and 21% of older hearing-impaired adults own hearing aids (Jerger *et al.*, 1995).

Many older adults try to hide the fact that they have difficulty hearing – often due to a denial of the aging process, fear of serious concern, or acknowledgment that hearing devices "imply" old age. The rejection of hearing aids is often associated with the high cost of hearing aids, difficulty in manipulating the controls, and/or the perception that they call attention to the handicap (Jerger *et al.*, 1995).

Background noise can complicate listening for many adults and becomes far more problematic for those with a hearing impairment. Often, those with hearing aids cannot effectively separate the speech of the person from the competing background noise, which results in confusing sounds, turning off the hearing aid and, potentially, rejection of the hearing aid.

Recent advances in hearing aid technology include the use of digitally programmable hearing aids with circuitry that can reduce background noise or keep sounds from being over amplified. These technologies have benefitted most, but not all hearing aid users.

When working with older adults, it is not unusual to encounter individuals with hearing loss. Just as there were some recommended strategies for working with patients with impaired vision, the following recommmendations are for working with patients with impaired hearing.

Communication strategies

The following list of strategies can help facilitate communication with individuals with hearing impairments.

1 Tailor conversations to the patient's hearing ability:
   - ask patient for best route for communication (lip readings, hearing aid, note writing, or combination);
   - ask patient which is their better ear, and direct your communication to that ear.
2 Periodically confirm that you are understood. You may need to do this by having the patient repeat the conversation back to you. Simply asking if you are understood may illicit a "yes" when this is actually not the case.
3 Reduce as much background sound as possible (e.g., saliva ejector, music, intercom, staff chatter, running water).
4 Keep face and lips visible (well-lit) while speaking. Facial expressions and gestures can be helpful.

Speaking through a mask muffles sounds and prevents the patient from being able to see your lips forming the words.

5 Obtain patient's attention with light touch or signal before beginning to speak (e.g., tap shoulder, lightly touch their arm, or point to self).

6 Speak clearly, in a low frequency, slightly louder than usual. Slowing speech slightly improves clarity and allows for more processing time.

7 When possible, reduce the use of words starting with "f, s, t, and p"; and, when using these words, be sure to enunciate slowly and clearly.

8 Use simple, short sentences and avoid technical terms.

9 Use the tell–show–do approach when using a new type of instrument – especially those with vibration.

10 If the individual does not understand, rephrase rather than repeat your message.

11 Be sure you are understood before moving onto a new topic.

12 Use written information if communication breaks down.

13 Print common questions with yes/no answers with a large font, laminate the page and keep it easily accessible. Patients can read and point to the answer.

14 Keep two dry-erase boards easily accessible; one for patient and one for dental team.

The following list provides guidelines on management of those with hearing aids (not digital).

1 Unless you are trying to identify if a hearing aid is functional, avoid putting hands next to the hearing aid as this can produce feedback from the aid and cause it to squeal or whistle. This is caused by the amplified sound produced from the hearing aid going back into the aids microphone, thus getting reamplified. This does not occur with digital hearing aids as they can account for the feedback.

2 If someone is wearing a hearing aid, make sure that it is turned on and operational.

3 The patient may need to turn the hearing aid off during a procedure because of your closeness and the office sounds (e.g., handpiece) can be disturbing.

Also note that, although generally unintentional, one of the most hurtful responses to a hard-of-hearing person's request to repeat something is "never mind, it's not important." This response implies that the elder isn't important enough to include/repeat to. Similarly, when the need to repeat or experiencing *non sequitur* responses occurs, it is important to remain positive so as not to add to the negative perceptions of older adults.

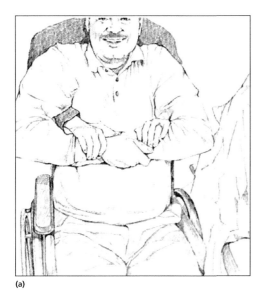
(a)

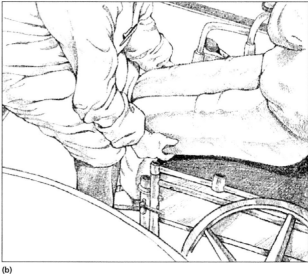
(b)

Figure 5.7 The two-person transfer. (a) First clinician stands behind the patient. (b) Second clinician initiates the lift. From the US Department of Health and Human Services (2009).

Mobility

Although the issues surrounding vision and hearing impairment are key concepts requiring a professional's attention, mobility and fall risk are also important issues to consider when treating older adults. It is important to reduce the risk of falls in the office both to reduce potential liability issues and to ensure patients remain safe. According to the Centers for Disease Control and Prevention (CDC), every year 33% of adults aged 65+ fall. For adults aged 65+ falls are the most common cause of nonfatal injuries and hospital admissions for trauma (CDC, 2013).

Sometimes it may be necessary to transfer a patient from their wheelchair to the dental chair. Resources and guidance are available from the National Institute of Dental and Craniofacial Research (https://www.nidcr.nih.gov). There you can find step by step instructions regarding patient transfers as reproduced below (US Department of Health and Human Services, 2009).

Six steps to a safe wheelchair transfer

Step 1: Determine the patient's needs

Ask the patient or caregiver about:
- Preferred transfer method
- Patient's ability to help
- Use of special padding or a device for collecting urine
- Probability of spasms
  Reduce the patient's anxiety by announcing each step of the transfer before it begins

Step 2: Prepare the dental operatory

Remove the dental chair armrest or move it out of the transfer area. Relocate the hoses, foot controls, operatory light, and bracket table from the transfer path. Position the dental chair at the same height as the wheelchair or slightly lower. Transferring to a lower level minimizes the amount of strength necessary during the lift.

Step 3: Prepare the wheelchair

Remove the footrests. Position the wheelchair close to and parallel to the dental chair. Lock the wheels in place and turn the front casters forward. Remove the wheelchair armrest next to the dental chair. Check for any special padding or equipment.

Step 4: Perform the two-person transfer (Fig. 5.7)

Support the patient while detaching the safety belt. Transfer any special padding or equipment from the wheelchair to the dental chair. *First clinician*: Stand behind the patient. Help the patient cross his arms across his chest. Place your arms under the patient's upper arms and grasp his wrists. *Second clinician*: Place both hands under the patient's lower thighs. Initiate and lead the lift at a prearranged count (1–2–3–lift). *Both clinicians*: Using your leg and arm muscles while bending your back as little as possible, gently lift the patient's torso and legs at the same time. Securely position the patient in the dental chair and replace the armrest.

Step 5: Position the patient after the transfer

Center the patient in the dental chair. Reposition the special padding and safety belt as needed for the patient's comfort. If a urine-collecting device is used, straighten the tubing and place the bag below the level of the bladder.

Step 6: Transfer from the dental chair to the wheelchair

Position the wheelchair close to and parallel to the dental chair. Lock the wheels in place, turn the casters forward, and remove the armrest. Raise the dental chair until it is slightly higher than the wheelchair and remove the armrest. Transfer any special padding. Transfer the patient using the two-person transfer (see step 4). Reposition the patient in the wheelchair. Attach the safety belt and check the tubing of the urine-collecting device, if there is one, and reposition the bag. Replace the armrest and footrests.
  By transferring patients properly you will avoid injury to yourself, your staff and your patients.

Osteoarthritis or degenerative joint disease

Osteoarthritis (OA) or degenerative joint disease (DJD) is a progressive pathologic change in the hyaline cartilage and underlying bone of a joint. It is the most common type of arthritis. The joints most commonly affected are knees, hips, hands and the spine. Osteoarthritis in weight-bearing joints has the greatest impact on older adults, affecting movement and the ability to care for themselves.

The prevalence of OA increases with age, with 34% of those aged 65+ and almost 100% of those aged 80+ effected. Individuals with OA often experience pain, joint stiffness, swelling, and loss of function. Although there is no cure for OA, managing symptoms aids in improving function.

Managing mobility issues

Geriatricians use mobility as an indicator of how well an older adult thrives. Addressing mobility issues in the practice enables one to envision how a patient will physically interact in the environment. Mobility concerns include potential physical barriers that a patient may encounter in the dental office. There is a fine line between the office that "complies" and the one that is welcoming. For instance, if a patient utilizes a wheelchair, then ramps or elevators and doorways that can accommodate the wheelchair are needed. Addressing a patient's psychologic and physical needs

will ensure space in the waiting room where a person in a wheelchair can blend in and not be stuck in the middle of the room ringed by "normal chairs."

The waiting room is an area of the office that sets the tone for the visit and is important (Figs 5.8 & 5.9), just as a staff that is well trained in working with older adults is important. A warm and welcoming environment should include chairs that are comfortable and stable for people to sit. They should be of appropriate height and have broad arm support. The arms are a significant part of the chair and should extend a bit

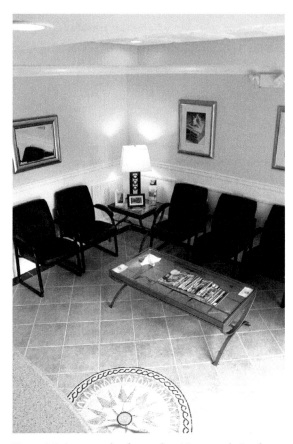

Figure 5.9 An example of a good waiting area design for older patients. Notice the overhead lighting and the task lighting. The chairs have arms and although cushioned for comfort but are not overstuffed and difficult to get up from. There are no throw rugs and there is emergency lighting should power be lost. One thing to notice is the glass table tops that have sharp corners. Either a bumper around the edge of the table or a rounded edge may be more friendly to older adults should someone bump into the table. Courtesy of Michael Dental Care.

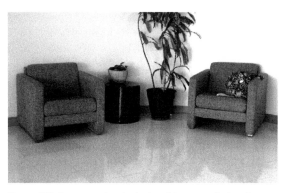

Figure 5.8 An example of a bad waiting area design for older patients. This waiting area has deep chairs that are low to the ground. While there is good ambient light there is no task lighting for reading. The floors are highly reflective and will be slippery if they get wet. There is no place to put down any papers. The only small table has a plant on it. There is much room for improvement in this waiting area. Courtesy of Ruth S. Goldblatt.

beyond the depth of the seat so as to be comfortable and stable enough to support a person as they sit and stand. Overstuffed chairs may be welcoming for some but are a strain for older adults to use.

The following box provides management suggestions that cover many areas of concern for older adults in your practice – not only vision, hearing, and mobility. The suggestions provide ideas that, while they can be specific, when taken together provide a common thought pattern when treating older adults. We consider the overall feeling in an office of importance, as patients often notice the little things that make their experience at a doctor's office much more pleasant and inviting.

Management strategies for patients with mobility limitations

1. Train staff to safely transfer a patient in and out of the dental chair. Attentive team members allow patients to feel safe and cared for and not an imposition on the practice.
2. When dependent upon a walker or cane, patients often need to know where that assistive device will be when they are in the dental chair and many prefer to have their device in their line of vision. Consider placing a small hook nearby so their cane can be hung and in their sight.
3. When seating or dismissing a patient to the dental chair, raise the chair so the seat is a little higher than their hip joint. This will help individuals to stand alone to get in and out of the dental chair by themselves. It reduces the rocking often seen when an older person is trying to stand, and it helps to maintain their dignity.
   a) If you do need to assist someone to stand, place your feet in front of the patient's feet just while they are in the motion of standing – toe-to-toe, to stabilize them. Your feet will prevent the patient's from slipping out from under them while standing.
   b) If patient is using a walker with wheels, make sure the brakes are locked as they stand.
   c) Orthostatic hypotension is a common side effect of medications, especially antihypertensives. Make sure the patient are stable before they start walking. Have them look you in the eye so you know they are stable and comfortable.
4. For those treating many individuals who use wheelchairs, having a wheelchair lift in the office is a useful addition to the practice.
5. All areas (bathrooms, hallways, and at least one operatory) needs sufficient room to allow wheelchairs and scooters to enter doorways, turn corners, and turn around.
6. Handrails are needed on ramps longer than six feet and need to be on both sides of ramps and stairs.
7. Stairs and ramps need to be marked with contrasting colored, nonstick treads or paint to help those with visual impairments to distinguish where one step ends and another begins.
8. Use levers rather than doorknobs and faucets, to assist use by those with diminished hand strength.
9. Use grab bars in the restroom, around the toilet.
10. Have an internal alert system in the restroom, for emergency use (e.g., a pull string that sets off an alarm or triggers an emergency light at the front desk area).
11. Have longer hoses in dental operatory that are accessible to wheelchairs, for patients unable to transfer to the dental chair.
12. Keep floors clear of water and tubing to reduce fall risks.
13. Waiting room furniture needs to include textures to help provide tactile clues for identification.
    a) Avoid upholstery and floor coverings with stripes or checks as they can be visually confusing.
    b) Use chairs with broad, stable arms that extend past the seat so that the patient can lean on them when standing or sitting.
    c) Use brightly colored accessories, to create contrast and make furniture easier to locate.
14. Have large print books such as *The Reader's Digest* available in waiting areas.
15. Keep signs at eye level and have exits clearly marked.
16. Use nonskid surfaced flooring, and remove or secure scatter rugs.
17. Use no-glare products to clean and polish furniture and flooring.
18. Keep furniture and children's toys out of main traffic areas.
19. Use adjustable blinds to reduce glare from natural lighting.
20. Provide task lighting on desks or tables to write on instead of clipboards.

Electronic health records

As the electronic health records become more popular, older adults and individuals with impaired vision may be challenged by: (i) the technology; (ii) visualizing the monitor and/or keyboard; (iii) utilizing the mouse or touchscreen; (iv) understanding how to use computer appropriately. Computers and electronic health records may be viewed as a nightmare for a person with poor eyesight and/or stiff hands. As screen resolution increases, text size and icons are often reduced. Fortunately, many computers provide a wide range of options to change these "features" and make computers accessible for the those with visual or physical limitations. Most computers have tools that enhance visibility and accessibility as listed below.

1 *Screen resolution*: A high screen resolution is best; however, a high resolution reduces the size of everything and text becomes very hard to read. Hence, it may help to reduce the screen resolution. To retain sharpness and visibility, you can also increase the DPI (dots per inch). Tutorials can be found for your particular software by using the help function for each particular software. Many web sites are designed so that you can adjust the font size on the home page with the click of a mouse.

2 Increase the contrast and/or use larger text and icons to enhance readability.

Case study

Revisiting Mrs. Gonzalez

Let's revisit Mrs. Gonzalez's scenario that started this chapter to identify where senior-friendly awareness might have had the appointment ending in a more positive fashion:

1 *Transportation.* Ask about patients' transportation options during the initial telephone call. The dental team needs to be aware of any issues related to the timing of appointments. This can help question whether the number of appointments is going to be an issue, and if so, the treatment plan may need to be redesigned. In general, patients appreciate fewer visits when transportation is difficult to attain. Staff can help patients arrange pick-up time with the driver, van service, or taxi.

2 *External – physical environment:*
   a) Have a ramp with side rails so patients have an easy alternative to steps.
   b) Have an electric door assist with touchpad control to open the door outside of the building and at the office entrance.
   c) Have doorbells to allow patients to notify staff if assistance is needed outside.
   d) Use easy-to-read signage outside the office for visual recognition.

3 *Waiting/reception area:*
   a) Have welcoming, attentive staff present to assist patients when they enter and when they need to complete paperwork. Make sure staff members are aware of all new patients, that they know to make eye contact close to the patient, to introduce themselves, and to escort the patient into the operatory with a smile.
   b) Have large print nonglare forms for patients who need them.
   c) Have a well-lighted (task lighting) desk or work area for patients to complete forms.
   d) Have comfortable hard-back chairs with broad arms in waiting area.

4 *Hallways.* These need to be uniformly well lit with no slippery floors and no throw rugs.

5 *Office space:*
   a) Restrooms, operatories, and office need to be well-marked.
   b) Keep patient assistive devices in their line of sight when possible, or alert patient to where it will be located.
   c) Have staff offer patient assistance with movement and seating.
   d) Train staff to identify and respond appropriately to individuals with hearing and/or vision problems.

Addressing these age-related issues can make dental offices more senior friendly and can lead to better quality patient relationships and the provision of quality oral health care. Dental visits are more relaxed and productive when patients don't arrive at the operatory confused, stressed, and anxious.

Conclusion

A senior-friendly office is designed to specifically appeal to an aging demographic without alienating those in other age groups. This concept is similar to the development of a vehicle's blind-spot detector or systems designed to allow a car to back into a parking space without assistance from the driver.

As we age, our senses become less acute and require more input to reach threshold. Age-related changes to hearing and vision have the most notable changes and the greatest impact on one's life.

Older adults have many interactions with healthcare providers. By having an office that is aware of and sensitive to the common issues that seniors face, you will be able to provide care in an environment that is positive and comfortable for all involved.

References

Arditi, A. (2014) *Effective Color Contrast. Designing for People with Partial Sight and Color Deficiencies.* http://www.lighthouse.org/accessibility/design/accessible-print-design/effective-color-contrast. Accessed March 18, 2014.

CDC (Centers for Disease Control and Prevention) (2013) *Falls Among Older Adults: An Overview.* From http://www.cdc.gov/homeandrecreationalsafety/falls/adultfalls.html. Accessed March 18, 2014.

Cooper, B.A. (1986) The use of color in the environment of the elderly to function. *Clinics in Geriatric Medicine,* **2**(1), 151–63.

Department of Justice (2010) *2010 ADA Standards for Accessible Design.* From http://www.ada.gov/regs2010/2010ADAStandards/2010ADAstandards.htm. Accessed March 18, 2014.

Department of Justice (2011) *Fact Sheet: Highlights of the Final Rule to Amend the Department of Justice's Regulation Implementing Title II of the ADA.* http://www.ada.gov/regs2010/factsheets/title2_factsheet.html. Accessed March 18, 2014.

Department of Justice (2014) *Information and Technical Assistance on the Americans with Disabilities Act.* http://www.ada.gov. Accessed March 18, 2014.

Dillon, C.F., Qiuping G., Hoffman, J.J. & Chia-Wen, K. (2010) *Vision, Hearing, Balance, and Sensory Impairment in Americans Aged 70 Years and Over: United States, 1999-2006. NCHS Data Brief, Number 31, April 2010.* From http://www.cdc.gov/nchs/data/databriefs/db31.htm. Accessed March 18, 2014.

Federal Interagency Forum on Aging Related Statistics (2010) *2010 Older Americans: Key Indicators of Well-Being.* From http://www.agingstats.gov/Main_Site/Data/Data_2010.aspx. Accessed March 18, 2014.

Jerger, J., Chmiel, R., Wilson, N. & Luchi, R. (1995) Hearing impairment in older adults: new concepts. *Journal of the American Geriatrics Society,* **43**(8), 928–35.

Lighthouse International (2014) Web site. http://www.lighthouse.org. Accessed March 18. 2014.

Maylahn C., Gohdes, D.M., Blamurugan, A. & Larsen, B.A. (2012) Age-related eye diseases: an emerging challenge for public health officials. *The Eye Digest.* From http://www.webcitation.org/63MvNQy6m. Accessed March 17, 2012.

National Eye Health Education Program (2007) *Eye Health Needs of Older Adults. Literature Review.* From https://nei.nih.gov/nehep/research/The_Eye_Health_needs_of_Older_Adults_Literature_Review.pdf. Accessed March 18, 2014.

National Eye Institute (2014a) *Facts About Age-Related Macular Degeneration.* From http://www.nei.nih.gov/health/maculardegen/armd_facts.asp#1. Accessed March 18, 2014.

National Eye Institute (2014b) *Facts About Diabetic Retinopathy.* From http://www.nei.nih.gov/health/diabetic/retinopathy.asp. Accessed March 18, 2014.

National Eye Institute (2014c) *Glaucoma.* From http://www.nei.nih.gov/nehep/programs/glaucoma/index.asp. Accessed March 18, 2014.

Orr, A.L. (1998) *Issues in Aging and Vision: A Curriculum for University Programs and In-Service Training.* American Foundation for the Blind Press, New York, NY.

Pew Research Center (2010) *Baby boomers retire.* From http://pewresearch.org/databank/dailynumber/?NumberID=1150. Accessed March 18, 2014.

Pratt, S.R., Kuller, L., Talbott, E.O. *et al.* (2009) Prevalence of hearing loss in black and white elders: results of the Cardiovascular Health Study. *Journal of Speech, Language, and Hearing Research,* **52**, 973–89.

US Department of Health and Human Services (2009). *Wheelchair Transfer. A Health Care Provider's Guide,* NIH Publication No. 09-5195. From http://www.nidcr.nih.gov/NR/rdonlyres/6C7E21C3-ED54-46F8-ADBC-2373AC03C0E5/0/Wheelchair.pdf. Accessed March 18, 2014.

Vision Aware (2012) *Resources for Independent Living with Vision Loss.* From http://www.visionaware.org. Accessed November 2, 2012.

PART 3

Decision Making and Treatment Planning

CHAPTER 6

Geriatric Patient Assessment

Mary R. Truhlar

Department of General Dentistry, School of Dental Medicine, Stony Brook University, Stony Brook, NY, USA

Introduction

> The value of the geriatric assessment is that it provides a basis for treatment decisions and the prediction of treatment tolerance in the frail elderly patient.

This chapter is designed for the reader to develop an understanding of how to assess the older adult patient, why a focus on function is important, which tools are useful for incorporating into the dental office visit, and strategies to enhance communication and understanding with older patients. The importance of a "geriatric" assessment has long been recognized and classically described as "a multidisciplinary evaluation in which the multiple problems of older patients are uncovered, described, and explained, if possible, and in which the resources and strengths of the person are cataloged, need for services assessed, and a coordinated care plan developed to focus interventions on the person's problems" (AGS Public Policy Committee, 1989). The value of a "geriatric" assessment versus a traditional patient assessment lies in the recognition that many times "usual" care may not meet an elderly patient's needs. Despite the fact that the majority of elderly live independently, disability and dependency rises steadily with increasing age and must be part of the equation when developing any course of patient care.

A geriatric assessment is essential to the establishment of a realistic, well-planned, and beneficial course of dental treatment. The development of the tools and an approach to the individual assessment is base on the findings of measures of oral health status in older adult population assessments. The Geriatric Oral Health Assessment Index (GOHAI), a self-reported oral health assessment index, developed by Atchinson and Dolan (1990), gave the dental profession one of its first tools to measure oral health in the geriatric population. Ongoing population assessments give insight into changing population characteristics, the accuracy of developing diagnostic tools, as well as assess the effectiveness of implemented treatment modalities. Despite progress in the development of generally applicable assessment tools, the discipline of geriatrics is confounded by the innate population characteristic of increasing individual variability that naturally occurs with aging. The older adult/geriatric population is heterogeneous – ranging from physically fit, healthy, active, engaged elders to medically complex, frail, isolated individuals living either independently or with assistance in their own homes or in long-term care facilities. Age is only a number; it does not reflect ability or functionality. Therefore, a geriatric assessment should be an essential part of every older patient examination with the goal of efficiently and effectively collecting information that facilitates diagnosis, suggests interventions, is a predictor of outcomes and future needs, and takes into consideration the concerns and desires of the patient and/or caregiver. The key is to identify and become familiar with a select group of short screening assessments and communication strategies that will assist in establishing not only the patient desires and dental diagnosis, but will provide an appraisal of the patient's capacity to tolerate as well as the prognosis of a selected course of dental treatment.

Common geriatric conditions that must be considered in the head, neck, and oral examination of the older adult are covered in Section 4. As for the domains of general medical health, psychologic, social, and physical function, a number of geriatric assessment models and definitions exist to evaluate status and are discussed in other sections of this book. When utilizing any assessment in the older population it needs to include evaluation of the caregiver and environmental concerns with an emphasis on the optimization of independent function supporting an increase in "active" life expectancy. In assessing functional health and dental service utilization in community-dwelling elderly, Dolan *et al.* (1998) concluded that even in a well-educated older population, impaired functional status is associated with lower levels of dental service utilization. *To summarize, the geriatric assessment represents a "shift in focus" from a disease specific evaluation to a function-oriented evaluation, with the understanding that small changes in function can make a big difference in quality of life for patients and their caregivers.*

Case study 1

A patient with an otherwise healthy oral cavity presents with asymptomatic mandibular incisors with mobility of II–III and requests the fabrication of a bilateral mandibular removable partial denture. In a healthy young adult patient the treatment discussion would most likely involve long-term treatment options, given the demonstrated high oral disease risk and the desire to fabricate a prosthesis that will not require retreatment in the near future. However, if the patient was an octogenarian, consideration should be given to retaining the teeth. The patient demonstrates lower disease risk due to longevity of retention of the dentition and the teeth have a reasonable chance of remaining for the patient's life expectancy. In addition, retention of the teeth will provide the patient with less surgical trauma and increased comfort in function and esthetics when the denture is not in the patient's mouth.

This chapter presents the components of a "function-oriented assessment" as they apply to the older adult in the dental office setting. These components facilitate the establishment of a realistic dental treatment plan relative to the patients overall well-being and capacity. The following components will be addressed in order listed.

- *Communication status*: Ability to express, see, hear, and/or understand the provider or information presented.

- *Physical status*: Independence in Activities of Daily Living (ADLs) and Instrumental Activities of Daily Living (IADLs).
- *Mobility status*: Fine and gross motor abilities.
- *Mental status*: Memory and cognitive ability.
- *Nutritional status*: Malnutrition and dehydration.
- *Social support*: Ability to engage assistance needed.
- *Medical status and consultation*: Ability to medically tolerate the procedure.

Communication status

Communication is assessed when a patient first encounters the staff and strategies to establish and maintain effective communication are essential in developing a productive doctor–patient relationship. The older patient benefits tremendously from an environment that supports communication. This includes well-lit rooms, minimal extraneous noise, and minimal interruptions during conversation. The technique of establishing the initial relationship is intuitive and straightforward, but not always put into practice. Introduce yourself by name, address the patient by last name (until invited to do otherwise), and avoid "terms of endearment"such as "dear" or "sweetheart." Sit at eye level facing the patient directly, speak slowly in a deep tone, ask open-ended questions, such as "What would you like me to do for you?" and allow ample time for the patient to answer. Whenever possible, try to communicate with the patient without your mask on. The mask muffles sounds, and also precludes the patient being able to see and/or read your lips. Rephrase and summarize to ensure the patient and provider have a similar understanding of the information exchanged. *It should not be assumed that the geriatric patient needs sensory accommodations; however, they should be offered.* Inquire about visual deficits and be prepared to offer and have available larger print material, including business cards, brochures, care instructions, and educational as well as reception room leisure material. For the hearing impaired individual, increase voice volume according to need and ensure extraneous noise is monitored. Generally, the hearing in one ear is better than the other. Ask the patient in which ear they have better hearing, and speak into that ear. Do not shout. Patients with hearing impairments often perceive speech sounds as muffled; shouting only makes the muffled sounds louder, not clearer. Also, facilitate and encourage the use of assistive devices, such as hearing aides and corrective eyewear, and be prepared to provide written copies of important discussions with contact information on a routine basis. (See Chapter 5 for additional discussion of sensory impairments.)

Physical status

Evaluation of the independence in homecare is evaluated with a review of the patient's ability to perform ADLs and IADLs. There are six basic ADLs: dressing, eating, ambulation, toileting, transferring (being able to move from the bed to a chair), and hygiene (grooming and bathing). The higher function IADLs consist of the community interactions of shopping, housekeeping, accounting/managing finances (writing checks, balancing a checkbook), food preparation, telephone use, medication dosing, and transportation. Some type of disability is reported by approximately 40% of adults aged 65 and older, and, as shown in Fig. 6.1, the rate of limitations in activities among persons aged 85 and older is much higher than those for individuals aged 65–74 (US Department of Health and Human Services, 2011).

A person's ability to perform ADLs is very indicative of the prognosis for the progression of oral disease and the ability to maintain oral health. In addition to the impact of disabilities on social, psychologic, and interpersonal factors, diminishing ADLs impact a person's ability to comply with treatment instructions and oral home care. Technical procedures may require in-office evaluation and modification due to physical and medical conditions and personal assistance may need to be identified to complete tasks. Patients can be assessed for "preclinical disabilities" (developing, but not "clinically evident" disability) by asking about perceived difficulties (Fried *et al.*, 2001). Fried and colleagues concluded from their cross-sectional study that there appears to be a preclinical stage of physical disability which precedes onset of task difficulty (disability) (Fried *et al.*, 2001). In a cross-sectional study of community-dwelling elderly women, these authors concluded that there appears to be a preclinical stage of physical disability that precedes the onset of task difficulty. Recognition of this stage provides a basis for identifying older adults at risk of becoming disabled and provides the practitioner with a window of opportunity to introduce devices and techniques, giving the patient the opportunity to accommodate before the onset of the disability. Limitations in the higher level IADLs can be used to identify subtle functional losses in otherwise high functioning patients. These subtle losses are frequently overlooked and undervalued in the complete geriatric assessment, but can provide valuable information on patient capacity and give indication of the overall treatment prognosis.

Mobility status

Evaluation of a person's mobility is integral to the geriatric assessment and is assessed in the review of ADLs. However, falls and gait disorders, which are so common among the elderly, should be reviewed and monitored separately because they are closely related to greater functional impairment and are a major cause of patient morbidity and mortality (Centers for Disease Control):

- Approximately one-third of elderly fall each year representing a major cause of nursing home placement.
- One out of three adults aged 65 and older falls each year but less than half talk to their healthcare providers about it.

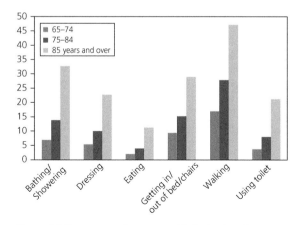

Figure 6.1 Percentage of persons with limitations in activities of daily living by age group: 2009. From US Department of Health and Human Services (2011), p. 15.

• Among older adults (those aged 65 and older), falls are the leading cause of injury death. They are also the most common cause of nonfatal injuries and hospital admissions for trauma.
• In 2010, 2.3 million nonfatal fall injuries among older adults were treated in emergency departments and more than 662 000 of these patients were hospitalized/institutionalized.
• Twenty to thirty percent of people who fall suffer moderate to severe injuries, such as lacerations, hip fractures, or head traumas. These injuries can make it hard to get around or live independently, and increase the risk of early death.

Concomitant medical risk factors such osteoarthritis, cataracts, neuropathy, foot problems, cerebral vascular accidents, pain, peripheral vascular disease, and neuromuscular weakness need to be noted and accommodated. Fall risk assessment commences with observation of the patient as they ambulate from the reception area to operatory and continues with the question "Have you fallen in the past year?" Any elicited concerns should be discussed with the patient and caregiver and referred for a further evaluation. The easily administered "Get Up and Go Gait Assessment" (see box below) can used to further document findings for referral (*Herman et al.*, 2011).

Get Up and Go Gait Assessment

The test procedure is relatively simple. Subjects are asked to stand up from a standard chair (seat height about 18 inches), walk a distance of 10 feet (marked on the floor) at a comfortable pace, turn, walk back and sit down. Subjects are permitted to use routine walking aids and are instructed not to use their arms to stand up. No physical assistance is given. The time to complete the task is measured with a stopwatch. Timing commences on the command "Go" and stops when the subject's back is positioned against the back of the chair after sitting down. Usually the task is performed twice. Shorter times indicate better performance. A suggested cutoff point of 13.5 seconds serves as a threshold for identifying persons with an increased risk of falling.

Managing mobility concerns in the office should be part of routine practice. Carefully selecting and placing signs and providing adequate lighting in each room will aid in supporting ambulatory independence and minimizing any visual disorientation or mental confusion of the elderly patient. When selecting office decor choose firm, standard-height chairs with arms for support. Cushioned chairs and sofas may be comfortable, but they create more difficulty for older adults to stand up from a seated position. Set up office furniture to promote and facilitate access and minimize obstacles. In addition, the operatory should accommodate and be equipped for wheelchair patients or those who use walkers. Bathrooms should contain safety bars on the wall. Railings in hallways provide elders with additional stability. Hardwood, tile, or laminate floors present less opportunity for tripping than carpeting. Use of scatter rugs should be avoided, as should loose wires and cords in the operatory. (See Chapter 5 for more tips on creating a Senior Friendly Office.)

Mental status

An older individuals mental status is an integral determinant of the patient's capacity to successfully complete a given course of dental therapy.

Case study 2

An edentulous 85-year-old white male presents for the fabrication of a maxillary and mandibular complete dentures. His spouse accompanies the patient and explains to the providing resident doctor that her husband has successfully worn dentures for many years but has recently been losing weight with a diminishing appetite due to ill-fitting dentures. The health history and questioning completed by the wife produces negative medical or physical findings. The dental examination confirms ill-fitting and poorly retentive dentures in an otherwise asymptomatic healthy oral cavity. On completion of the fabrication of the new dentures, the patient and his spouse return for multiple adjustment visits and are very unhappy with the prostheses, citing inability to eat and no return of a previously hearty appetite. A second opinion from a supervising doctor was requested.

Following several minutes reviewing the patient's concerns, it became obvious that the spouse was doing all the talking for the patient. The wife was asked to accompany the resident doctor to another area while the supervising doctor engaged the patient in conversation. The patient was asked and answered

---

numerous questions regarding the morning's events at his home. The wife answered the same questions in the separate area. When none of the answers matched the supervising doctor opened the conversation to include a discussion the husbands cognitive and memory status. The wife, who had so ably covered her husbands diminishing mental function, was now asked to face her husband's cognitive deterioration. She was informed of the vital role of cognition and memory in adapting to and functioning with new oral prostheses and the impact of mental status on the appetite.

In addition to providing the additional follow-up visits necessary for the patient to accommodate to the new dentures, the patient and his caregiver wife were referred for appropriate medical evaluation and support.

2 If the person can complete this task, they are then asked to draw a clock. The clock should include the shape, the numbers, and the hands in the correct position
3 The person is then asked to repeat the words from the first part of the test. If the person can repeat all three words the person is not "probably suffering from dementia." If the person is unable to repeat any of the words, they might be categorized as mildly cognitively impaired. If the person cannot draw the clock or if it looks abnormal (Fig. 6.2) they would fall into the category of "probably" suffering from mild cognitive impairment.

The above example illustrates an informal memory assessment. There are a number of well-validated cognitive assessments to document cognitive deterioration, including the widely used Folstein's Mini-Mental State Examination (MMSE) and easily performed Mini-cog Assessment (Borson *et al.*, 2003). These examinations assess the executive functions of orientation, registration, recall, attention, calculation, language, and visuospatial skills. The Mini-cog Assessment is a brief test with a reasonable sensitivity and specificity (Osterberg *et al.*, 2002). The Mini-cog Assessment consists of a three-item recall test (immediate and delayed) and a Clock Drawing Test (CDT). The Mini-cog takes around three minutes to perform and the results obtained are that cognitive impairment falls in three qualitative categories: is absent, probable, or present, rather than a numerical scale. This adds to its simplicity as a screening test, but means the test has no value in either monitoring disease progression or rating severity because there is no metric for comparison (Hattori *et al.*, 2008).

Individuals can also fail to pass the Mini-cog Assessment due to complications from other illness or medical therapies. Therefore, it is necessary to refer patients with abnormal findings for appropriate medical evaluation.

When an individual presents or is newly diagnosed with impaired cognition plan to manage the dental treatment in consultation with their physicians and caregivers. Due to the progressive nature of many dementias, patients should be considered in their best condition at each visit and obtainable diagnostic tests and treatment should not be deferred or delayed. Do as much as possible as soon as possible.

The three-minute Mini-cog Assessment

This test consists of three parts:
1 The examiner names three objects and then asks the person being tested to repeat them back (e.g., tree, house, banana). If the person cannot repeat the three objects after a few tries (cannot learn them), a medical consultation is required

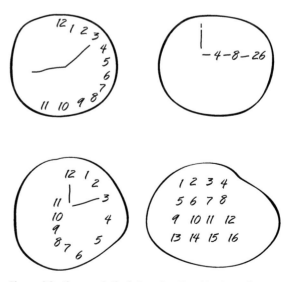

Figure 6.2 Abnormal Clock Drawing Test (CDT) results from Mini-cog Assessment.

With the passage of time, providing treatment will become more challenging for the patient and the provider. Educational material, referral information, and support of caregivers should be readily available. In addition, be familiar with the patients advanced directives when the treatment plan includes behavioral management with sedation or general anesthesia.

Nutritional status

Screening for nutritional status, malnutrition, and dehydration, is an essential and frequently overlooked part of a comprehensive geriatric dental assessment. Minimal information obtained should include questions regarding an unexplained diminished appetite, discomfort of the oral cavity during ingestion of food, restricted diet and food consistency, limited liquid consumption or decreased frequency of urination, and unintentional weight loss. Positive answers or information should be evaluated and correlation to positive findings on oral examination should be addressed. The causes such as lack of caregiver support in use of assistive devices or oral disease altering function (i.e., insertion of prosthesis, pain, infection, dry mouth, lack of dentition, or ill-fitting prosthesis) can be identified and discussed during the preliminary visit. Research studies looking for a link between perceived masticatory ability, condition of dentition and/or dental prostheses, and malnutrition remains debated and it is generally agreed that there is great individual variability (Altenhoevel *et al.*, 2012). The research of Altenhoevel and colleagues found that impairments in masticatory function documented by clinical exam (dental status, denture quality, and condition) and interview (stated problems, symptoms, and discomfort) may lead to food avoidance and a higher incidence of digestive complaints, but showed no significant relationship to actual nutritional status, as demonstrated by the Mini Nutritional Assessment (MNA) (Woodford & George, 2007). Therefore, unexplained changes in nutritional status, all of which can result in precipitous changes in overall well-being, require immediate evaluation and management in consultation with the patient's physician.

Social support

A focused social assessment, including identifying individuals the patient consents to have informed of findings and treatment, is invaluable part of the examination. The availability of a personal support system greatly increases the successful management of all patients, but is essential when working with a vulnerable elderly patient. The social system for a vulnerable older patient supports the scheduling of appointments, facilitates solutions to transportation and access, and assists with the management, communication, and coordination between multiple healthcare providers. Individuals in the support system provide the much needed confirmation and reinforcement of examination findings and treatment considerations and facilitate the successful implementation and follow-up of dental care. *Attention must be given by the provider to strategically utilize but not overburden the members of the support system.*

Case study 3

An 84-year-old woman begins to cry when instructed by a dental hygienist that she should be using an electric toothbrush to clean her husband's teeth because the manual brushing she is performing is not adequate. The flustered hygienist attributes the wife outburst to the increasing stress associated with her husbands escalating dementia. She dismisses the patient and wife, telling them "everything will be OK" and to schedule a return for a follow-up evaluation and further dental cleaning. At the front desk the wife confides in the receptionist that she is not sure if she can return because she finds these dental visits too demanding.

Realizing that the importance of maintaining the patient's schedule of care, the office staff pursued this last statement and the wife, grateful to have a concerned listener, conveyed the following information. She has been the sole caretaker for her husband since his diagnosis of Alzheimer's disease 3 years ago. At this time it takes her about 4 hours to assist her husband with dressing, bathing, and toileting every morning. The thought of any change or addition to this already taxing regimen was unimaginable to her.

Having this information in hand, the dental team was now much more prepared to commence a conversation that would investigate ways to strengthen the patient's social support system, assist an aging spouse, and develop a realistic care plan to address his oral health needs.

Medical status

Age-related changes, increase in the incidence of systemic disease, and greater medication use all combine to predispose the elderly population to pathologic changes in their medical and oral health. *Unlike disease in youth, disease in old age is characterized by multiplicity, iatrogenicity, chronicity, and duplicity of presentation.* This type of presentation increases the complexity of case management and challenges the accuracy of diagnosis and treatment decisions.

Case study 4 (Fig. 6.3)

The dental images from this patient case demonstrate the characteristics of disease presentation in the elderly (*multiplicity, iatrogenicity, chronicity, and duplicity*). Unlike a younger patient, this patient presents with none of the usual symptoms of infection; pain, lymphadenopathy, swelling, fever, or erythema. This medically vulnerable older patient presented with vague symptoms and a functional complaint of food impaction. In recognizing the confounding factors of the presentation of disease in the elderly, the practitioner is better able to a comprehensive assessment, accurate diagnosis and prognosis, and viable and beneficial treatment options.

Given the complex nature and presentation of medical–dental disease in the elderly, it is imperative that dentists working with the frail elderly have a solid working knowledge of systemic diseases, associated classes of pharmacologic therapy, and the implications to oral health and medical stability (De Rossi & Saughter, 2007). Four major areas of concern in medically managing the dental treatment of an older patient are: increased risk of infection, risk of uncontrolled bleeding, risk of drug actions and interactions and actions, and the patient's ability or capacity to tolerate the dental treatment (Ship, 2002).

Adverse drug reactions (ADR) are the most common cause of iatrogenic illness in hospital and affect 20–25% of community elderly annually. Up to 10–15% of all hospital admissions for the elderly are drug-related problems and 28% are preventable. Common symptoms include confusion, nausea, loss of balance, change in bowel pattern, falls, and sedation. These symptoms are often overlooked or may be treated as disorders and treated with additional medications.

Risk factors for ADR are:
- Advanced age;
- Female gender;
- Lower body weight/frailty;
- Hepatic or renal insufficiency;
- Polypharmacy;
- Prior drug reactions.

The elderly patient's ability or capacity to tolerate physiologic stress and therefore dental treatment can be viewed as "homeostenosis" – the progressive restriction of homeostatic reserve that occurs with aging in every organ (Fig. 6.4).

A well-written succinct consultation to address the patient's medical status is a very important part of the dental assessment of a medically complex patient.

KEY POINTS OF THE MEDICAL CONSULTATION

1 It is a consultation, not a medical clearance (exception may be for sedation/general anesthesia).
2 The consultation is for medical or medication issues that require attention, either prior to starting, during, or after dental treatment, or to address a previously unrecognized medical issue.
3 The consultation is not intended to confirm dental–medical treatment protocols that the providing dentist should be familiar with and conversant in. The providing dentist should be up to date in current premedication guidelines and standards of care, and comfortable with and prepared to discuss and implement them.
4 A well-written medical consultation is focused on relevant issues and questions:
   a) Briefly states pertinent medical history, medications, and allergies;
   b) Overviews intended dental treatment;
   c) Details medical concerns regarding dental treatment;
   d) Requests additional medical information or medical tests needed for dental treatment decisions;
   e) Concludes with a statement such as "please advise," avoiding statements requesting "medical clearance." The decision to treat, modify treatment, or not treat the patient is made by the dental provider in consultation with the appropriate members of the patient's healthcare team.

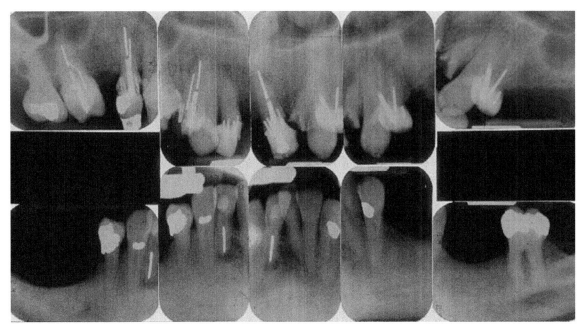

Figure 6.3 Dental images from patient case demonstrating the characteristics of disease presentation in the elderly (see Case study 4 and text for more details).

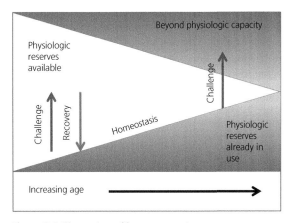

Figure 6.4 Illustration of homeostenosis.

assessment of physical, cognitive, and social aspects of the patient's well-being. These components of the geriatric dental assessment should be briefly reviewed at every visit, as they change more frequently in the frail elderly and represent barriers to maintaining good oral health.

Summary

The comprehensive geriatric dental assessment includes a focused function-oriented evaluation, it promotes wellness and independence, it uses strategies that enhance communication, and it includes

---

DISCUSSION QUESTIONS (FOR CASE STUDY 5, P. 69)

1 Why is a "geriatric" assessment important?
2 Identify key features of a "geriatric" assessment.
3 Review the following case study regarding Mrs. F. and consider the following questions:
   a) What are your concerns related to the presentation and future management of this patient?
   b) What additional information is needed to complete your assessment of this patient?
   c) What is the next step?

Case study 5

"Mrs. F."

Mrs. F. is a 76-year-old widow who presents to the dental office for an initial assessment. She has not seen a dentist in over a year and wants to have her teeth "cleaned" for her granddaughter's wedding. The receptionist informs the dentist that Mrs. F. arrived with her son, who filled out the registration and data forms, and will return in an hour to pick her up.

- The medical form reports Mrs. F. is under the care of an internal medicine physician and was last seen two months ago. Positive responses on the medical history form include a fall, resulting in hospitalization, a left hip replacement in 2009, atrial fibrillation, and hearing impairment.
- *Medications listed include*: Coumadin® (warfarin) 5 mg every day, Aricept® (donepezil hydrochloride) 10 mg every day, and a multivitamin.
- *Allergy noted*: Penicillin.

Mrs. F. is pleasant and agreeable and confirms the above information. She does not add additional details when asked and is anxious to continue so she can her teeth cleaned. She reports a dental history of regular examinations and cleanings, and her dental exam generally supports this statement. Her reported home hygiene regimen includes daily manual brushing and mouth rinse (unsure of type or brand) with occasional flossing. Clinical and radiographic dental examination findings are:

a) *Head and neck exam*: within normal limits (WNL).

b) Mrs. F. retains 80% of her dentition with two recurrent carious lesions and an asymptomatic nonrestorable tooth no. 3.

c) She demonstrates fair oral hygiene (OH), mild generalized gingivitis, moderate plaque, probing depths 3–4 mm, isolated recession of 1–2 mm, no mobility, and generalized moderate staining.

In explaining to Mrs. F. the need to consult with her internist, she doesn't understand what her physician has to do with her dental treatment, as they have never been involved in the past. When given her dental diagnosis and treatment needs, in addition to the dental cleaning, she requests the presence of her son. She becomes very agitated in learning that he is not currently present and wants to return to the reception area to find him.

References

AGS Public Policy Committee (1989) Comprehensive geriatric assessment. *Journal of the American Geriatrics Society*, **37**, 473–4.

Altenhoevel, A., Norman, K., Smoliner, C. & Peroz, I. The impact of self-perceived masticatory function on nutrition and gastrointestinal complaints in the elderly. *The Journal of Nutrition, Health & Aging*, 2012, **16**(2), 175–8.

Atchinson, K. & Dolan, T.A. (1990) Development of the geriatric oral health assessment index. *Journal of Dental Education*, **54**(11), 680–7.

Borson, S., Scanlan, J.M. & Chen, P., *et al.* (2003) The Mini-cog as a screen for dementia: validation in a population-based sample. *Journal of the American Geriatrics Society*, **51**, 1451–4.

CDC (Centers for Disease Control and Prevention) (2014) *Injury Prevention and Control (WISQARS)*. From http://www.cdc.gov/injury/wisqars/facts.html. Accessed March 19, 2014.

De Rossi, S.S. & Slaughter, Y.A. (2007) Oral changes in older patients: a clinician's guide. *Quintessence International*, **38**, 773–80.

Dolan, T.A., Peek, C.W., Stuck, A.E. & Beck, J.C. (1998) Functional health and dental service use among older adults. *Journal of the American Geriatrics Society*, **53A**(6), M413–18.

Fried, L., Young, Y., Rubin, G. & Bandeen-Roche, K. (2001) Self-reported preclinical disability identifies older women with early declines in performance and early disease. *Journal of Clinical Epidemiology*, **54**(9), 889–901.

Hattori, Y., Mito, Y. & Wantanabe, M. (2008) Gastric emptying rate in subjects with experimentally shortened dental arches: a pilot study. *Journal of Oral Rehabilitation*, **35**, 402–7.

Herman, T., Giladi, N. & Hausdorff, J.M. (2011) Properties of the "Timed Up and Go" test: more than meets the eye. *Gerontology*, **57**(3), 203–10.

Osterberg, T., Tsuga, K., Rothenberg, E., *et al.* (2002) Masticatory ability in 80 year old subjects and its relation to intake of energy, nutrients and food items. *Gerontology*, **19**, 95–100.

Ship, J.A. (2002) Geriatrics. In: *Burket's Oral Medicine: Diagnosis and Treatment* (eds. M.S. Greenberg & M. Glick), pp. 605–22. Decker, Hamilton, ON, Canada.

US Department of Health and Human Services (2011) *A Profile of Older Americans*. From http://www.aoa.gov/Aging_Statistics/Profile/2011/docs/2011profile.pdf. Accessed April 18, 2014.

Woodford, H.J. & George, J. (2007) Cognitive assessment in the elderly: a review of clinical methods. *QJM; monthly journal of the Association of Physicians*, **100**(8), 469–84.

CHAPTER 7

Treatment Planning and Oral Rehabilitation for the Geriatric Dental Patient

Peter Y. Kawamura[1] and Mary R. Truhlar[2]

[1]Department of Veterans Affairs Medical Center, San Francisco, CA, USA
[2]Department of General Dentistry, School of Dental Medicine, Stony Brook University, Stony Brook, NY, USA

Introduction

Many patients, including the elderly (or their families) will seek dental care because something in their mouth changed. It is not uncommon to hear a functional complaint from an older patient such as "My tooth broke," "My denture doesn't fit anymore and it hurts," or "My mom/dad isn't eating well and we think that her/his teeth don't fit right …". Due to a number of reasons; finances, lack of dental insurance, overwhelming medical care issues, inconvenience of transportation; the older patient more frequently than their younger counterpart is likely to not have regular dental care for an extended period of time (Dolan *et al.*, 2005; Kiyak & Reichmuth, 2005). The clinical picture is disheartening: missing nonreplaced teeth; moderate–severe gingival inflammation; multiple carious lesions frequently at the margins of crowns and on root surfaces; ill-fitting and poorly maintained prosthesis; retained roots; moderate oral debris and calculus; and malocclusion secondary to lack of oral maintenance and rehabilitation. The dismal appearance of the patient's clinical situation is frequently compounded by: a complex medical presentation with multiple diagnoses and polypharmacy; families who share the financial and social burdens of care and want "only what is really necessary" and "nothing complex"; and a providing dentist who has a limited available skill set in the management of the medically complex frail elderly.

As daunting as it may seem, providing dentistry for the older patient really relies on some fundamental clinical skills and tasks, that are in the repertoire of most dentists. The providing dentist also needs to possess additional skills in geriatric patient assessment and be comfortable managing the associated medical, physical, cognitive, and social findings. The *clinical dental procedures* for restoring individual teeth do not change from patient population to patient population; what does change is the *approach to overall case management.*

Diagnostic studies to facilitate planning and treatment

Diagnostic casts mounted in maximal intercuspal position (MIP) or centric occlusion (CO) is a fundamental and necessary step for any patient needing more than operative dentistry and single crowns within an existing dentition. Any time bridges, implants, partial, or complete dentures are contemplated, an accurate, three-dimensional, replica of the dentition and occlusion, i.e., diagnostic casts, will enable proper planning, temporization, and definitive restorations to be done. The mounted casts serve as a medico-legal record of the initial presentation of the patient and should not be altered or marked. Additionally, the patient who allows you to make two alginate impressions and an occlusal record during the early stages of diagnosis and treatment planning probably will allow you to work

---

KEY POINTS

- The patient's existing dental treatment can serve as an indication of the importance of good oral health for this patient. This is a good starting point for conversations and decision-making when dementia, physical limitations in effective oral health home care, or family priorities complicates the picture.

- More time needs to be spent upfront asking questions, setting priorities, and developing an understanding of treatment goals with the patient and/or caregiver. This will facilitate a focused and timely course of treatment.

- Recognize early the important confounding issues/problems and develop a phased and sequenced approach that is amenable to modification as needed. This will minimize patient, caregiver, and clinician frustration when working with medically frail and labile patients.

- Emphasize the value of hygiene prevention visits. Ongoing dental hygiene visits with reinforcement of home-care instruction to the patient and/or caregiver and application of preventive agents, such as fluoride varnish, is essential to maximizing the environment for the placement of dental restorations, as well as maintaining the patient's oral health.

- Consider the full range of available treatment modalities when planning the oral health management of an older adult. Incorporate dental implant options into treatment planning to expand and facilitate opportunities to effectively restore the patient's function and esthetics.

---

in his or her mouth. So in addition to diagnostic value, study casts also have predictive value in terms of the ability of patients to comply with treatment requirements.

A full intraoral set of photographs *(front face (no smile), front face (smiling), profile view, front view of teeth in occlusion and lips retracted, left side view with intraoral mirror, right side view with intraoral mirror, maxillary occlusal view with mirror, and mandibular occlusal view with mirror)* is invaluable to document various clinical conditions and provide a solid medico-legal record of the patient's initial presentation. Tooth shades and positions can be determined from photographs and incorporated in future prostheses. Be sure to obtain a signed informed consent to photograph the patient.

An assessment of the patient's temporomandibular joints, maximal intraoral opening, and number of functional pairs of occluding teeth should be made. Popping, clicking, crepitus, tendency for dislocation, and deviations in movements need to be recorded. Maximal intraoral opening, along with patient cooperation, is important in evaluating access to the posterior teeth. The number of *functional pairs of teeth* is critical to establish, as these are the teeth the patient has been functioning with and will continue to habitually use whether or not they wear prostheses.

Besides the radiographic data that panoramic and bitewing images provide, the process of obtaining images yields invaluable information about the patient's ability to follow directions, remain still for prolonged periods, and to endure the discomfort of intraoral films/sensors. Especially with the use of rigid digital sensors, the patient who tolerates the imaging procedure will probably tolerate the dentist probing, manipulating and working in his or her mouth. Cone beam computerized tomography (CBCT) imaging should be considered for a definitive three-dimensional radiographic assessment of the patient who has more complex restorative needs, anatomical deviations, or head and neck pathology concerns.

Planning for dental treatment in the older adult

In a general dental practice, the focus is on restoring dentition and function in healthy ambulatory patients. When an older patient presents with multiple health issues, the focus shifts to maximizing function and esthetics while managing the patient safely within his or her physiologic limitations.

Following are some key questions focusing on oral function that can facilitate the assessment and planning process.

Can the patient chew foods of the desired consistency?

Much of the joy of eating and joy of life comes from eating the variety of foods one wants. Patients often talk about looking forward to biting into "that juicy steak" or "cob of corn" once their teeth are fixed or they get their new dentures. While foods can be ground or pureed to facilitate swallowing, the natural consistency of the food will provide the most satisfying eating experience. Oral rehabilitation should be directed at maximizing the patient's masticatory efficiency.

Does the patient choke or have swallowing problems?

Choking and swallowing problems (dysphagia) while eating can indicate that the patient has not masticated and moistened the food bolus sufficiently to swallow safely. Patients tend to have a set number of chewing strokes before they swallow, so if there is an abrupt change in their ability to grind the food bolus into a "swallowable" mass, they can potentially have problems in the initial oral phase of swallowing. In addition, residual effects of strokes and neuromuscular diseases of movement such as Parkinson's disease and multiple sclerosis, can affect the swallowing process. Special attention needs to be directed to fabrication of prostheses, as well as insuring that these patients have a protected airway when receiving dental treatment. One way to protect the airway is to place an opened gauze pad that drapes over the oropharynx and extends out of the mouth. The patient may need to be positioned in a semi-reclined position instead of a more fully reclined position. The saliva ejector will need to be positioned in the most dependent position in the mouth to collect fluids. The high volume suction needs to be used to catch all aerosols and large volumes of fluids as they are generated to minimize choking and swallowing issues during treatment.

Can the patient manage a prosthesis?

Inserting and removing a removable denture requires the dexterity and coordination to correctly position, seat, and remove the prosthesis. Patients will often bite the denture into place and, if it is not correctly positioned, they will break or bend denture clasps or connectors. Removing the denture can be a problem if a patient is arthritic or can only use one hand and cannot unseat retentive clasps. In addition, care needs to be exercised with the patient with tactile sensory deficits, as they may be unable to sense where the prosthesis is in their mouth. If the patient cannot demonstrate that he or she can manage a prosthesis, then caregivers need to become involved in placing, removing, and cleaning the prosthesis and also insuring that the patient's abutment teeth are properly debrided and maintained. It is important to include appropriate and timely caregiver training and education in insertion, removal, and cleaning of prostheses, as well (see the "Can the caregiver(s) manage prosthesis?" section later in this chapter).

Case study

A cast partial denture was fabricated for a patient who was wheelchair bound following a severe stroke. He came in one day several weeks after delivery of the partial denture complaining that it was not fitting well. When asked, he demonstrated that he used his right hand to seat the denture (his left side was paralyzed) and his left lower lip got stuck under one of the clasps. "See?" he said, "It doesn't fit right." When asked, "Can you feel your lip being pinched by the denture?" he answered "No, I can't feel anything on the left side."

Can the patient tolerate the prosthesis?

Wearing dentures is a skill that is developed over time and requires a certain amount of patience, endurance, and tolerance. The following obstacles need to be overcome for successful denture use: adjusting to lack of tooth proprioception to enable the patient to know where the food bolus is; tongue, cheeks, and lips must develop coordinated and restricted movements to effectively hold the dentures in place; chewing efficiency/force is drastically reduced compared to natural teeth; speech and swallowing need to be re-learned or modified; there is a tendency to gag if the dentures extend over sensitive tissues; the mucosa is easily traumatized by uneven denture surfaces. There is no boilerplate way of designing the prosthesis to ensure patient tolerance and acceptance. A thorough examination of intraoral anatomy and identification of factors that will impact denture use will allow for the design of a prosthesis that best adapts to the patient's functional limitations. Examples include:

- "I" bar clasps may not work for the patient with arthritis who cannot get their fingertips under this type of clasp and may benefit from the use of a bulkier Akers/circumferential clasping.
- Flanges may need to be modified for the patient learning to tolerate a new prosthesis and acrylic can be added slowly to gradually accustom the patient to the bulk and extensions of the denture.
- Denture adhesive can be used to assist in controlling the retention and stability of the new denture. As the patient becomes more skillful in tolerating the dentures less of the adhesive may be needed.
- Gaggers may not tolerate the palate of a maxillary denture and can do well with a palate-less prosthesis retained by two or more dental implants.

Can the caregiver(s) manage prosthesis?

When the patient cannot manage the denture, the caregiver needs to be involved in the insertion, removal, and care of the prosthesis. The caregiver needs to be instructed in the various tasks that need to be done and must be able to *demonstrate back* these skills. Teaching the caregiver to manage the prosthesis is important but more important is the process of *empowering* the caregiver to become involved with the oral care for the patient. Often the caregiver wants to help the patient but feels powerless to do so because the patient "wants to do it themselves". Discussions with the patient and caregiver should be together and the caregiver can be "assigned" a role in helping the patient. In this setting, the patient may be more willing to allow the caregiver to assist because the doctor has "authorized" the caregiver to participate in oral care.

Which teeth are most strategic for patient to maintain?

When treating the medically frail elderly, inevitably a circumstance will arise in which the provider is prioritizing the retention and restoration of teeth. All teeth are important to the patient's function and/ or esthetics; however, treatment planning should give priority to retaining and preserving the following teeth, with accompanying rationale:

Teeth in occlusion These are the teeth the patient uses for chewing and incising food and have adapted their jaw movements to maximize their contact.

Teeth structure that can provide proprioception These teeth/roots enable the patient to know where they are masticating and to more selectively position the food bolus for mastication.

At least one tooth on either side of each arch, preferably in same coronal plane These teeth provide cross arch retention and stability for removable prostheses. Retaining teeth in the same coronal plane helps to create predictable axes of rotations.

Teeth with periodontal support Selection of teeth with good periodontal support, recognizing that with an adequate hygiene regimen, teeth with loss of attachment bone support can still be maintained and provide function, esthetics, and proprioception.

Teeth requiring restoration of coronal structure Depending on the functional and esthetic role of the tooth, coronal damage can be repaired with pins and troughs and grooves to replace lost structure. Use of composite resins and resin-modified glass ionomer materials have improved in functional strength and ease of application since they were originally introduced. Composite resin materials are providing greater occlusal wear characteristics and packable and flowable consistencies allow for easier manipulation and placement. Resin-modified glass ionomer restorative materials (RMGI), especially light cured, combine the benefits and ease of use of resins and the inherent bonding and fluoride-release characteristics of glass ionomers.

Maxillary and mandibular central or lateral incisor These teeth help to support the upper lip and minimize the collapsed midface appearance, the *"old person"* look. For families dealing with the imminent loss of a loved one, retaining these teeth can help support the patient's established appearance and avoid added feelings of loss, grief, and guilt for the family.

Cuspids These teeth are the longest rooted teeth, one of the last teeth to be lost under natural circumstances, and have traditionally served as overdenture abutments. They form what has often been referred to as the "cornerstones" of the dental arch, provide proprioception, help define the smile line, and establish the occlusal plane. The extraction of cuspids needs careful attention and planning to avoid extensive buccal plate loss and increased dental arch morbidity post-surgically. Used as overdenture abutments, they can protect the maxillary anterior edentulous ridge from excessive trauma from remaining mandibular anterior teeth. In the mandibular arch they can serve to stabilize and retain partials or overdentures that would otherwise be dislodged by cheeks, tongue, and lips.

Bicuspids, especially with opposing tooth contact When not "lone standing," these teeth help to provide posterior support, can be used to retain partials, and are easier for the patient to access for hygiene procedures than molar teeth.

The lone standing molar tooth The lone standing molar can serve as a denture abutment, a critical posterior stop, and can provide valuable proprioception even if opposing artificial denture teeth. A domed molar root will functionally turn a potential Kennedy class II distal extension situation into a Kennedy class III tooth bound edentulous space by providing an occlusal stop for the partial.

Maxillary anterior roots that oppose mandibular anterior teeth Retaining maxillary tooth roots opposing intact mandibular dentition will protect the maxillary ridge from trauma and prevent combination syndrome – where repeated trauma from mandibular anterior teeth causes excessive resorption of the edentulous anterior ridge. This leaves flabby gingival tissues, no residual ridge alveolar bone, and fibrotic enlarged maxillary tuberosities.

Can a patient function with a shortened dental arch?

The shortened dental arch (SDA), i.e., one in which there is an intact anterior region but with a reduced number of occluding pairs of posterior teeth, can

provide adequate masticatory efficiency for many patients. Witter *et al.* (1999) reported that "the shortened dental arch concept is based on circumstantial evidence: it does not contradict current theories of occlusion and fits well with a problem-solving approach." For a subset of our patient population this concept offers some important advantages and may be considered a strategy to reduce the need for complex restorative treatment in the posterior regions of the mouth. Armellini and von Fraunhofer (2004) reviewed the literature on the SDA and reported that various studies showed that masticatory efficiency is not impaired significantly with decreased posterior occlusion, that perceived reductions in function and changes in food preferences were acceptable to patients in one study, that SDAs with the presence of 20 or more "well-distributed" teeth did not lead to alterations of food selection, and that there is impaired masticatory ability or shifts in food selection when there are less than 10 pairs of occluding teeth (Armellini & van Fraunhofer, 2004). Similar support for the SDA concept was documented in a 2006 review of the literature by Kanno and Carlson (2006). They concluded that there were no clinically significant differences between subjects with SDAs of three to five occlusal units and complete dental arches regarding variables such as masticatory ability, signs and symptoms of temporomandibular disorders, migration of remaining teeth, periodontal support, and oral comfort. In addition, they noted that the SDA concept was accepted by dentists but not widely practiced. These reviews supported the restorative approach that the use of the SDA comprising anterior and premolar teeth generally fulfills the requirements of a functional dentition.

What is the patient's disease trajectory and can I maintain his or her oral status along this trajectory?

The concept of "disease trajectory" comes from palliative care and refers to the common courses and patterns of decline in the end stages of many diseases. (See Chapter 2 for additional information on palliative care.) Lunney *et al.* (2002, 2003) reviewed four theoretical trajectories of dying: sudden death; terminal illness; organ failure; and frailty. These models were used to examine the patterns of decline in their study population, which drew decedent data from four areas of the country. They found that the patterns of decedents were very similar to the theoretical models and offered a fifth pattern, one in which "individuals experience a steady decline in function but at a moderately high level of performance" (Lunney *et al.*, 2002). They noted that "end of life care must also serve those who become increasingly frail, even without a life threatening illness" (Lunney *et al.*, 2003).

Understanding disease trajectory can be very useful when applied to management of the geriatric patient. It facilitates the organization of your findings, and enhances the ability to recognize issues that need to be dealt with immediately and delineate treatment sequencing. A paper by Elstad and Torjuul (2009) discussed the temporal characteristics of sickness: the immediacy of patient suffering, the basic continuity of life through sickness and health care, and the indeterminism and precariousness of sickness. Managing the frail elderly and the progressively declining patient often involves doing less and less, at a time when the patient needs more attention to maintain their oral status. Understanding the patient's disease trajectory, the intermittent and/or progressive nature of his or her oral disease activity, and developing management strategies to minimize oral decline/damage will enable the patient to preserve their dental restorations, minimize periodontal infections, and minimize the development of new dental pathologies.

Treatment planning: issues and approaches

Separating out the patient's issues or problems will help you demystify and uncomplicate the often tangled mass of problems that present to you in the geriatric patient. Issues and problems can conveniently be divided into two groups: (i) global or nondental; and (ii) dental. The global issues tend to impact the patient's overall care and management, often affecting the extent and timing of dental care. Taken together, all the recognized issues provide a more complete picture and assessment of the patient's problems and help providers recognize the diversity of medical, mental status, functional, social, and dental issues that need to be addressed to make dental care successful.

Approaches to manage each problem or issue should be as simple and straightforward as possible and help to clarify tasks for dental staff and family members. Taken together, all the approach strategies provide comprehensive management tools to help staff treat the patient and to help the patient get the most out of dental care.

Global issues and approaches

Separating out each of the patient's "global" or nondental issues and determining how to manage each will significantly help to make the overall management of the "complex, medically compromised" patient less formidable. Table 7.1 lists some common global issues and some possible approaches.

Table 7.1 Common global issues and some possible approaches

Issue	Approach
Congestive heart failure	Check at each visit for disease control. Any exacerbations? Medications unchanged? Taking medications regularly? No change in symptoms?
Angina with exertion	Have nitroglycerin present on countertop for immediate access.
Confusion (dementia)	Have family member or caregiver present as a familiar/calming/influential face.
	Determine best time of day to treat patient. Avoid late afternoons as the confused patient may "sundown" (become increasingly confused at the end of the day)
Wheelchair for mobility	Have sliding board present for transfers. Identify patient's strong side: this is the side the patient will lead with when getting in and out of the dental chair
Unstable/brittle diabetes	Ask patient for glucometer readings at each visit
	Have glucose source ready for immediate use
	Ask if patient took medications and when their last meal was
Coumadin use	INR (internationalized normalized ratio) before any surgical procedure
Parkinson's disease	Arrange appointments when the patient is most functional and alert after his or her medications
	Keep patients semi-reclined to avoid choking/aspiration

Table 7.2 Common dental issues and possible approaches

Issue	Approach
Multiple root decay	Restore with resin-modified glass ionomer. Treat with fluoride varnish every three months
Severe gingival inflammation with heavy oral debris	Use a three-headed toothbrush, develop patient/caregiver skills in using this brush Increase recall frequency to every 3 months with fluoride varnish
Decay at crown margins	Restore with glass ionomer or resin-modified glass ionomer. Advise patient/caregiver that new crown(s) may be needed
Broken teeth with residual roots	Consider root canal treatment and doming residual root Extractions
Loss of abutment tooth for partial	Consider implant with attachment to provide retention, stability, and support to existing prosthesis
Loss of posterior support	Develop occlusion for shortened dental arch

Dental issues and approaches

Recognizing dental problems and solutions is much more in the realm of the practicing dentist. Often the geriatric patient will present with multiple carious lesions, especially on root surfaces and at crown margins. While the damage may be extensive, the dentist should always evaluate which teeth are most strategic for the patient (see the "Which teeth are most strategic for patient to maintain?" section earlier in this chapter) and put the most effort into restoring these teeth. These will generally be the teeth the patient will function with regardless of whether they wear a prosthesis or not. These will also generally be the teeth that are most cleansable or accessible to oral hygiene by the patient or caregiver. Dental issues and approaches must always be considered in relation to the patient's disease trajectory. As the patient becomes less able to maintain daily oral care, the restorations need to be more accessible, cleansable, and easily managed by patient and caregiver. Table 7.2 lists some common dental issues and possible approaches.

Treatment planning: important goals

Unlike restorative practices with healthy ambulatory patients where treatment goals are generally more procedure driven, treating the geriatric patient more often involves tailoring procedures and treatments to the patient's physiologic, psychologic and functional limitations. A mesial-occlusal (MO) composite on tooth no. 12 in the confused patient in a wheelchair becomes a monumental task – time consuming, production limiting, frustrating for doctor, staff, and family members, and fraught with unpredictable turns in events that can prevent completion of the restoration.

For these and other frail elderly patients it is critical to redefine what a successful patient outcome of treatment would be. **Patient success**, then, may mean sitting long enough for oral debridement of half of the mouth, or successful use of an acrylic partial with class 2 mobile abutments, consistent low levels of oral debris at the gumline and interproximally without new caries and minimal gingival inflammation, or the ability to wear a complete denture all day with denture adhesive. While none of the above might be considered a **dental success** or a traditional expected dental outcome, each can be successfully achieved and maintained.

Treatment goals and decisions should be reviewed with the patient and caregiver and generally should address the following important areas:

> **Important areas to be addressed for treatment goals and decisions**
>
> - Treat emergent issues as soon as possible, avoiding the "let's wait and see" attitude to minimize ongoing pathologies
> - Make infection control, i.e., minimizing or eliminating decay, gingival/periodontal inflammation, endodontic/pulpal infections, and the removal of hopelessly damaged or abscessed teeth, a fundamental goal of management
> - Minimize disruptions in function to enable confused patients to successfully keep using their dentures, to minimize potential swallowing problems, and to maintain consistent dietary intake
> - Maintain anterior esthetics

- Maintain functional tooth pair contacts so the patient can continue to masticate
- Empower the caregiver to assist or finish up oral care started by the patient
- Create stable endpoints/phases in the treatment process to enable the patient to function, have reasonable esthetics and to prevent recurrent infections in the event that there is a catastrophic illness, injury, or situation that would keep the patient from continuing treatment
- Design partials with additional rests and embrasure-style clasping to allow for functional prostheses in the event that abutment teeth are lost
- Consider acrylic partial dentures that can have denture teeth easily added as natural teeth are lost

Implant restorations for the elderly

In the older adult, dental implants provide the ability to anchor crowns and dentures in an oral environment that is often more hostile to restorations and dental prostheses and more prone to caries due to diminished presence of saliva and/or reduced fine oral motor function. Implant treatment also enables the restoration of edentulous spaces without involving adjacent teeth which may have multiple restorations or may be intact and unrestored. As noted by Weber: "They also facilitate treatment decisions, which are more typically needed for the older patient: teeth with reduced periodontal support, endodontic, or structural deficiencies, which may have a good to fair prognosis if left alone, but would not make predictable abutments for prosthetic devices, can be maintained without compromising the prognosis of the planned restorations" (Weber, 2008). However, patients and families are often reluctant to consider this treatment option due to finances or concerns about exposing the older patient to a surgical procedure. In 2010, a short-term retrospective pilot study examined implant integration and bone resorption at a mean of 32 months post-insertion in medically compromised elderly. The study found that implant therapy in older adults with well-controlled systemic disease should not be considered to be a high-risk procedure relative to the type of implant supported prosthesis, surgical procedure associated with implant placement, or presence of systemic

disease (Hyo-June et al., 2010). The dependent elderly can also benefit from implant treatment with minimal impact on gingival health. In a study of 32 Swedish elderly (selected from an initial group of 3041 eligible for subsidized dental care), Olerud and colleagues found that the subjects were satisfied with their implants and that their natural teeth and implants show[ed] few signs of oral diseases. The authors did note that there has been a change in attitudes toward dental implants among the Swedish elderly, "… even at older ages, people wish to avoid removable dentures" and they expected "… an increase in dependent elderly people with implants will be a reality in the future." Additionally, "… since the number of edentulous individuals will decrease in the future, more elderly individuals will have a combination of natural teeth and implants" (Olerud et al., 2012). Implant treatment does, however, tend to be expensive: the implant and restorative parts, the surgical procedure, and the restorations can be cost-prohibitive for many patients. Interestingly, in the competitive dental marketplace one can see prices for implants and procedures slowly decreasing. Perhaps with more widespread use and acceptance in the future, the costs of implant treatment will be more accessible to more elderly dental consumers.

Implant treatment is restoratively driven and therefore requires meticulous preplanning and teamwork. The reader is referred to Stanford's article for a broad review on dental implants in geriatric dentistry in the general practice (Stanford, 2005).

The learning curve for providing implant therapy is steep and requires ongoing continuing education and practice. However the possibilities are numerous and can provide creative restorative solutions that are biomechanically sound.

One implant can serve as a root form anchor to support a single crown (Fig. 7.1a,b), or serve as an abutment to hold a partial in place (Fig. 7.2a,b). A single implant serving as an abutment for a partial provides retention (resistance to vertical displacement), stability (resistance to horizontal or lateral displacement), and support (resistance to tissueward movement) of the partial. The resilience of the attachment allows for rotation of the distal extension portion of the partial and acts as a stress-releasing element (Fig. 7.2a,b).

Two implants can retain an implant retained/tissue supported overdenture or serve as abutments for an

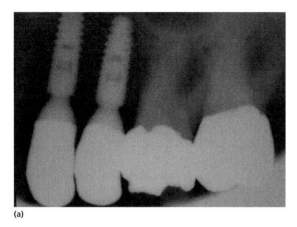

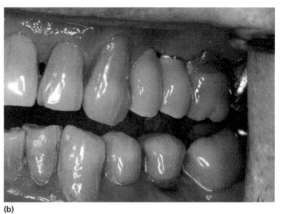

Figure 7.1 (a,b) Single implants used as root form anchors for porcelain fused to metal crowns (PFMs).

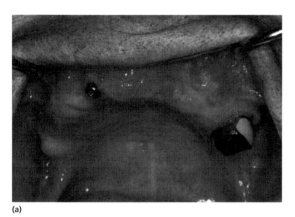

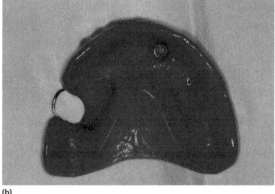

Figure 7.2 (a,b) Single implant placed on the upper right to retain and support a partial denture.

implant fixed bridge (Fig. 7.3). A bar, e.g., Hader bar, attached to the two implants will have retentive clip assemblies in the overdenture (Fig. 7.4a,b). The McGill University symposium on the efficacy of overdentures for the treatment of edentulous patients developed a consensus statement which supports the use of two dental implants with mandibular overdentures. "The evidence currently available suggests that the restoration of the edentulous mandible with a conventional denture is no longer the most appropriate first-choice prosthodontics treatment. There is now overwhelming evidence that a two-implant overdenture should become the first choice of treatment for the edentulous mandible." (Feine & Carlsson, 2003).

Two implants can also be used in the maxilla to retain a maxillary complete denture especially in

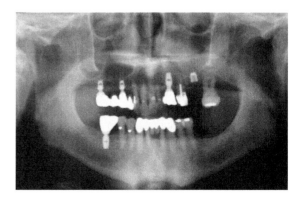

Figure 7.3 Multiple implants support an implant fixed bridge, upper right, and crowns. Note the anterior cantilever pontics at tooth sites no. 6 and no. 11, which are kept out of occlusion to minimize lateral forces.

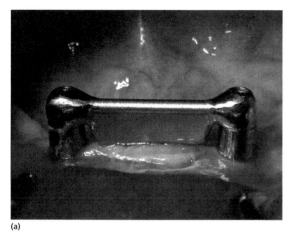

(a)

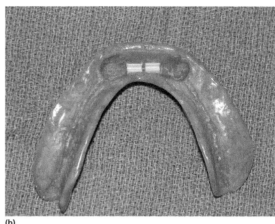

(b)

Figure 7.4 (a,b) Two implants with a bar and clip attachment system.

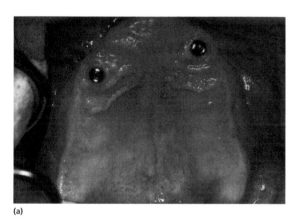

(a)

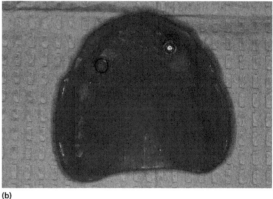

(b)

Figure 7.5 (a,b) Two maxillary implants to retain a maxillary complete denture. Note that the full palate will provide tissue support and that the denture flanges have been constructed to help maximize conventional denture retention.

patients who are xerostomic and who have poorly retentive dentures (Fig. 7.5a,b).

Three or four implants can serve as abutments for an implant retained and supported overpartial or overdenture (Fig. 7.6a,b,c). These prostheses are implant retained and supported, creating no tissue pressure.

Treatment planning: important goals

While treatment options and patient presentations are multiple and varied, the treatment plan for the individual patient needs to be *rational and appropriate* for his or her situation and the provider's clinical skills and knowledge. Ettinger and Berk (1984) proposed the concept of "rational dental care". They

explained that, "… individualized care should occur only after all the modifying factors have been evaluated and that this approach is much more appropriate for older patients than 'technically idealized dental care" (Ettinger, 2006). Various modifying factors need to be considered before treatment (Ettinger 2006). Consider these as the dentist's "due diligence":

- The patient's desires and expectations.
- The type and severity of the patient's dental needs.
- How the patient's dental problems affect his or her quality of life.
- The patient's ability to tolerate the stress of treatment (his or her mental and medical statuses as well as mobility).
- The patient's ability to maintain oral health independently.

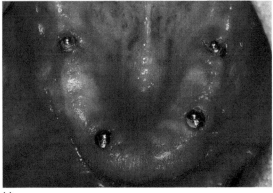

(a)

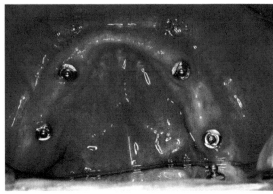

(b)

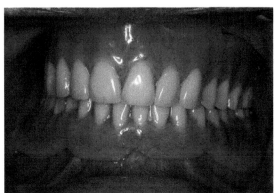

(c)

Figure 7.6 (a,b) Four implants in the maxillary arch and four implants in the mandibular arch. Implant overdentures were constructed that are totally implant supported with no tissue support. (c) Four implants in each arch with retentive ball attachments and gold caps used to retain and support maxillary and mandibular overdentures.

- The probability of positive treatment outcomes.
- The availability of reasonable and less-extensive treatment alternatives.
- The patient's financial status.
- The dentist's ability to deliver the care needed (skills and available equipment).
- Other issues (e.g., the patient's life span, family influences and expectations, and bioethical issues).

Conclusion

Treatment planning and oral rehabilitation for the geriatric patient provides an environment that may be more challenging for the oral health professional. The challenges are generally not procedural or technical challenges. Older adults may present with medical complexities, physical and cognitive limitations, financial concerns, and individual and family expectations. Organizing your system of data collection to provide a consistent method of evaluation of all appropriate treatment options and the patient's ability to tolerate dental treatment, and engaging family/caregivers when indicated will lead to the most successful possible outcome in restoring esthetics and function.

DISCUSSION QUESTIONS

1 Which diagnostic studies are important in developing an appropriate treatment plan for a geriatric patient, and why?
2 What medical conditions can lead to choking and swallowing problems? How should treatment be modified to address these issues? What other conditions might contribute to choking and swallowing issues?
3 Create a checklist of critical questions to use in assessing how to proceed with a treatment plan for the geriatric patient.
4 Describe what adaptations need to be considered by a patient in adjusting to his or her first dental prosthesis (partial or complete)? What advice would you give to a patient upon inserting the first prosthesis?

References

Armellini, A. & von Fraunhofer, A. (2004) The shortened dental arch: a review of the literature. *The Journal of Prosthetic Dentistry*, **92**(6), 531–5.

Dolan, T.A., Atchison, K. & Huynh, T.N. (2005) Access to dental care among older adults in the United States. *Journal of Dental Education*, **69**(9), 961–74.

Elstad, I. & Torjuul, K. (2009) Continuity of nursing and the time of sickness. *Nursing Philosophy*, **10**(2), 91–102.

Ettinger, R.L. (2006). Rational dental care: Part 1. *Has the concept changed in 20 years? Journal – Canadian Dental Association*, **72**(5), 441–5.

Ettinger, R.L. & Beck, J.D. (1984). Geriatric denal curriculum and the needs of the elderly. *Special Care in Dentistry*, **4**(5), 207–13.

Feine, J.S. & Carlsson, G.E. (eds.) (2003). *Implant Overdentures: The Standard of Care of Edentulous Patients.* Quintessence Publishing, Chicago, IL.

Hyo-Jung, L., Young-Kyun, K., Jin-Young, P., *et al.* (2010) Short-term clinical retrospective study of implants in geriatric patients older than 70 years. *Oral Surgery, Oral Medicine, Oral Pathology and Oral Radiology*, 2010, **110**, 442–6.

Kanno, T. & Carlsson, G.E. (2006) A review of the shortened dental arch concept focusing on the work by the Käyser/Nijmegen group. *Journal of Oral Rehabilitation*, **33**(11), 850–62.

Kiyak, H.A. & Reichmuth, M. (2005) Barriers to and enablers of older adults' use of dental services. *Journal of Dental Education*, **69**(9), 975–86.

Lunney, J., Lynn, J. & Hogan, C. (2002). Profiles of older Medicare decedents. *Journal of the American Geriatrics Society*, **50**, 1108–12.

Lunney, J., Lynn, J., Foley, D., *et al.* (2003) Patterns of functional decline at the end of life. *JAMA: The Journal of the American Medical Association*, **289**, 2387–92.

Olerud, E., Hagman-Gustafsson, M.L. & Gabre, P. (2012) Oral Status, oral hygiene, and patient satisfaction in the elderly with dental implants dependent on substantial needs of care for daily living. *Special Care in Dentistry* **32**(2), 49–54.

Stanford, C.M. (2005) Application of oral implants to the general dental practice. *Journal of the American Dental Association*, **136**(8), 1092–100.

Weber, H.-P. (2008) Implant dentistry as an approach to tooth replacement for older adults. In: *Improving Oral Health for the Elderly* (eds. I.B. Lamster & M.E. Northridge), pp. 303–25. Springer, New York.

Witter, D.J., van Palenstein Helderman, W.H., Creugers, N.H. & Käyser, A.F. (1999) The shortened dental arch concept and its implications for oral health care. *Community Dentistry and Oral Epidemiology*, **27**(4), 249–58.

CHAPTER 8

Informed Consent for the Geriatric Dental Patient

Jessica De Bord

Children's Village, Yakima, WA, USA; Department of Pediatric Dentistry, University of Washington, Seattle, WA, USA

Informed consent

Informed consent is a concept that recognizes that individuals have the right to make decisions about their health care. The idea of informed consent is rooted in autonomy. Autonomy is the notion that individuals have a right to self-determination (Eyal, 2011). In the context of health care, autonomy means that people have the right to adequate information in order to understand their condition and treatment choices, and the right to use that information to make healthcare decisions (Eyal, 2011). These rights create corresponding obligations on the part of the healthcare provider to provide such information to patients, and to respect their patients' healthcare choices. If healthcare providers do not uphold these obligations, they have violated patients' rights. Informed consent is a necessary factor in providing quality care (Brody, 1989).

Background

Informed consent is a relatively new concept. Historically, health care was more paternalistic, in that healthcare providers decided the best course of action or treatment, and their patients complied. However, under the auspices of healthcare research, many inappropriate and unethical medical studies were conducted. A prototypical example is the Tuskeegee Syphilis Experiment, in which African-American men with syphilis were neither treated nor even informed of their condition so that researchers could observe the progression of their disease (Coleman *et al.*, 2005). Another example of an ethical violation in research was a study conducted at the Jewish Chronic Disease Hospital in which elderly patients were injected with live cancer cells without their knowledge to study that disease (Coleman *et al.*, 2005). Ethical violations such as these, that dramatically infringed on the rights of people participating in healthcare research, illustrated the pressing need to have potential research participants understand what the research was, along with any potential risks and benefits. Armed with this information, individuals could then decide in an educated manner whether they wanted to participate in a given study. This concept then migrated from research to health care in general (Beauchamp, 2011). The application in general health care for patient permission to perform health services became known as "informed consent." It recognized that people are autonomous, have the right to receive information, to make decisions, and deserve to have their values, beliefs, and priorities honored when receiving health care.

Informed consent is important because patients have a right to make choices about themselves and their health care. For patients to make educated/informed choices, it is necessary that their provider gives them the adequate and appropriate information with which to do so. If a provider makes unilateral decisions about a patient's health care, does not provide the patient with adequate information to

Geriatric Dentistry: Caring for Our Aging Population, First Edition. Edited by Paula K. Friedman.

© 2014 John Wiley & Sons, Inc. Published 2014 by John Wiley & Sons, Inc.

Companion website: www.wiley.com/go/friedman/geriatricdentistry

make an informed decision, or proceeds with the *assumption* that the patient has consented, the provider has violated the patient's right to autonomy and to make his or her own healthcare decisions.

In clinical practice, it is not uncommon for practitioners to think of informed consent as simply a piece of paper to be signed prior to treatment; however, true informed consent is a process that involves an ongoing conversation between the provider and patient (Brody, 1989). It involves the provider giving the patient adequate information with which to make an informed decision. Ideally, the patient understands the condition requiring treatment, the benefits and the risks of the proposed or recommended treatment, as well as the alternative treatment choices and their risks and benefits. Of particular note is that part of a patient's understanding necessarily includes understanding the risks and benefits of declining treatment entirely. Additionally, providers should communicate to their patients, in clear and appropriate terminology, the provider's thought process that led to the recommended treatment (Brody, 1989). The patient ought to have the opportunity to ask questions and have to have them answered (Brody, 1989). For example, if a patient has an odontogenic infection, the provider should explain, in understandable terms, that the infection exists and what caused it. Then, if the recommended treatment is root canal therapy, this should be explained to the patient, including information about why preserving the tooth is the treatment of choice; what would be involved with the therapy, including facts such as the need for a crown following the treatment; and an explanation of the chances that the root canal therapy could fail. The provider would also be obligated to inform the patient that extraction, with or without placement of an implant, would be an alternative method of treatment, and explain both the risks of extraction and the implications of tooth loss. Again, declining treatment is an option, and the risks of that choice – in this case the risk of leaving an infection untreated – also need to be explained. With this understanding, the patient would be able to make a choice that is informed and would be able provide knowledgeable consent for treatment.

When the informed consent process has taken place, it is critical to adequately document the process in the dental record. Having the document that the patient signed providing consent is important, but is, in and of itself, inadequate documentation. The chart note should document the relevant facts of the provider's conversation with the patient, including the explanation of the condition, the recommended treatment, its risks and benefits, possible alternative treatments, their risks and benefits, and the risks of no treatment. The patient's decision should be documented; and should, ideally, include a comment on the patient's reasoning for this decision. For clarity of understanding and risk management purposes, the patient should sign the informed consent form.

Informed consent for geriatric patients

Many geriatric patients are competent to make their own healthcare decisions, and the informed consent process should be carried out in the typical fashion. The default assumption is that individuals are competent until proven otherwise (Kluge, 2005). It is not uncommon for healthcare providers to assume that patients are competent when they agree with the healthcare provider and incompetent when they disagree with the healthcare provider; however, this is not the case. A rational and autonomous person can disagree with a healthcare provider or refuse the proposed treatment; similarly, an incompetent person can agree with the healthcare provider and treatment plan. Agreement with the proposed treatment does not necessarily mean the patient is a competent decision-maker, and disagreement does not mean that they are incompetent.

In the USA, decisions for incapacitated patients account for half of the decisions about life-sustaining treatment for patients in nursing homes, and three-quarters of the decisions for patients with life-threatening illness who are hospitalized (Rid & Wendler, 2010). When geriatric adults are not competent to make healthcare decisions on their own, there are alternatives to the traditional informed consent process, including surrogate decision-makers and advanced directives (Jawarska, 2009). These concepts are important to the dental provider for two reasons. First, it is important to be aware of how to go about providing dental care and making treatment decisions for older adults who are not competent. Secondly, the dental provider should be aware of the patient's wishes and healthcare directives should there be a medical emergency, so that the dental team is able to provide treatment in a fashion compatible with the patient's wishes, and to provide emergency response personnel with appropriate and complete information.

When an older adult is not competent to make decisions, another individual must make healthcare decisions for him or her. That person is called a surrogate decision-maker (Jawarska, 2009). Surrogate decision-makers are either designated by the patient through a durable power of attorney, or, if none is designated, state statues name next-of-kin as surrogates should the patient become incapacitated with no named surrogate (Rid & Wendler, 2010). A surrogate decision-maker typically makes healthcare decisions based on one of two standards, either the substituted judgment standard or the best interest standard (Dunn et al., 2011; Jawarska, 2009). Using the substituted judgment standard, a decision-maker attempts to make a decision based on what he or she believes the individual would have decided for him or herself, if competent (Dunn et al., 2011; Jawarska, 2009). Using the best interest standard, the decision-maker makes healthcare choices based on what is in the best interest of the individual at the time (Dunn et al., 2011; Jawarska, 2009). Data show that the challenge to surrogate decision-makers is that surrogates do not make the decisions that the patients would make for themselves approximately one-third of the time (Scheunemann et al., 2012).

A person who was once competent, which is the case with many older adults, may have an advance directive. Advance directives may simply name the surrogate decision-maker, or they may delineate specific details regarding healthcare preferences (Jawarska, 2009). Advance directives may include Do Not Resuscitate (DNR) orders declining cardiopulmonary resuscitation (CPR), or other types of preferences, but traditional advance directives are frequently limited (Hickman et al., 2010). Even when patients have preferences regarding life-sustaining treatment, they may elect to have procedures done to mitigate pain and improve their quality of life, and these orders should not dissuade clinicians from providing palliative care. One of the challenges of advance directives is that they may not provide guidance for the specific medical situation that presents itself (Scheunemann et al., 2012). A type of advance directive, that attempts to mitigate the limitations of traditional advance directives, is the Physician Orders for Life-Sustaining Treatment (POLST) program (Hickman et al., 2010). In addition to wishes regarding CPR, this system details healthcare preferences, including preferences regarding specific interventions, antibiotic use, and artificial nutrition. It is a standardized program, designed to facilitate the coordination of care across settings (Hickman et al., 2010). However, it is still difficult for patients to truly predict what they would want in a hypothetical situation because they cannot predict the future specific medical situation and the associated emotional and social contexts (Sundore & Fried, 2010). Therefore, patients are encouraged to not only designate a surrogate, but to engage in conversations with clinicians and surrogates about their values regarding health, and to consider giving surrogates leeway to make decisions in light of the relevant information when a specific circumstance presents itself (Sundore & Fried, 2010).

Informed consent is an important process for healthcare providers and their patients, including older adults. When an older adult is not competent to make decisions for themselves, a surrogate decision-maker may be engaged to make healthcare decisions for them. This surrogate may be designated by the patient in a durable power of attorney, or by the state, predicated on that state's statutes. Additionally, the patient may have an advance directive to ensure that their healthcare wishes are known. Dental providers should be aware of who the surrogate decision-maker is for the patient and know of any advance directives, both for making decisions with regard to dental care and so that healthcare preferences can be honored when the patient is in the dental setting.

Case study 1

An older adult presents as a new patient. He displays symptoms of dementia. He is shabbily dressed, has poor hygiene, and you suspect poor nutrition. He was dropped off at the appointment by a friend and he reports that he has a relative that checks on him occasionally.

Case study 1 questions

1 How do you go about getting consent for treatment for this patient?
2 What other people or organizations might you want to engage for this patient?

Case study 2

You have an elderly patient who has dementia and is not able to make decisions. Prior to becoming incapacitated, she appointed her daughter as her healthcare proxy. She has multiple missing teeth, and multiple carious teeth. Due to her behavior she will not likely be able to tolerate partial or complete dentures. Her daughter would like all the teeth restored and implants placed under general anesthesia.

Case study 2 questions

1 What factors would you consider in making your treatment recommendations?
2 How would you go about the informed consent process with the patient's daughter?

Case study 3

Your patient is a veteran with cancer and has a POLST, which includes a DNR. He has elected to not receive treatment for his cancer due to a poor prognosis and the side effects of the treatment. He would like to spend his remaining months with his family and with a good quality of life. He has multiple unrestorable teeth that are causing him pain and interfering with his ability to eat. He would like them extracted to mitigate the pain and allow him to eat comfortably, and he would like to have the procedure done under general anesthesia, for which there is no medical contraindication. The anesthesiologist is hesitant to provide intravenous sedation since the patient has a DNR.

Case study 3 questions

1 What are the concerns with providing anesthesia to someone with a DNR?
2 Should the patient's desire to not have life-saving treatment for his cancer prevent him from having a procedure under general anesthesia to mitigate his pain and improve his quality of life? Are there alternatives treatment and/or pain control modalities that could be considered?

References

Beauchamp, T.L. (2011) Informed consent: its history, meaning, and present challenges. *Cambridge Quarterly of Healthcare Ethics*, **20**, 515–23.

Brody, H. (1989) Transparency: informed consent in primary care. *The Hastings Center Report*, **19**, 5–9.

Coleman, C.H., Menikoff, J.A., Goldner, J.A., *et al.* (2005) *The Ethics and Regulation of Research with Human Subjects.* Lexis Nexis, Newark, NJ.

Dunn, L.B., Hoop, J.G., Misra, S., *et al.* (2011) "A feeling that you're helping": proxy decision making for Alzheimer's research. *Narrative Inquiry in Bioethics*, **1**(2), 107–22.

Eyal, N. (2011) Informed consent. In: *The Stanford Encyclopedia of Philosophy*, Fall 2012 edn (ed. E.N. Zalta). From http://plato.stanford.edu/archives/fall2012/entries/informed-consent/. Accessed March 21, 2014.

Hickman, S.E., Nelson, C.A., Perrin, N.A., *et al.* (2010) A comparison of methods to communicate treatment preferences in nursing facilities: traditional practices versus the physician orders for life-sustaining treatment program. *Journal of the American Geriatrics Society*, **58**, 1241–8.

Jawarska, A. (2009) Advance directives and substitute decision-making. In: *The Stanford Encyclopedia of Philosophy*, Summer 2009 edn. (ed. E.N. Zalta). From http://plato.stanford.edu/archives/sum2009/entries/advance-directives/. Accessed March 21, 2014.

Kluge, E.W. (2005) Competence, capacity, and informed consent: beyond the cognitive-competence model. *Canadian Journal on Aging*, **24**, 295–304.

Rid, A. & Wendler, D. (2010) Can we improve treatment decision-making for incapacitated patients? *Hastings Center Report*, **40**, 36–45.

Scheunemann, L.P., Arnold, R.M. & White, D.B. (2012) The facilitated values history: helping surrogates make authentic decisions for incapacitated patients with advanced illness. *American Journal of Respiratory and Critical Care Medicine*, **186**, 480–6.

Sundore, R.L. & Fried, T.R. (2010) Redefining the "planning" in advance care planning: preparing for end-of-life decision making. *Annals of Internal Medicine*, **153**, 256–61.

CHAPTER 9

Evidence-Based Decision Making in a Geriatric Practice

Mary R. Truhlar

Department of General Dentistry, School of Dental Medicine, Stony Brook University, Stony Brook, NY, USA

Introduction

Evidence-based decision making is defined as:

> The conscientious, explicit and judicious use of current best evidence in making decisions about the care of individual patients
>
> (Sackett *et al.*, 1996).

Older adults, generally considered persons over the age of 65 years, comprise a distinct population that often provides diagnostic and therapeutic challenges to clinicians. Practitioners working with this cohort need the skills to search and critically evaluate the literature, problem solve, and make evidence-based decisions in the care of patients. The practice of evidence-based medicine integrates individual clinical expertise with the best available external clinical evidence from systematic research. Taken one step further it integrates the best research evidence with clinical expertise and patient values (Sackett *et al.*, 2000). In applying evidence-based decision making (EBDM) to the field of dentistry The American Dental Association (ADA) Center for Evidence-Based Dentistry defines it as the process of finding relevant information in the dental literature to address a specific problem, using some simple rules of science and common sense to quickly judge the validity of health information, and finally the application of the information to answer the original clinical question (ADA: http://ebd.ada.org/about.aspx).

Twenty-five years ago we got our news and information from a few universal sources; today both

> **KEYPOINT**
>
> A medically complex and pharmalogically challenging population, such as the older adult, greatly benefits from the combined use of practitioner expertise, research evidence, and patient values when making decisions in a clinical healthcare setting.

the dental professional and patient get an abundance of information from many sources. *The dental profession is no longer the only or the main source of dental healthcare information for our patients.*

Evidence-based decision making provides practitioners with an approach for the management of information and facilitates the translation of scientific evidence into clinical practice decisions, thus supporting the delivery of quality patient care. The term "information overload" is frequently applied to the experience of managing today's data influx; however, too much data may not be the real issue. Complaints about "too many books" emerged during the course of the 18th century in England, France, and Germany (Blair, 2010). The late 18th-century reader felt themselves to be overwhelmed by the number of books being printed. The anxiety felt in the later part of the 18th century was related to a rapid increase in new print titles, an increase of about 150% over 30 years. Today we are not so dissimilar, we find ourselves to be overwhelmed by meteoric rise in emails and digital communications. Wellmon (2012) believes that much of the way that we deal with the information around us have their antecedents throughout history, and the real issue lies not in the sheer volume of information but in a perceived inability to manage new information. Therefore, developing a technique to manage, distill, and analyze information would greatly enhance our ability to remain current and conversant in patient care.

The process

Evidence-based decision making in clinical practice begins with a clearly defined question related to patient care. The second step consists of efficiently accessing established sources of relevant topic information. This is followed by a critical appraisal of the evidence. Implementation of the findings is followed by continuous re-evaluation and assessment with the goal of maintaining a constant state of best practice.

Sites for online EBDM tutorials

- ADA Center for Evidence-Based Dentistry (http://ebd.ada.org/)
- CEBM – Centre for Evidence Based Medicine (http://www.cebm.net/)
- CEBD – Centre for Evidence Based Dentistry (http://www.cebd.org)

Sources of evidence

In "searching for the truth" an array of information can be obtained from diverse sources. Primary sources include clinical trials, cohort and case-controlled studies, and case reports. Secondary sources include systematic reviews, reviews of literature, meta-analysis, evidence-based journals, and evidence-based clinical guidelines (e.g., ADA). Web-based sources cover all the domains and offer point of care tools.

Scholarly articles/communications, whether in a hard copy or online format, present substantiated research and academic discussion among professionals and are an appropriate source for EBDM. There are popular and readily available communications that fall into a gray area. In these sources it is frequently difficult to distinguish research-based

material from unsubstantiated "expert" information given by a distinguished editorial panel. Popular communications such as dental magazines designed to inform and entertain may contain some research-based evidence but are not considered rigorous enough for EBDM. Trade communications that reach out to practitioners in specific industries to share market and production information are for business purposes and should be viewed in this manner.

KEYPOINT

In the practice of geriatric dentistry, where medical issues frequently interface with the provision of dental care, the systematic review (SR) can provide a good overview of the studies related to a given topic area (e.g., Is there a scientifically based reason to recommend prescribing antibiotic premedication for patients with joint replacements?)

A well-written systematic review provides the practitioner with a quick and encompassing look at the state of scientific research on a specific clinical question. An SR synthesizes the results from multiple studies addressing the same question by: statistically combining and distilling large quantities of data, evaluating the quality of each study and overall evidence in an objective manner, and concluding with an organized review of clinically useful information. In contrast, the case study and expert opinion provide less robust evidence, which frequently is limited to observational data reflecting the sentiment "We do this in my practice."

Sources for systematic reviews

- **Cochrane Library: Collaboration – Oral Health Group** (International) (http://www.ohg.cochrane.org)
- **TRIP database** (UK) (http://www.tripdatabase.com/)
- **DARE (Database of Abstracts and Reviews of Effects)** (UK) (http://www.crd.york.ac.uk/crdweb/)
- **NICE (National Institute of Clinical Excellence)** (UK) (http://www.nice.org.uk/)
- **AHRQ (Agency for Healthcare Research and Quality)** (USA) (http://www.ahrq.gov)
- **PubMed** (USA) (http://www.ncbi.nlm.nih.gov/)

Critical appraisal of the evidence

Reviewing the evidence requires a method to assess the statistical and clinical significance as well as the applicability of the material presented. A journal's "impact factor" (IF) is a good starting point for evaluation of the quality articles it contains. Not all journals are created equal or are perceived as being equal, and the impact factor can be used as a tool to rate a journal's importance within its field. It can serve as an indication of how reliable an article may be; however, it should not be used to assess the importance of individual articles, nor as a measure of an individual investigator's relevance. Impact factor is calculated yearly for journals and indexed in Thomson Reuters's Journal Citation Reports© (http://go.thomsonreuters.com/jcr/). This is the most universally used and understood journal rating system. Impact factor is a numerical measure of a scientific journal's average number of citations of recent articles. Citations can include but are not limited to articles, reviews, meeting proceedings, or notes. Editorials or letters-to-the-editor are not included. The larger the IF value, the more important the journal is considered.

KEYPOINT

Impact factor = the number of articles published in 2009 and 2010 that were cited by journals during 2011 / the total number of citable items published by the journal in 2009–2010. For example, if a journal has an IF of 10 for 2011, that means each article published in 2009 and 2010 received an average of 10 citations.

The validity of IF is impacted by several factors including the fact that most investigators cite their own articles; the current popularity of the field of study; and if a survey of experts feel it shows limited correlation to actual journal quality. However, it remains the gold standard for rating a journal's contribution to scientific literature. Table 9.1 lists the journals of interest to a geriatric practice.

In addition to knowing the source quality, a series of screening questions should be applied to the communication to further determine rigor and relevance of the material. Depending on the information type (e.g., SR, review of literature, meta-analysis, case report), the questions will vary.

The following questions would be most applicable for a SR

- Was the question clear and concise?
- Were the studies reviewed appropriate to the question?
- Was the quality of the studies addressed?
- Was it a comprehensive literature review?
- Was it an up-to-date review?
- Was there a reasonable presentation and interpretation of the studies results?
- Were all study outcomes considered and addressed?
- Can the studies reviewed be applied to your local cohort or location?
- Was a risk/benefit ratio addressed?

Implementation of an evidence-based geriatric dentistry practice

The goals of EBDM are to quickly sort through a vast amount of information, to know how and when to ask challenging questions of others, to keep up-to-date on current research findings, and to offer the best, scientifically supported care to your patients. However, having the desire to execute EBDM does not necessarily ensure that it fits into a busy geriatric practice. To assist in accomplishing these goals it is essential to develop and establish a practical approach to facilitate the incorporation and continued use of this practice style.

KEYPOINT

Consider a "divide and conquer" approach to make the process less cumbersome and more rewarding.

Identify information specialists in your practice, group, or study club and assign specific topics to interested persons and have them report findings and initiate discussions. Approach dental colleagues and sales representatives with systematic review-type

Table 9.1 Journals of interest to a geriatric practice sorted by impact factor*

Abbreviated journal title	ISSN	2010 total citations	Impact factor	5-Year impact factor	Immediacy index	2010 articles	Cited half-life	Eigenfactor® score	Article Influence® score
J Dent Res	0022-0345	13 593	**3.773**	4.389	0.437	229	>10.0	0.02257	1.296
J Am Dent Assoc	0002-8177	5458	**2.195**	2.282	0.281	121	>10.0	0.00876	0.667
J Oral Rehabil	0305-182X	3509	**1.462**	1.739	0.343	108	8.5	0.00614	0.520
Oral Surg Oral Med	1079-2104	10 429	**1.417**	–	0.167	408	>10.0	0.01659	
J Dent Educ	0022-0337	1978	**1.018**	–	0.277	130	7.0	0.00281	

* Courtesy of Thomson Reuters's 2010 Journal Citation Report©.

questions, challenge low-level evidence, and seek systematic reviews from independent, unbiased sources to support clinical practice decisions.

When presenting the evidence to the patient or caregiver recognize the need to be concise, while being informative. Be prepared with the resources to answer questions in the face of a rapidly growing information age, as well as being able to guide older adult patients and caregivers in the decision-making process.

KEYPOINT

Research has shown that when faced with two choices people make effective decisions; however, given three or more choices they are less effective in decision making and tend to defer to "What they have always done" (Redelmeier & Schafir, 1995).

EBDM in practice

EBDM case study 1

Case study 1: the situation

An older female patient presents with mitral valve prolapse and aortic stenosis. She is scheduled for a hip replacement surgery in 6 weeks. The patient asks: "My orthopedic surgeon has explained that I will need antibiotics prior to dental treatment following my surgery. I have previously been given antibiotics for my heart and then I was told I did not need to take them anymore. Why do I need antibiotics again?"

Case study question

1 Is there a scientifically based reason to recommend or not recommend the prescribing antibiotic premedication for the prevention of systemic bacteremia post-invasive dental procedures?

The following communications would serve as a good starting point for discussion with the patient.

Communications containing the current
guidelines/information statements
Cardiac
Reference no. 1 Wilson, W., Taubert, K.A., Gewitz, M., *et al.* (2007) AHA [American Heart Association] Guideline. Prevention of infective endocarditis. *Circulation*, 2007, **116**, 1736–54. From 10.1161/CIRCULATIONAHA.106.183095.

Orthopedics
Reference no. 2 American Association of Orthopedic Surgeons (2012) *Information Statement: Antibiotic Prophylaxis for Bacteremia in Patients with Joint Replacements, Feb 2009.* Update December 7, 2012. From http://www.aaos.org/research/guidelines/PUDP/dental_guideline.asp.

Systematic review of studies relevant to post-dental
procedure infective endocarditis
Reference no. 3 'Oliver, R., Roberts, G.J., Hooper, L. & Worthington, H.V. (2008) Antibiotics for the prophylaxis of bacterial endocarditis in dentistry. *Cochrane Database of Systematic Reviews*, Issue **4**. Art. no. CD003813. DOI: 10.1002/14651858.CD003813.pub3.

Objective To determine whether prophylactic antibiotic administration compared to no such administration or placebo before invasive dental procedures in people at increased risk of infective endocarditis (IE) influences mortality, serious illness, or IE incidence.

Search strategy, data collection, and analysis for this SR A search was run on MEDLINE (1950 to June 2008) and adapted for use on the Cochrane Oral Health, Heart and Infectious Diseases Groups' Trials Registers, as well as the following databases: CENTRAL (The Cochrane Library 2008, Issue 2); EMBASE (1980 to June 2008); and the *meta*Register of Controlled Trials (to June 2008).

Study inclusion criteria Due to the low incidence of IE, cohort, and case-control studies with suitably matched control or comparison groups were considered.

The intervention The administration of antibiotic compared to no administration before a dental procedure in people considered at increased risk of IE. Cohort studies should follow those at increased risk and assess for outcomes. Case-controlled studies should match people who had developed IE with those at similar risk but who had not developed IE.

Outcomes of interest Mortality or serious adverse event requiring hospital admission; development of IE following any dental procedure in a defined time period; development of IE without prior dental procedure; adverse events to the antibiotics; and cost factor associated with the provision of antibiotics.

Data collection and analysis Two authors independently reviewed selected studies for inclusion, assessed quality, and extracted data related to the outcomes of interest.

Results One case-controlled study met the inclusion criteria. The study collected all the IE cases in the Netherlands over a 2-year period, finding a total of 24 people who developed IE within 180 days of an invasive dental procedure and had required antibiotic prophylaxis according to current guidelines because of increased risk of endocarditis due to a pre-existing cardiac problem. Controls attended local cardiology outpatient clinics for similar cardiac problems, had undergone an invasive dental procedure with no sequela within the past 180 days, and were matched by age with the cases. There was no significant effect of antibiotic prophylaxis on the incidence of IE. No randomized cohort studies met the inclusion criteria.

Authors' conclusions This SR identified only one case-controlled study that met inclusion criteria. There remains no clear evidence that antibiotic prophylaxis is effective or ineffective against IE in people who are at risk and undergo an invasive dental procedure.

Clinical implications There is a lack of evidence to support published guidelines or discuss whether the potential harms and costs of antibiotic administration outweigh any beneficial effect. Practitioners need to discuss the dilemma of antibiotic prophylaxis with their patients before a decision is made about administration.

Position papers relevant to post-dental procedure joint infections

Reference no. 4 Little, J.W., Jacobson, J.J., Lockhart, P.B., for American Academy of Oral Medicine (2010) The dental teatment of patients with joint replacements: a position paper from the American Academy of Oral Medicine. *Journal of the American Dental Association.* **141**(6), 667–71. This position paper was written with the support of the leadership of the American Academy of Oral Medicine (AAOM) in response to the February 2009 American Academy of Orthopaedic Surgeons (AAOS) information statement in which the organization "Recommends that clinicians consider antibiotic prophylaxis (AP) for all total joint replacement patients prior to any invasive procedure that may cause bacteremia."

Methods The authors reviewed the literature on this subject as it relates to the AAOS's February 2009 information statement. The paper was reviewed and approved by the leadership of the AAOM and dental experts on this subject.

Results The risk of patients' experiencing drug reactions or drug resistant bacterial infections and the cost of antibiotic medications alone do not justify the practice of using antibiotic prophylaxis (AP) in patients with prosthetic joints.

Authors' conclusions The authors identified the major points of concern for a future multidisciplinary, systematic review of AP use in patients with prosthetic joints. In the meantime, they conclude that the new AAOS statement should not replace the 2003 Joint Consensus Statement. Until this issue is resolved, the authors suggest dentists consider the following three options: inform their patients with prosthetic joints about the risks associated with AP use and let them decide; continue to follow the 2003 guidelines (AP for the first 2 years post-surgery); or suggest to the orthopedic surgeon that they both follow the 2003 guidelines.

Cleghorn, B. (2010) Joint replacement prophylaxis: review of AAOM Position Paper. *JCDA: Canadian Dental Association.* Issue **4**.

Discussion Cleghorn supports the well-researched stance taken by Little *et al.* (2010) in the *JADA* position paper. "This recent *JADA* article [which is a position paper of the AAOM] recommends that a systematic review of antibiotic prophylaxis use in patients with total joint replacements be undertaken. Until this systematic review is performed, the authors recommend that the February 2009 AAOS information statement not replace the 2003 ADA/AAOS guidelines." He concurs with Little *et al.* (2010) that the February 2009 AAOS Information Statement has resulted in concern in the dental community with respect to the increase use of AP for patients with total joint replacements. He notes that the February 2009 AAOS Information Statement was developed without the involvement of organized dentistry or other nonorthopedic medical specialties and did not provide an evidence-based rationale for a return to the pre-2003 guidelines.

Reference no. 3 Jevsevar, D., Abt, E. (2013) AAOS-ADA clinical practice guideline 2012. Prevention of orthopaedic implant infection in patients undergoing dental procedures. *The Journal of the American Academy of Orthopaedic Surgeons.* **21**(3) 195–7.

Discussion Authors continue to find that there is an "identified need for further research in this area to provide clear evidence regarding the correlation between dental procedures and joint infections in patients with orthopaedic implants."

EBDM case study 2

Case study 2: the situation

An older female patient presents with complaint of burning of the tongue and foul taste increasing over the past several months. The patient asks, "What can I do to improve this situation?"

Case study question

1 Are there scientifically based recommendations for the management of patients with burning mouth syndrome?

The following communications would serve as a good starting point for discussion with the patient.

Systematic review relevant to the management of "burning mouth syndrome"
The systematic review that follows is the most recently available but is seven years out-of-date. This gap in the advancement of research is acknowledged by an expert in the field in the second 2010 review article.

Reference no. 1 Zakrzewska, J.M., Forssell, H. & Glenny, A.-M. (2005) Interventions for the treatment of burning mouth syndrome (review). *Cochrane Database of Systematic Reviews,* Issue 1. Art. No. CD002779. DOI: 10.1002/14651858. CD002779.pub2.

Authors' objective To determine the effectiveness and safety of any of the numerous interventions versus placebo for relief of symptoms and improvement in quality of life for patients with the complaint of burning mouth syndrome (BMS). This term is applied to a burning sensation in the mouth, most frequently the tongue, in patients where no underlying dental or medical causes are identified and no oral signs are found. Sufferers frequently show evidence of anxiety, depression, and personality disorders. Reported prevalence rates in general populations vary from 0.7 to 15% and at highest risk are peri- and post-menopausal women.

Search strategy, data collection and analysis for this review A search was run on the Cochrane Oral Health Group Trials Register (October 20, 2004), CENTRAL (The Cochrane Library 2004, Issue 4), MEDLINE (January 1966 to October 2004), and EMBASE (January 1980 to October 2004). *Clinical Evidence,* Issue no. 10, 2004 (BMJ Publishing Group Ltd), conference proceedings, and bibliographies of identified publications were searched to identify the relevant literature.

Study inclusion criteria Randomized controlled trials (RCTs) and controlled clinical trials (CCTs) that compared a placebo against one or more treatments in patients with BMS.

The intervention All treatments that were evaluated in placebo-controlled trials.

Outcomes of interest Relief of burning/discomfort.

Data collection and analysis Two authors independently reviewed selected studies for inclusion, assessed quality, and extracted data related to the outcomes of interest.

Results Nine studies met inclusion criteria. Diagnostic criteria for BMS were not always clearly reported. The interventions examined were antidepressants (2), cognitive behavioral therapy (1), analgesics (1), hormone replacement therapy (1), alpha-lipoic acid (3), and anticonvulsants (1). Of the nine studies, three interventions demonstrated a statistically significant reduction in BMS symptoms: all three alpha-lipoic studies, the one anticonvulsant clonazepam study, and the one cognitive behavioral therapy study. Only two of these studies reported using blind outcome assessment. None of the other treatments examined in the included studies demonstrated a significant reduction in BMS symptoms.

Authors' conclusions There is little research evidence that provides clear guidance for those treating patients with BMS. Studies, of high methodologic quality, need to be undertaken in order to establish effective forms of treatment. There is insufficient evidence to show the effect of painkillers, hormones, or antidepressants for BMS; however, there is some evidence that learning to cope with the disorder, anticonvulsants, and alpha-lipoic acid may offer some relief. More research is needed.

Position paper relevant to the management of BMS
Reference no. 2 Epstein, J. (2010) Burning mouth syndrome. Review of Zakizewska, J.M. *et al.* "Interventions for the treatment of burning mouth syndrome." *JCDA: Canadian Dental Association*, Issue 4.

Discussion Epstein updates the well-researched Zakrzewska *et al.* (2005) Cochrane Review entitled "Interventions for the treatment of burning mouth syndrome." He states that this review "Effectively summarizes the evidence base for BMS up until 2005." The review applied stringent inclusion criteria for studies on BMS, resulting in limited guidelines for clinical care. The review presented significant results from studies using the following interventions for the management of BMS: cognitive behavioral therapy, clonazepam therapy, and alpha-lipoic acid therapy. Five years later, of these three interventions, clonazepam continues to shown promise. Although alpha-lipoic acid did show potential benefit, more recent studies are not as supportive and the original study on cognitive behavioral therapy had poorly defined outcome measures. The state of our knowledge for the management of chronic BMS has not significantly advanced from 2005 and there remains a pressing need for more controlled studies with adequate sample sizes to validate the outcome measures.

Conclusion

As demonstrated in these case studies, the application of EBDM in clinical practice is particularly relevant to the medically complex geriatric population. The use of systematic reviews can assist the practitioner in implementing an evidence-based practice. Utilizing a focused clinical question in "PICO" format that identifies the **p**opulation: an **i**ntervention, a **c**omparison (if appropriate), and an **o**utcome; the SR presents an excellent research strategy that utilizes several databases, details selection criteria, assures independently performed reviews by more than one individual, discusses and summarizes results, and interprets the evidence with discussion, application, implications, and future research needs for clinical practice.

References

Blair, A. (2010) *Too Much to Know: Managing Scholarly Information before the Modern Age*. Yale University Press, New Haven, CT, p. 15.

Cleghorn, B. (2010) Joint replacement prophylaxis: review of AAOM Position Paper. *JCDA: Canadian Dental Association*, Issue 4.

Epstein, J. (2010) Burning mouth syndrome. Review of Zakizewska, J.M. *et al.* "Interventions for the treatment of burning mouth syndrome." *JCDA: Canadian Dental Association*, Issue 4.

Jevsevar, D., Abt, E. (2013) AAOS-ADA clinical practice guideline 2012. Prevention of orthopaedic implant infection in patients undergoing dental procedures. *The Journal of the American Academy of Orthopaedic Surgeons.* 21(3) 195–7.

Little, J.W., Jacobson, J.J., Lockhart, P.B., for American Academy of Oral Medicine (2010) The dental teatment of patients with joint replacements: a position paper from the American Academy of Oral Medicine. *Journal of the American Dental Association*, 141(6), 667–71.

Oliver, R., Roberts, G.J., Hooper, L. & Worthington, H.V. (2008) Antibiotics for the prophylaxis of bacterial endocarditis in dentistry. *Cochrane Database of Systematic Reviews*, Issue 4. Art. no. CD003813. DOI: 10.1002/14651858. CD003813.pub3.

Redelmeier, D.A. & Schafir, E. (1995) Medical decision making in situations that offer multiple alternatives. *Journal of the American Medical Association*, 273, 301–5.

Sackett, D.L., Rosenberg, W.M.C., Gray, J.A.M., *et al.* (1996) Evidence based medicine: what it is and what it isn't. *British Medical Journal*, 312, 71–2.

Sackett, D.L., Straus, S., Richardson, W., *et al.* (2000) *Evidence-Based Medicine: How to Practice and Teach EBM*. Churchill Livingstone, London.

Wellmon, C. (2012) Why Google isn't making us stupid … or smart. *The Hedgehog Review*, **14.1**, Spring 2012.

Wilson, W., Taubert, K.A., Gewitz, M., *et al.* (2007) AHA [American Heart Association] Guideline. Prevention of infective endocarditis. *Circulation*, 2007, **116**, 1736–54. From http://dx.doi.org/10.1161/CIRCULATIONAHA.106. 183095. Accessed March 24, 2014.

Zakrzewska, J.M., Forssell, H. & Glenny, A.-M. (2005) Interventions for the treatment of burning mouth syndrome (review). *Cochrane Database of Systematic Reviews*, Issue 1. Art. No. CD002779. DOI: 10.1002/14651858. CD002779.pub2.

PART 4

Common Geriatric Oral Conditions and their Clinical Implications

CHAPTER 10

Root Caries

Dick Gregory and Susan Hyde
School of Dentistry, University of California, San Francisco, CA, USA

Introduction

Dental caries (tooth decay) is a transmissible infection caused by specific bacteria (*Streptococcus mutans*, *Streptococcus sobrinus*, lactobacilli, and others) that colonize tooth surfaces, feed on carbohydrates, and produce acids as waste products. These acids dissolve the mineral content of the tooth, and if not halted or reversed, a carious lesion (cavity) is formed (Featherstone *et al.*, 2012).

The risk for dental caries persists throughout life. A dynamic balance exists between pathologic factors that promote caries and protective factors that inhibit it. Pathologic factors include acid-producing bacteria, frequent consumption of fermentable carbohydrates, poor oral hygiene, as well as subnormal salivary flow and composition. Protective factors include normal salivary function, fluoride, daily thorough oral hygiene, casein phosphopeptide-amorphous calcium phosphate paste (GC's Tooth Mousse®, MI Paste®, and Recaldent®), and extrinsic topical antibacterial substances (Featherstone *et al.*, 2012).

Carious lesions are termed either primary (new lesions on previously unrestored surfaces) (Fig. 10.1) or secondary (new caries around existing restorations) (Fig. 10.2). They occur on the crowns of teeth and exposed root surfaces. Periodontal disease (gum disease), results in loss of gingival (gum) attachment and exposure of the tooth's root surface. The root comprises the biologic structures cementum and dentin. Root surface cementum and dentin are more susceptible to cavitation because they are less mineralized than enamel ,the biologic material that comprises the crown of the tooth, and begin to demineralize at a higher salivary pH.

Older adults are retaining an increasing number of natural teeth, and nearly half of all individuals aged over 75 have experienced root caries. Root caries is a major cause of tooth loss in older adults, and tooth loss is the most significant negative impact on oral health-related quality of life for the elderly (Saunders & Meyerowitz, 2005). A false perception exists among dental professionals and policy-makers that dental caries is, for the most part, only active in younger people. Several of the clinical, social, and behavioral changes common to aging predispose older adults to the highest rates of decay are discussed below. The need for improved preventive efforts, and treatment strategies for this population is acute. Better clinical surveillance by public health agencies will drive decisions about oral health policy and education (Dye *et al.*, 2007; Griffin *et al.*, 2004).

Prevalence and risk factors

The prevalence of untreated root caries is 12% for adults aged 65–74 and 17% for those aged over 75 (Dye *et al.*, 2007). African Americans and Mexican Americans experience more oral health problems, including dental caries, throughout the life course. Lower educational attainment is also strongly associated with increased oral health problems at all ages and across all races.

Aging is often associated with changes in oral morphology, chronic systemic disease such as diabetes,

Geriatric Dentistry: Caring for Our Aging Population, First Edition. Edited by Paula K. Friedman.
© 2014 John Wiley & Sons, Inc. Published 2014 by John Wiley & Sons, Inc.
Companion website: www.wiley.com/go/friedman/geriatricdentistry

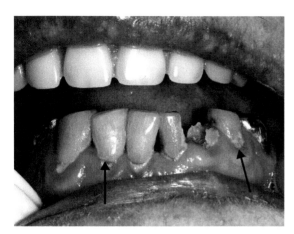

Figure 10.1 Primary root caries under heavy plaque accumulation: teeth nos. 22–27.

and decreasing dexterity, making personal oral hygiene more difficult, particularly for the oldest and most frail individuals. The pain of arthritis and neuropathies make it difficult to grasp or manipulate a manual toothbrush. Patients with dementia experience a higher prevalence of caries than those without dementia, and the rates are related to dementia type and severity. Individuals needing assistance with oral hygiene and whose caregivers have difficulties providing effective oral care experience the highest rates (Rethman *et al.*, 2011).

Another risk factor that often accompanies aging is patients taking multiple medications. More than 500 medications have the potential to decrease salivary flow, which leads to xerostomia (dry mouth) and subsequently dental caries. Other social and behavioral factors that contribute to the higher frequency of root caries in older adults include lack of a perceived need for dental treatment and a history of smoking and alcohol consumption (Featherstone, 2004; Featherstone *et al.*, 2007; ten Cate & Featherstone, 1991).

Good oral hygiene is also compromised by existing dental restorations and the presence of oral prostheses and appliances. Wearing a removable partial denture is associated with higher rates of dental caries. It is unclear whether this is due to the initial high caries rate that resulted in tooth loss or if the denture has a role in causing caries due to increased root surface exposure on the abutment teeth, food impaction, and plaque accumulation.

Caries risk assessment

Understanding factors and behaviors that directly or indirectly impact caries pathogenesis offers opportunities to reduce the caries burden of the aging population. Caries Management By Risk Assessment (CAMBRA) is a conservative and effective approach to prevention and treatment of the disease across the life course (Featherstone, 2004). Caries pathogenesis is recognized as a balance between protective factors (fluoride, calcium phosphate paste, sufficient saliva, and antibacterial agents) and pathologic factors (cariogenic bacteria, inadequate salivary function, poor oral hygiene, and dietary habits – especially frequent ingestion of fermentable carbohydrates) (Featherstone, 2004). Correctly assessing caries risk can identify a therapeutic treatment regimen for effectively managing the disease by reducing pathologic factors and enhancing protective factors, resulting in fewer carious lesions (Featherstone, 2004). With accurate risk assessment, noninvasive care modalities (chlorhexidine rinse and fluoride rinse or varnish) can be used proactively to prevent carious lesions and therapeutically to remineralize early carious lesions. Restorative procedures for more advanced lesions can be conservative, preserving tooth structure and benefiting patient oral health (Featherstone, 2004).

CAMBRA has proven to be a practical caries risk assessment methodology and a systematic and effective approach to caries management. Targeted antibacterial and fluoride therapy based on salivary microbial and fluoride levels has been shown to favorably alter the balance between pathologic and protective caries risk factors. Caries risk assessment with aggressive preventive measures and conservative restoration has been shown to result in a reduced two-year caries increment compared to traditional, nonrisk-based dental treatment. Altering the caries balance by reducing pathologic factors and enhancing protective factors, namely antimicrobial (for example, chlorhexidine) and fluoride rinses, reduced caries risk and resulted in fewer carious lesions. Readers are encouraged to further familiarize themselves with this research and CAMBRA methodology (Featherstone *et al.*, 2012).

For the older adult population the etiology and pathogenesis of dental caries are known to be multifactorial, but the interplay between intrinsic and extrinsic factors is still not fully understood. Caries

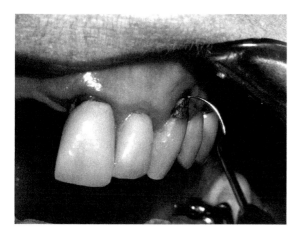

Figure 10.2 Tooth no. 11 shows secondary caries apical to a root carious lesion previously restored with amalgam.

research commonly tests an intervention for a single pathologic factor; however, it is observed that effective caries control requires a comprehensive and coordinated approach. The predictors of root caries most frequently reported in the literature are caries history, number of teeth, and plaque index (Topping *et al.*, 2009). In addition to the pathologic factors mentioned in the introduction to this chapter, patients with one or more existing carious lesions are at risk for additional new carious lesions in the future (Fig. 10.2). Simply restoring a single lesion does not reduce the bacterial loads in the rest of the mouth.

Dental plaque is a complex biofilm constantly forming and maturing. It consists of microorganisms and extracellular matrix including cariogenic acid-producing bacteria. In high caries-risk individuals the bacterial challenge must be lowered to favorably alter the caries balance. Patients with moderate to high levels of mutans streptococci and lactobacilli require targeted antibacterial treatment and fluoride to combat growth and remineralize tooth surfaces (Featherstone *et al.*, 2012). Recommended regimens are described in the next paragraph.

Evidence-based clinical recommendations generally favor fluoride-containing caries preventive agents; however, chlorhexidine-thymol varnish has also been shown to be effective in the treatment of root caries (Tan *et al.*, 2010). A 38% solution of silver diamine fluoride (SDF) applied annually (Saforide®, Bee Brand Medical, Japan), or 5% sodium fluoride varnish applied every 3 months (Air Force Medical

Service, 2007), or 1% chlorhexidine varnish applied every 3 months (Ivoclar Vivadent Corporate, 2014), have all been found more effective in preventing new root caries than giving oral hygiene instruction alone (Slot *et al.*, 2011). Recent recommendations for the prevention of primary root caries called for the professional application of 38% SDF solution annually and 22,500 ppm sodium fluoride varnish applications every 3 months to prevent secondary root caries (Rosenblatt *et al.*, 2009).

There is questionable evidence that xylitol and sorbitol gum can be used as an adjunct for caries prevention (Tan *et al.*, 2010). Cariogenic bacteria prefer six-carbon sugars or disaccharides and are not able to ferment xylitol, depriving them of an energy source and interfering with growth and reproduction. Systematic reviews of clinical trials have not provided conclusive evidence that xylitol is superior to other polyols such as sorbitol (Gluzman *et al.*, 2013) or equal to that of topical fluoride in its anti-caries effect (Mickenautsch & Vengopal, 2012).

Pathologic factors versus protective factors

Diet

A lifetime of caries and/or periodontal disease frequently results in tooth loss. In addition to the reduced masticatory function accompanying tooth loss, it is also common for older adults to experience a diminished ability to taste food. The resultant dietary shift from complex to simple sugars promotes caries. Cariogenic bacteria metabolize sucrose, glucose, fructose, and cooked starches to produce organic acids that dissolve the mineral content of enamel and dentin. The amount, consistency, and frequency of consumption determine the rate and degree of demineralization. Some medications and dietary supplements containing glucose, fructose, or sucrose also contribute to caries risk (Tan *et al.*, 2010).

Genetic susceptibility

There appears to be variation in individual susceptibility to caries. Intrinsic host factors related to the structure of enamel, immunologic response to cariogenic bacteria, and the composition of saliva play key roles in modulating the initiation and progression of the disease. Genetic variation of the host factors may contribute to an increased risk for dental caries; however, the evidence supporting an inherited susceptibility to caries is limited. Utilizing the human genome sequence to improve understanding of a genetic contribution to caries pathogenesis will provide a foundation for future research (Shuler, 2001).

Saliva

Saliva contains many important caries-protective components, such as calcium, phosphate, and fluoride, which are essential to tooth surface remineralization. Salivary proteins and lipids form a protective pellicle on the tooth surface, while other proteins bind calcium, maintaining saliva as a super-saturated mineral solution. Bicarbonate, phosphate, and peptides in saliva provide a critical pH-buffering function. With age, the amount of saliva remains stable; however, saliva becomes thicker due to a reduction in serous flow relative to the mucous component, resulting in decreased lubrication or perceived decreased moistness.

Fluoride

Other than the pre-eruptive mineralization of the developing dentition, systemic benefits of fluoride are minimal. The anti-caries effects of fluoride are primarily topical in adults. The topical effect is described as a constant supply of low levels of fluoride at the biofilm/saliva/dental interface being the most beneficial in preventing dental caries. Therapeutic levels of fluoride can be achieved from drinking fluoridated water and the use of fluoride products (toothpaste, rinse, gel, varnish). Fluoride can inhibit plaque bacterial growth, but more significantly, fluoride inhibits demineralization and enhances remineralization of the tooth surface (Featherstone et al., 2012).

The most widely used forms of fluoride delivery have been the subject of several systematic reviews, providing strong evidence supporting the use of dentifrices, gels, varnishes, and mouth rinses for the control of caries progression. Dentifrices with fluoride concentrations 1000 ppm and above have been shown to be clinically effective in caries prevention when compared to a placebo treatment. More evidence is needed to determine the benefits of the combined use of two modalities of fluoride application as compared to a single modality (Pessan et al., 2011). Considering the currently available evidence and risk benefit aspects, brushing twice daily with a fluoride containing dentifrice is one of the most effective ways to control caries. However, brushing alone does not overcome a high bacterial challenge, and additional fluoride therapy should be targeted towards individuals at high caries risk. Frequent topical application of fluoride appears to be a successful treatment for incipient root caries lesions by remineralizing decalcified structure, irrespective of the type of fluoride treatment used (Featherstone et al., 2012).

Chlorhexidine

The use of chlorhexidine for caries prevention has been a controversial topic among dental educators and clinicians. Chlorhexidine rinses, gels, and varnishes or combinations of these items with fluoride have variable effects in caries prevention, and the evidence is regarded as "suggestive but incomplete." The most persistent reductions of mutans streptococci have been achieved, in order of more effective to less effective, by chlorhexidine varnish followed by gels and, lastly, mouth rinses. While chlorhexidine has been widely used in Europe before gaining US Food and Drug Administration (FDA) approval, the only chlorhexidine-containing products currently marketed in the USA are 0.12% chlorhexidine mouth rinses. The preferred dosage regimen for rinsing is once a day with 5 cc of a 0.12% chlorhexidine gluconate solution for 1 week every month for a year (Featherstone et al., 2012). Patients should be informed of the likelihood of dark staining of their teeth during chlorhexidine use, and that the staining is easily removed during a dental prophylaxis. Bacterial testing should be used to monitor the clinical success of chlorhexidine therapy (Autio-Gold, 2008). Better antibacterial therapies for high caries-risk individuals are needed, and they must be combined with remineralization by fluoride (Featherstone et al., 2012).

Chlorhexidine is effective at reducing the bacterial challenge in high caries-risk individuals even when compliance is problematic. In the absence of regular professional teeth cleaning and oral hygiene instruction, chlorhexidine varnish may provide a beneficial effect for frail elders and patients with xerostomia (Autio-Gold, 2008). Cervitec®, a chlorhexidine-thymol varnish, may help to control established root lesions and reduce the incidence of new root caries among institutionalized elderly. It is the only nonfluoride caries agent to receive a favorable recommendation from a panel for caries prevention (Slot *et al.*, 2011).

Silver diamine fluoride

Recent interest in the antimicrobial use of silver compounds suggest that silver nitrate (SN) and silver diamine fluoride (SDF) are more effective at arresting active carious lesions and preventing new caries than fluoride varnish, and may be a valuable caries-preventive intervention. Possible mechanisms for SDF's clinical success include its antimicrobial activity against a cariogenic biofilm of *S. mutans* or *Actinomyces naeslundii* formed on dentin surfaces and slowing down the demineralization of dentin (Chu *et al.*, 2012). While SDF is available from international chemists online and has been shown to be as safe as fluoride varnish, effective for treating carious lesions, and is widely used in other countries, it does not currently have FDA approval.

Clinical decision making

Diagnosis of a carious lesion on a root surface raises ethical and practical questions. Can the lesion be remineralized with fluoride therapy or does it require a restoration? Is it an active or arrested carious lesion? Is the root caries causing or likely to cause any pain? How do the risks and benefits to the patient of not treating a carious lesion compare to those associated with restoring it? Does the patient have access to follow-up care?

If the lesion is to be restored, what technique and material will result in the best outcome for the patient? What is the patient's ability to maintain the restoration and what is the future caries risk? Systemic disease burden, xerogenic medications, diet quality, salivary function, manual dexterity, cognitive ability, the need for caregiver assistance, and access to care all contributes to caries risk.

The literature suggests that there is a fair agreement between visual/tactile appearance of caries and the severity/depth of the lesion. No single clinical predictor is able to reliably assess the activity of a carious lesion (Topping *et al.*, 2009). However, a combination of predictors increases the accuracy of lesion activity prediction for both primary coronal and root lesions. Three surrogate methods have been used for evaluating lesion activity (construct validity); all have disadvantages. If construct validity is accepted as a "gold standard," it is possible to assess the activity of primary coronal and root lesions reliably and accurately at one examination by using the combined information obtained from a range of indicators – such as visual appearance, location of the lesion, tactile sensation during probing, and gingival health (Topping *et al.*, 2009).

Treating root caries can be technically challenging. The location of the root caries may be difficult to access; it often may extend below the gingival margin, making it necessary to retract the gingiva with a clamp, pack retraction cord to expose the cervical margin of the lesion, or utilize laser or electrosurgery to recontour the gingiva and obtain access to the lesion. One important and relevant diagnostic consideration is, "What is the clinician's ability to successfully restore a particular carious lesion?" The location of the carious lesion on the tooth, the tooth's location in the mouth, and patient's ability to cooperate all contribute to the challenge of placing a successful restoration. How extensive and close to the pulp (nerves and blood vessels of the tooth) is the carious lesion? Other important questions to consider in the treatment of root caries include the following: How likely is a pulp exposure and the subsequent need for root canal therapy? Will the operator be able to achieve a dry field and have adequate visualization and access with a handpiece and/or instruments? Will conservative caries removal result in a better outcome for the patient than aggressive treatment?

Caries removal

Partial caries removal has been found to greatly reduce the risk of pulp exposure (Walls & Meurman, 2012). For asymptomatic teeth, partial caries removal generally results in no detriment to the patient from increased pulpal symptoms, decay progression under restorations, or premature loss of restorations (Walls & Meurman, 2012). When pulpal exposure is a concern in treating deep lesions, partial caries removal is the preferred approach (Walls & Meurman, 2012).

There is limited scientific evidence for laser treatment being as effective as a rotary bur for removing carious tissue. However, treatment time with lasers is prolonged

Box 10.1 Clinical tip

Steps in treating root caries with partial caries removal

In the absence of clinical symptoms of pulpal involvement, stepwise caries excavation to stained but firm dentin followed by the placement a thin liner of calcium hydroxide, or antimicrobials such as chlorhexidine-thymol varnish, or polycarboxylate cement combined with a tannin-fluoride preparation, are all effective in reducing bacteria and promoting remineralization of any carious dentin that remains after the stepwise excavation (Ricketts *et al.*, 2006).

compared to using a traditional handpiece, and to date no conclusions can be drawn regarding biologic or technical complications, or the cost-effectiveness of the method (Jacobsen *et al.*, 2011).

Restorative materials: amalgam, composite, glass ionomer

The longevity (failure rate, median survival time, median age) of silver amalgam fillings has been compared to direct composite (tooth-colored) fillings in permanent teeth. Amalgam fillings have been shown to have greater longevity than composite fillings; however, composites and their adhesives are frequently replaced by the next generation of materials with improved properties, making periodic revisions of these conclusions necessary (Antony *et al.*, 2008). Economic analyses report lower costs for amalgam fillings due to the higher complexity of and time needed to place composite fillings. Resin bonding to dentin or enamel requires adequate isolation and saliva contamination control. This is time consuming and often difficult to achieve in restoring root caries lesions at or near the gingival margin where most occur. Self-etching adhesives provide decreased clinical application time and reduce the risk of saliva contamination (Antony *et al.*, 2011).

A 2009 *Statement on Dental Amalgam* released by the American Dental Association Council on Scientific Affairs remains consistent with a more recent review of the international literature on amalgam toxicity (ADA, 2009). Various anecdotal complaints of systemic toxicity due to mercury

release from dental amalgam do not justify the discontinuation of amalgam use from dental practice or the replacement of serviceable amalgam fillings with alternative restorative dental materials (Uçar & Brantley, 2011). Available scientific data show that the mercury released from dental amalgam restorations does not contribute to systemic disease or systemic toxicologic effects. No significant effects on the immune system have been demonstrated with the amounts of mercury released from dental amalgam restorations, and only very rarely have there been reported allergic reactions to mercury from amalgam restorations (Uçar & Brantley, 2011). No evidence supports a relationship between mercury released from dental amalgam and neurologic diseases (Uçar & Brantley, 2011).

Glass ionomer, resin-modified glass ionomer, and composite resin have been compared in high caries-risk patients. Both glass ionomer and resin-modified glass ionomer restorations contain fluoride and release it into the saliva and adjacent tooth structure. While no significant difference in caries prevention between the two materials has been observed, reduction in new caries formation for glass ionomer and resin-modified glass ionomer restorations was more than 80% greater than for composite resin restorations in the treatment of cervical caries

Box 10.2 Clinical tip

Glass ionomer is particularly suitable for restoring root carious lesions. It has good esthetic and anti-cariogenic properties, allows for chemical bonding to teeth, and has gained wide acceptance in restoring carious lesions on the accessible buccal and lingual root surfaces. Minimally invasive techniques for restoring more difficult to access interproximal root surfaces with glass ionomer have been developed demonstrating a survival rate of 77.4% at 80 months. Caries removal, complete filling of the resulting cavity preparation, and marginal integrity as demonstrated by radiographic quality is the single most important predictor for restoration survival (Gilboa *et al.*, 2012; Ricketts *et al.*, 2006). When compared to amalgam, significantly less secondary caries has been observed at the margins of single-surface glass ionomer restorations in permanent teeth after 6 years (Mickenautsch *et al.*, 2010).

for head and neck radiation patients with xerostomia who did not adhere to a caries-preventive fluoride rinse protocol (McComb *et al.*, 2002; Uçar & Brantley, 2011).

Atraumatic restorative treatment

Atraumatic restorative treatment (ART) is an essential caries management technique for improving access to oral care. The approach, initiated 25 years ago in Tanzania, Africa, has evolved into a caries management concept for improving quality and access to oral care globally. Local anesthesia is seldom needed and only hand instruments are used to remove caries (Frencken *et al.*, 2012). ART uses a high-viscosity glass ionomer restoration to restore single-surface lesions in permanent posterior teeth, including root carious lesions. There appears to be no difference in the survival of single-surface high-viscosity glass-ionomer ART restorations and amalgam restorations in permanent posterior teeth including Class V root surface lesions (Frencken *et al.*, 2012).

Box 10.3 Future directions

Atraumatic restorative treatment (ART) is expected to play a significant part in essential caries management for the frail elderly, especially as additional scopes of practice are more widely included in an expanded clinical care team. One of the indications for the appropriate use of the ART approach is for the elderly who are homebound or living in institutions. More studies are needed to investigate the potential of ART in providing essential caries management in this population. However, field trials report two-year survival rates of 90% with no significant difference between ART restorations using high-viscosity glass ionomer and those produced through the traditional approach of complete caries removal using rotary instruments, and resulting in a higher risk of pulp exposure (Honkala & Honkala, 2002). Anecdotal clinical reports of dentists and expanded function hygienists and assistants providing onsite care for nonambulatory older adults provide support from the field for this clinical approach. More research is needed in a clinical randomized-controlled trial environment to provide systematic evidence for this approach.

Case study

The Director of Nursing in a local residential care facility requests a consultation with a dentist for Mrs. Switzer, who is 86 years old and has a fractured maxillary left lateral incisor. Mrs. Switzer was admitted to the facility 3 weeks previously with moderate Alzheimer's disease, depression, and severe hypertension. Mrs. Switzer attended her dentist 1 month before entering the facility but did not follow the dentist's recommendations for periodontal debridement, intracoronal restorations, and a fixed partial denture. Previous to this appointment, Mrs. Switzer had not seen a dentist for 2 years, although she claims to have visited her dentist frequently over the years before then. Consequently, she is referred to the care facility's dentist for further assessment and treatment of the fractured tooth.

The dentist examines Mrs. Switzer to confirm that the maxillary left canine has an asymptomatic, but complete, coronal fracture due to root caries (Fig. 10.3). He notes also that there is copious plaque and food debris throughout the teeth and mouth. On questioning, Mrs. Switzer reveals that she drinks tea sweetened with sugar constantly "for energy" and to be sociable in the facility, and she takes multiple medications for blood pressure, depression, and occasional memory loss. The dentist requests the radiographs taken before she entered the facility to determine the extent of the carious lesions (Fig. 10.4). A diagnosis is made of extensive root caries involving all previously restored teeth.

A treatment plan of extraction of the fractured maxillary left lateral incisor and replacement using an acrylic removable partial denture is made. The carious lesions are scheduled for restoration using resin-modified glass ionomer material. The patient's daughter is warned that excavation of the root caries might result in tooth fracture. If this occurs, then the fractured teeth would require extraction, denture teeth could be added to the acrylic removable partial denture in the maxilla, and/or an additional prosthesis would be needed for the mandible. Personalized diet and daily mouth care counseling is discussed with the patient, daughter, and nursing staff. Daily use of 0.2% neutral sodium fluoride is prescribed for prevention of root caries.

Courtesy of MacEntee *et al.* (2011).

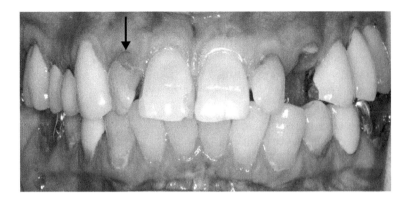

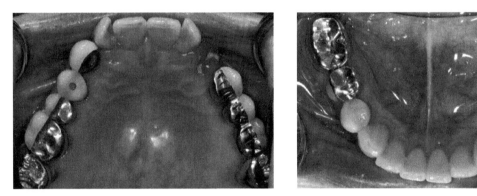

Figure 10.3 Root caries are clinically detectable on most remaining teeth. The clinical crown of tooth no. 11 is completely missing due to caries. Arrow shows an example of root caries.

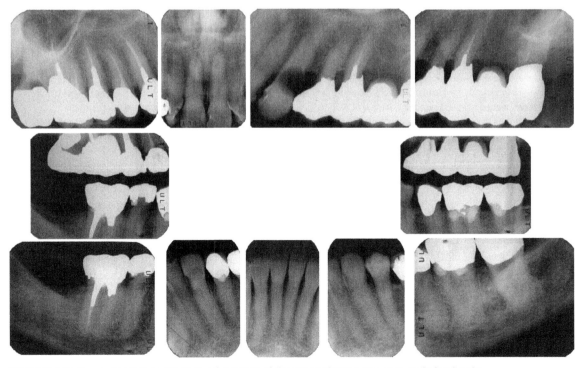

Figure 10.4 Radiographs taken to determine the extent of the carious lesions (see case study for details).

DISCUSSION QUESTIONS

1 Describe how a caries risk assessment and management methodology, such as CAMBRA, might be integrated into a clinical dental practice and what patient benefits could be expected.
2 Describe the clinical benefits of normal salivary function, and explain how reduced salivary flow impacts caries risk.
3 Explain how the older adult population keeping more of their teeth might affect your clinical practice, and what preventive and restorative options you might use.

References

ADA (American Dental Association) (2009) *Statement on Dental Amalgam*. ADA Council on Scientific Affairs. From http://www.ada.org/1741.aspx. Accessed April 18, 2014.

Air Force Medical Service (2007) *Synopsis of Fluoride Varnishes (Project 06-16) (2/07)* From http://www.afms.af.mil/shared/media/document/AFD-130327-445.pdf. Accessed March 23, 2014.

Antony, K., Genser, D., Hiebinger, C. & Windisch, F. (2008) Longevity of dental amalgam in comparison to composite materials. *GMS Health Technology Assessment*, **4**, Doc12.

Autio-Gold, J. (2008) The role of chlorhexidine in caries prevention. *Operative Dentistry*, **33**(6), 710–16.

Chu, C.H., Mei, L., Seneviratne, C.J. & Lo, E.C. (2012) Effects of silver diamine fluoride on dentine carious lesions induced by *Streptococcus mutans* and *Actinomyces naeslundii* biofilms. *International Journal of Paediatric Dentistry*, **22**(1), 2–10.

Dye, B.A., National Center for Health Statistics & National Health and Nutrition Examination Survey (2007) *Trends in Oral Health Status: United States, 1988–1994 and 1999–2004. Vital Health and Statistics*, **11**(248), 1–92.

Featherstone, J.D. (2004) The caries balance: the basis for caries management by risk assessment. *Oral Health & Preventive Dentistry*, **2**(Suppl 1), 259–64.

Featherstone, J.D., Domejean-Orliaquet, S., Jenson, L., *et al.* (2007) Caries risk assessment in practice for age 6 through adult. *Journal of the California Dental Association*, **35**(10), 703–7, 710–13.

Featherstone, J.D., White, J.M., Hoover C.I., *et al.* (2012) A randomized clinical trial of anticaries therapies targeted according to risk assessment (caries management by risk assessment). *Caries Research*, **46**, 118–29.

Frencken, J.E., Leal, S.C. & Navarro, M.F. (2012) Twenty-five-year atraumatic restorative treatment (ART) approach: a comprehensive overview. *Clinical Oral Investigations*, **16**(5), 1337–46.

Gilboa, I., Cardash, H.S. & Baharav, H. (2012) A longitudinal study of the survival of interproximal root caries lesions restored with glass ionomer cement via a minimally invasive approach. *General Dentistry*, **60**(4), e224–30.

Gluzman, R., Katz, R.V., Frey, B.J. & McGowan, R. (2013) Prevention of root caries: a literature review of primary and secondary preventive agents. *Special Care in Dentistry*, **33**(3), 133–40.

Griffin, S.O., Griffin, P.M., Swann, J.L. & Ziobin, N. (2004) Estimating rates of new root caries in older adults. *Journal of Dental Research*, **83**(8), 634–8.

Honkala, S. & Honkala, E. (2002) Atraumatic dental treatment among Finnish elderly persons. *Journal of Oral Rehabilitation*, **29**, 435–440.

Ivoclar Vivadent Corporate (2014) *Cervitec Plus*. From http://www.ivoclarvivadent.com/en/competences/all-ceramics/prevention-care/cervitec-plus. Accessed March 23, 2014.

Jacobsen, T., Norlund, A., Englund, G.S. & Tranaeus, S. (2011) Application of laser technology for removal of caries: a systematic review of controlled clinical trials. *Acta Odontologica Scandinavica*, **69**(2), 65–74.

MacEntee, M.I., Muller, F. & Wyatt, C. (eds.) (2011) *Oral Healthcare and the Frail Elder: a Clinical Perspective*. Blackwell Publishing, Oxford.

McComb, D., Erickson, R.L., Maxymiw, W.G. & Wood, R.E. (2002) A clinical comparison of glass ionomer, resin-modified glass ionomer and resin composite restorations in the treatment of cervical caries in xerostomic head and neck radiation patients. *Operative Dentistry*, **27**(5), 430–7.

Mickenautsch, S. & Yengopal, V. (2012). Effect of xylitol versus sorbitol: a quantitative systematic review of clinical trials. *International Dental Journal*, **62**(4), 175–88.

Mickenautsch, S., Tyas, M.J., Yengopal, V., Oliveira, L.B., *et al.* (2010) Absence of carious lesions at margins of glass-ionomer cement (GIC) and resin-modified GIC restorations: a systematic review. *The European Journal of Prosthodontics and Restorative Dentistry*, **18**(3), 139–45.

Pessan, J.P., Toumba, K.J. & Buzalaf, M.A. (2011) Topical use of fluorides for caries control. *Monographs in Oral Science*, **22**, 115–32.

Rethman, M.P., Beltrán-Aquilar, E.D., Billings, R.J., *et al.* (2011) Non-fluoride caries-preventive agents: executive summary of evidence-based clinical recommendations. Dental Association Council on Scientific Affairs Expert Panel on Non-fluoride Caries-Preventive Agents. *Journal of the American Dental Association*, **142**, 1065–71.

Ricketts, D.N., Kidd, E.A., Innes, N. & Clarkson, J. (2006) Complete or ultraconservative removal of decayed tissue in unfilled teeth. *The Cochrane Database of Systematic Reviews*, **3**, CD003808.

Rosenblatt, A., Stamford, T.C. & Niederman, R. (2009) Silver diamine fluoride: a caries "silver-fluoride bullet." *Journal of Dental Research*, **88**(2), 116–25.

Saunders, R.H. Jr. & Meyerowitz, C. (2005) Dental caries in older adults. *Dental Clinics of North America,* **49**(2), 293–308.

Shuler, C.F. (2001) Inherited risks for susceptibility to dental caries. *Journal of Dental Education,* **65**(10), 1038–45.

Slot, D.E., Vaandrager, N.C., Van Loveren, C., *et al.* (2011) The effect of chlorhexidine varnish on root caries: a systematic review. *Caries Research,* **45**(2), 162–73.

Tan, H.P., Lo, E.C., Dyson, J.E., *et al.* (2010) A randomized trial on root caries prevention in elders. *Journal of Dental Research,* **89**(10), 1086–90.

ten Cate, J.M. & Featherstone, J.D. (1991) Mechanistic aspects of the interactions between fluoride and dental enamel. *Critical Reviews in Oral Biology and Medicine,* **2**, 283–96.

Topping, G.V., Pitts, N.B. & International Caries Detection and Assessment System Committee (2009) Clinical visual caries detection. *Monographs in Oral Science,* **21**, 15–41.

Uçar, Y. & Brantley, W.A. (2011) Biocompatibility of dental amalgams. *International Journal of Dentistry,* 981595.

Walls, A.W. & Meurman, J.H. (2012) Approaches to caries prevention and therapy in the elderly. *Advances in Dental Research,* **24**(2), 36–40.

CHAPTER 11

Periodontal Disease

Saroj Gupta

Department of Periodontics, University of Maryland, Baltimore, MD, USA

Introduction

This chapter will review periodontal disease, one of the two most prevalent diseases of the oral cavity, the other being caries. We will address many of the facts and myths associated with periodontal disease.

Older people are increasingly retaining their natural teeth, but are at higher risk of oral disease accompanying increased longevity, with potential impact on quality of life. Maintenance of oral health may not have been a priority among elders for many reasons, including lack of coverage from Medicare (Medicare does not cover dental services for any elders) and Medicaid (coverage for adults varies from state to state, is limited to low-income individuals, and often provides no or minimal dental services for adults), or coverage from other third-party sources. Even private dental insurance often does not extend into retirement As a result of limited or nonexisting access to dental services, adults often resort to a hospital emergency room for their dental care, or neglect it entirely.

Throughout the life span, teeth remain at risk for the two most prevalent oral diseases – dental caries and periodontal disease. (See Chapter 10 for a discussion of root caries.) Older adults are at risk for new and recurrent decay that is untreated in approximately 30% of dentate adults. They are at increased risk for root caries because of both increased gingival (i.e., gum) recession that exposes root surfaces and increased use of medications that produce xerostomia (i.e., dry mouth). Approximately 50% of persons aged over 75 years have root caries affecting at least one tooth. Approximately 25% of older adults have loss of tooth-supporting structures because of advanced periodontal disease. Without early prevention and control interventions, these progressive conditions can necessitate extensive treatment to treat and prevent infection and restore function (CDC, 2003).

Self-ratings of health have been associated with functional ability. These associations suggest that older persons who report poorer general health are at increased risk for limited dexterity, mobility, and tolerance of stress; such factors can compromise abilities to maintain oral hygiene, visit a dental office, or tolerate treatment. These persons likely will need caregiver assistance and innovative strategies to maintain daily self-care, obtain regular oral assessments, and receive primary and secondary prevention services (CDC, 2003). Older persons usually require coordinated health care offered by different healthcare professionals due to high prevalence of complex chronic disease and psychologic disorders during aging, including depression, frailty, diabetes, cardiovascular and neurodegenerative disease (Fig. 11.1)

Compared with younger persons, the current cohort of older adults likely experienced higher rates of dental caries and tooth extraction as young adults and is more likely to have lost all their teeth. Patients with a history of smoking comprise approximately half of all cases of periodontal disease in the USA. The higher prevalence of tooth loss among smokers may be closely associated with the well-recognized adverse effects of cigarette smoking (Van Dyke & Sheilesh, 2005).

Geriatric Dentistry: Caring for Our Aging Population, First Edition. Edited by Paula K. Friedman.

© 2014 John Wiley & Sons, Inc. Published 2014 by John Wiley & Sons, Inc.

Companion website: www.wiley.com/go/friedman/geriatricdentistry

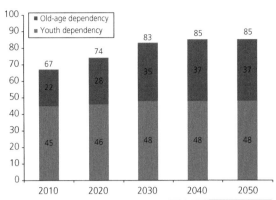

Total dependency = ((Population under age 20 plus population aged 65 and over) / (Population aged 20–64)) × 100.
Old age dependency = (Population aged 65 and over / Population aged 20–64) × 100.
Youth dependency = (Population under age 20 / Population aged 20–64) × 100.

Figure 11.1 Dependency ratios for the USA, 2010–2050. From US Census Bureau (Vincent & Velkoff, 2010).

Box 11.1 Age-related risk factors of periodontal disease

- Diminished general health, including functional impairments
- Diminished immune system
- Medication side effects
- Depression
- Memory decline
- Reduced salivary flow
- Change in financial status

Epidemiology of periodontal disease

Periodontal disease has a higher prevalence in older adults than any other age group. However, periodontal disease is not a direct result of aging. The old beliefs concerning periodontal disease were: (i) everyone was equally susceptible to periodontal disease; (ii) gingivitis progresses to periodontitis with resulting bone and tooth loss; and (iii) susceptibility to periodontitis increased with age (Burt, 2005). Epidemiologic studies of periodontitis have disproved all of these beliefs. Studies have shown that the majority of adult populations are affected by moderate periodontitis, but that only a small proportion, 5–15%, of any population suffers from severe generalized periodontitis, with these numbers holding true among both well-treated and

Box 11.2 Myths about periodontal disease

- Everyone is equally at-risk for periodontal disease
- Gingivitis progresses to periodontitits with resulting bone and tooth loss
- Susceptibility to periodontitis increases with age

underserved populations. The individuals most susceptible to periodontitis had signs dating back to teenage and adolescent years (Burt, 2005). The belief that gingivitis progresses to periodontitis has been disproved since the 1980s; a notable 3-year longitudinal study of patients with gingivitis showed that most of the patients were resistant to further clinical attachment loss (CAL) and development of periodontitis (Burt, 2005; Listgarten *et al.*, 1985).

The role of periodontal disease in oral health/overall health

Periodontal disease is an inflammatory disease caused by gram-negative anaerobic bacteria from dental plaque displaying virulent properties and increasing pro-inflammatory cytokines. Periodontal disease progresses to periodontitis when the inflammation extends to the periodontal ligament and alveolar bone which lead to loss or recession of gingival tissue, decrease in alveolar bone mass, tooth mobility/tooth loss, and potentially edentulism (Chung *et al.*, 2011).

These pro-inflammatory cytokines, notably tumor necrosis factor (TNF), interleukin-1 beta (IL-1β), and interleukin-6 (IL-6), associated with periodontal disease are noteworthy because they also have associations with many other chronic inflammatory diseases such as *rheumatoid arthritis, osteoporosis, myeloma, type II diabetes and atherosclerosis*; all of these diseases and conditions have been traced back to the same or similar etiologic onset of the inflammation (Chung *et al.*, 2011). Further, *Actinobacillus actinomycetemcomitans, Porphyromonas gingivalis* and other bacteria originating from plaque in the oral cavity can travel to other areas of the body and have been linked to infections of the endocardium, meninges, mediastinum, vertebrae, hepatobiliary system, lungs, urinary tract, and prosthetic joints (Dumitrescu, 2010). Plaque bacteria have been associated with systemic implications in the cardiovascular and nervous systems. For the dental examiner it is important to know and understand this information in order to comprehensively treat the patient. Many of the chronic inflammatory diseases have established associations with oral inflammation and thus these associations have placed the dental examiner in an important position to identify possible systemic diseases from a routine oral exam. If other systemic diseases are suspected the dental clinician can then work with the medical profession to discuss the findings and determine the best treatment plan for the patient.

Senescence of tissue

An etiologic component attributed to the higher prevalence of periodontal disease in older adults is a result of biologic aging or senescence of the periodontium. All tissues undergo certain changes as a result of aging: reduction in vascularity, elasticity, and reparative capacity are some of the common manifestations of aging, generally noticed in tissue. Periodontal tissues are no exception to this rule and may show signs of atrophy as age advances.

Gingival fibroblasts (GF) are the main cellular component responsible for synthesizing periodontium. The influences of oral bacteria on the GF are an important factor in periodontal disease and will be discussed in more detail later in the chapter. But studies have shown that aging GFs have an increased rate of intracellular phagocytosis, throwing off the homeostasis balance between degradation and synthesis, and leading up to a fivefold decrease in collagen production. In addition, aging GFs have increased DNA methylation, which reduces mRNA levels and further decreases collagen synthesis (Huttner *et al.*, 2009). The decreased collagen synthesis leads to dekeratinization and overall weakening of the gingiva. The oral epithelium thins and forms irregularly, which decreases the physical barrier ability of the epithelium to keep out pathogenic bacteria (Huttner *et al.*, 2009). The periodontal ligament, anchoring tooth to alveolar bone and serving as cushion during chewing, is composed of many types of cells that differentiate to affect the entire periodontium. Aging periodontal ligaments show decreased number of cellular components and, like

the gingival epithelium, its structure becomes irregular. Periodontal ligament cells differentiate into osteoblasts and osteoclasts involved in alveolar bone homeostasis. With age there is reduced osteoblast chemotaxis and osteoclast differentiation to osteoblast resulting in decreased alveolar bone density, an indicator of periodontal disease in itself (Huttner *et al.*, 2009). Of note in aging periodontal ligaments is the large amount of cytokines produced in response to mechanical stress, such as prostaglandin E2 (PGE2), IL-1β, and plasminogen activator. As periodontal disease is an inflammatory disease in response to cytokines caused by plaque biofilm bacteria, this is a significant observation.

Healthy gingiva of younger adults has been associated with simple, supragingival plaque biofilm (1–20 cell layers), and mainly consists of gram-positive, aerobic, and facultative aerobic bacteria with very few gram-negative bacteria. In comparison, older adults with no history of gingivitis displaying overall healthy oral conditions show an increased number of gram-negative bacteria directly related to inflammatory responses (Dumitrescu, 2010). Several of these gram-negative bacteria are associated with gingivitis and periodontitis including *P. gingivalis* and *Fusobacterium nucleatum*. The presence of these anaerobes in older adults is believed to be a result of aging and the body's natural decline in immune responses leading to a greater susceptibility to periodontal disease.

Identifying periodontal disease

Periodontal disease is an inflammatory disease with clear visual signs. When triaging the patient, the examiner needs to be able to identify visual differences between healthy versus diseased tissue. The color of normal, healthy soft tissues of the oral cavity, including the gingiva, tongue, and palate, should be coral-pink and, depending on the complexion of the individual, may contain areas of melanin pigmentation. The texture of the gingiva should be smooth or have a stippling consistency like the rind of an orange. A thorough clinical exam also includes checking for ulcers, lesions, cancers, or tumors of the oral cavity as well as the contours of the underlying bone. It is important to remember that older individuals with prior bone loss that have undergone periodontal therapy may have a significant amount of recession but maintain healthy gingiva, i.e, probing depths (PDs) of 1–3 mm, with no bleeding on probing (BOP).

Unhealthy gingiva displaying gingivitis is red, inflamed, and swollen, sensitive to touch, and bleeds on touching or probing (Figs 11.2 & 11.3). Patients presenting with periodontal disease may complain of pain, bleeding gums, spaces developing between teeth, bad breath, or areas of recession (Fig. 11.4). If gingivitis has been previously diagnosed it will be important to measure any further CAL or increases in PD. A pocket of 4 mm or greater is a sign of periodontal disease. Most gingivitis has been reported not to progress to periodontitis, but does need to be monitored and treated to control and reverse the effects. In recording PD and CAL it is also important to evaluate and record tooth mobility along with areas of gingival recession and root exposures (Fig. 11.1).

A review of the patient's medical and dental history can determine systemic diseases and medications that may contribute to periodontitis (Box 11.3 & Table 11.1). From a medical/dental history, it is important to identify the duration, progression and history of any previous gingivitis and/or periodontal disease, as older adult periodontitis is more a result of "lifetime of disease accumulation rather than an age specific condition" (Burt, 2005). If radiographs are available they are also useful for identifying further alveolar bone loss (Burt, 2005). It is especially important to look for patient and family histories of tobacco use and diabetes mellitus, as their link to periodontal disease is well established. For smokers, the odds of developing periodontal disease is related to smoking dosage and the extent of glycemic control in diabetes patients, with no difference between type 1 and type 2 diabetes mellitus (Van Dyke & Sheilesh, 2005). In addition, dementia/Alzheimer's disease, arthritis, Parkinson's disease, and coronary artery disease have all been linked to periodontal disease and should be noted in the health history (Buhlin *et al.*, 2011; Müller *et al.*, 2011). Medications that cause gingival hyperplasia (e.g., calcium-channel blockers, used to treat hypertension; and Dilantin®, used to treat epilepsy), also pose a potential problem for maintaining oral health. Gingival overgrowth can make

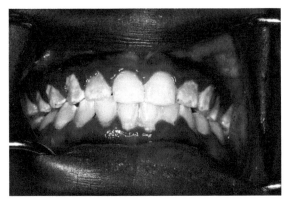

Figure 11.2 Patient with inflamed gingiva and plaque and tartar (calculus) build-up.

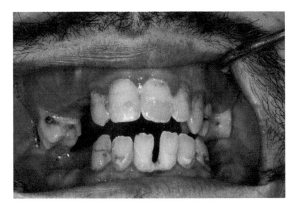

Figure 11.3 Patient displaying inflamed gingiva with plaque and tartar (calculus) build-up

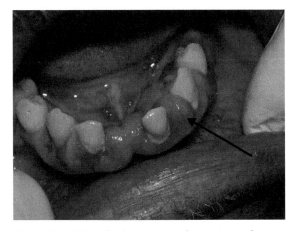

Figure 11.4 Patient displaying gingival recession and root exposure.

Table 11.1 Medications and symptoms as risk factors for periodontal disease

Medications	Symptoms
Antianxiety medications, Antihypertensives, Antidepressants, Anticholinergics, Calcium-channel blockers	Xerostomia, Oral mucositis, Gingival hyperplasia,
Cyclosporine, Dilantin®, Bisphosphonates, Cancer therapies	Osteonecrosis of jaw bone

Box 11.3 Health issues associated with periodontal disease and older adults

- Systemic diseases
- Arthritis/poor dexterity
- Cancer therapy
- Medications
- Genetics
- Tobacco use
- Poor nutrition
- Stress/depression
- Removable partial dentures
- Microorganisms

plaque removal difficult, which may lead to gingival inflammation. Severe cases of hyperplasia may completely cover the tooth surfaces and require repeated gingivectomy procedures.

Currently, CAL and PD are considered an adequate assessment of periodontal disease and combined with medical history, visual examination, and radiographs can further help to diagnose the presence of disease. If gingivitis and/or periodontal disease is diagnosed, it is important that follow-up evaluations be performed to determine whether the patient's condition is progressive (Armitage, 2003).

Cancer, cancer therapy, and periodontal disease

According to the American Society of Clinical Oncology, aging is the single greatest risk factor for developing cancer, as more than 60% of cancers in the USA occur in the over 65 age group. It is important to recognize that certain types of cancers, including the leukemia and other hematopoietic stem cell malignancies, can present with oral manifestations. Due to the reduction of normal white and red blood cells, the clinician may see petechial hemorrhages of the posterior hard palate and soft palate. Patients may also complain of spontaneous gingival bleeding, ulceration of mucosa, and serosanguinous discharge from the gingival sulcus. These symptoms may initially be mistaken as signs of periodontal disease and no associated with the underlying systemic etiology, especially if the cancer has not been diagnosed or the patient has not shared the diagnosis. These symptoms may also occur due to a significant reduction in white cells during chemotherapy.

Cognitive functioning

Alzheimer's disease, dementia, lower educational attainment, mild memory impairment, memory loss, and overall declining cognitive function have all been associated with periodontal disease and edentulism (Okamoto *et al.*, 2010; Stein *et al.*, 2007). Numerous studies have shown that older adults with dementia or Alzheimer's disease have a higher susceptibility to periodontal disease, most likely due to forgetting or the inability to maintain their own oral hygiene. In addition, older adults with edentulism show an association with memory loss (Siukosaari *et al.*, 2012). There may be an association between cognitive ability and periodontal disease. This relates to the hypothesis that the anaerobic bacteria of the plaque can enter the peripheral nervous system and make their way into the central nervous system where the lipopolysaccharide (LPS) can cause cytokine inflammation and virulent properties. Therefore, it is possible that preventing periodontal disease and tooth loss may have implications in maintaining the cognitive abilities in older adults.

Dexterity/functional issues

Conditions that affect dexterity and activities of daily living such as osteoarthritis, rheumatoid arthritis, injury, Parkinson's disease, or stroke may decrease the patient's ability to maintain adequate plaque control, increasing the risk for developing periodontal disease. One study found that persons with Parkinson's disease brushed their teeth less frequently and had longer intervals in between visits to the dentist as compared to the disease free control group (Mueller *et al.*, 2011). It may have been that the patients and/or their caregiver were simply neglecting their oral health and focusing on other aspects of their Parkinson's disease care and treatment, but both older adults and their caregivers need to maintain the oral health of the elderly who are experiencing difficulty with Activities of Daily Living (ADLs). Another study found that even at significant levels of existing periodontal treatment need – as measured by the Community Periodontal Index of Treatment Need (CPITN) index – there remain challenges and opportunities for patients to become aware of their periodontal status. Even at the most severe levels of disease, rating a 4 on a 4-point scale, with 1 being the healthiest and 4 reflecting the most severe disease state, only half of the elderly subjects reported gingival bleeding The other half still did not report any gingival bleeding despite the dental examiners' severe 4 rating according to the CPITN index and obvious bleeding (Siukosaari *et al.*, 2012). It was postulated that the deteriorating eyesight of the subjects caused them to simply not see the bleeding themselves and/or their brushing was too soft and inadequate for proper hygiene, thus not inducing bleeding. This highlights another factor that needs to be taken into account: older adults with impaired vision might not be able to adequately see their own oral hygiene status and, thus, not detect any signs of periodontal disease or bleeding if it occurs. In these situations electrical, vibrating, pulsating head toothbrushes should be prescribed, as they remove more plaque and improve oral hygiene better than manual toothbrushes without the need for the same fine motor movements.

Osteoporosis

Osteoporosis is characterized by a reduction in bone mass leading to weakened bones more susceptible to fractures. Periodontitis is characterized by the loss of connective tissue and alveolar bone. Therefore, the implications of osteoporosis as it relates to periodontitis cannot be overlooked as they have several common risk factors including age, smoking, and medications affecting healing (Dumitrescu, 2010). Studies directly linking osteoporosis to periodontal disease have shown mixed results, but most longitudinal studies have shown a positive correlation between alveolar bone mass and systemic bone mineral density. The association between periodontal disease and osteoporosis among healthcare providers is understood, but until more research is performed, there is insufficient evidence to assert causation in either direction (Koduganti, 2009).

Menopausal status

Another risk factor for periodontal disease is menopausal status in women. Post-menopausal women are at a high risk of osteoporosis. A recent study of post-menopausal women showed an inverse relationship between severe CAL (>5 mm) and bone mass density of the femur neck; as the severity of CAL increased, the bone mass density of the femur neck decreased. The results of this study did not look at osteoporosis specifically, but imply that if severe CAL is found during oral examination, the patient should also be advised to have her systemic bone health monitored due to the potential long-term implications (Gondim *et al.*, 2013). This study is significant because it shows a simple oral examination can be used, even without radiography available, to prevent or treat possible osteoporosis. For older adults in assisted living facilities, communal housing or who are bedridden, this is of particular importance due to the ease in using a perioprobe to measure CAL. But radiographs are also an extremely useful tool the dental examiner can use in identifying alveolar, maxillary, and mandibular bone resorption where, combined with other the other risk factors such as age, history, and smoking, periodontal disease and osteoporosis can be treated.

Studies have shown that after adjustment for variables such as age, race, socioeconomic status, and frequency of dental visits, that post-menopausal women receiving estrogen replacement therapies have much less BOP, CAL, and edentulism over time with higher jaw bone mass compared to women not receiving hormone therapy (Dumitrescu, 2010).

Implants and periodontal disease

Numerous studies have shown the effectiveness of dental implants in not only preventing alveolar bone resorption, but actually reversing the trend and causing alveolar bone formation (Dumitrescu, 2010). The literature and case reports of successful dental implants in osteoporotic patients have shown similar results as well and ruling out osteoporosis as a contraindication to dental implants. Osteoporosis is site specific, showing regenerative capabilities. If the local bone quality is sufficient to support the implant (types 1–3) the implant can be successful (Dao *et al.,* 1993; Dumitrescu, 2010; Friberg *et al.,* 2001).

Aspiration pneumonia

Aspiration pneumonia is the number one leading cause of death and the second most common cause of hospitalization among nursing home patients (Shay, 2002). Aspiration pneumonia is different than pneumonia as it is primarily caused by gram-negative anaerobes related to those found in dental plaque and the deep pockets of periodontal disease gingiva. Therefore, the oral hygiene of patients who are bedridden, in nursing homes, or suffer from chewing or swallowing dysfunction need to be carefully monitored. Tubes used to intubate or ventilate patients can cause pulmonary infections, as oral bacteria from the oral cavity may come into contact with the respiratory system. If possible, their oral health needs to be properly maintained, using suction tooth brushes at least two times per day along with cleaning the tubing coming into contact with the patients' mouth. It is generally understood that periodontal therapy will help reduce aspiration pneumonia by removing the gram-negative anaerobes, if this is a feasible treatment option for the patient (Shay, 2002).

Diet and nutritional changes

Periodontal disease can be a very painful condition due to the amount of inflammation and tissue destruction. As a result, patients may have difficulty chewing food leading to decreased caloric intake,

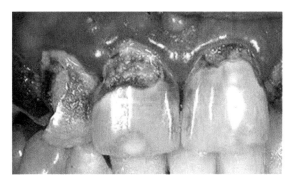

Figure 11.5 Patient with root caries.

subsequent weight loss, and/or nutrient deficiencies. The soft food selection of fermentable/refined carbohydrates, such as breads or pastries, combined with nutrient deficiencies can create an oral environment highly favorable to the development of more plaque. Increased plaque contributes to exacerbating periodontal disease. Aspirin can be prescribed for pain and inflammation, but periodontal therapy is needed to treat the periodontal disease and remove the plaque harboring the pro-inflammatory bacteria. Another significant problem associated with periodontitis is root caries due to recession. Gingival recession exposes the cementum-covered root surfaces. Cementum is softer than the enamel covering the crowns of teeth and roots are therefore more susceptible to decay. Cavities along the roots can lead to sensitivity and possible endodontic involvement (Figs 11.3 & 11.5). The ultimate consequence of periodontal disease is tooth loss, which can impair speech, affect the ability to eat, and decrease a patient's self-esteem.

There are many changes that occur as an individual ages, including a decrease in vitamin D and calcium absorption. This may be from gastrointestinal disorders, medications that prevent absorption, chronic alcohol abuse and is associated with low socioeconomic status. The resulting malnutrition may lead to decreased cell division, clot formation, and collagen synthesis and maturation. Aging may also contribute to increased phagocytic activity of immune system cells. These factors directly relate to the periodontal status of an individual and can mitigate healing after periodontal therapy. Further, older adults' nutritional status may change as a function of decreased olfactory sense. Since smell is closely associated with taste, a diminished olfactory sense may lead to unhealthy dietary changes. Painful dentures make it hard to chew and may cause shifts in nutrition towards soft foods and liquids leading to nutritional deficiencies. Also, decreased activity and mobility levels decrease metabolism, causing decreased appetite and increased susceptibility to malnutrition. All of these factors directly or indirectly may relate to periodontal disease.

Psychologic considerations

Stress and depression have both been found to adversely affect the periodontal status of patients. Stress has been related to the increased production of inflammatory mediators, which can increase the severity of the immune response to plaque bacteria. Older adults are subject to depression as their friends, family, and significant others pass away. Studies have shown that older adults living on their own have a higher occurrence of clinical depression compared to married couples living together (Dumitrescu, 2010). Depression can decrease immune function and compromise wound healing, which can lead to depression-induced memory loss. Patients who suffer from depression may also have a decreased response to periodontal therapy because of poor attitude, an inability to quit smoking, feeling overwhelmed with the treatment process, and overall poor compliance with the recommended treatment. Thus, it may be reasonable to infer that periodontal disease is associated with stress, anxiety, and depression (Dumitrescu, 2010). Socially isolated people are more at risk of oral disease and yet less likely to access care.

DISCUSSION QUESTIONS

1 What are systemic risk factors for periodontal disease?
2 How does periodontal disease contribute directly or indirectly to nutritional status?
3 What is the role of periodontal disease in the health status of nursing home residents?
4 Describe strategies for maintaining and improving periodontal health in frail elders?

References

Armitage, G. (2003) Diagnosis of periodontal diseases. *Journal of Periodontology*, **74**(8), 1237–47.

Buhlin, K., Mntyl, P., Paju, S., *et al.* (2011) Periodontitis is associated with angiographically verified coronary artery disease. *Journal of Clinical Periodontology*, **38**(11), 1007–14.

Burt, B. (2005) Position paper: epidemiology of periodontal diseases. *Journal of Periodontology*, **76**(8), 1406–19.

CDC (Centers for Disease Control and Prevention) (2003) Public health and aging: retention of natural teeth among older adults – United States, 2002. *MMWR Weekly*, **52**(50), 1226–9. From http://www.cdc.gov/mmwr/preview/mmwrhtml/mm5250a3.htm. Accessed March 26, 2014.

Chung, H.Y., Lee, E.K., Choi, Y.J., *et al.* (2011) Molecular inflammation as an underlying mechanism of the aging process and age-related diseases. *Journal of Dental Research*, **90**(7), 830–40.

Dao, T.T., Anderson, J.D. & Zarb, G.A. (1993) Is osteoporosis a risk factor for osseointegration of dental implants? *The International Journal of Oral Maxillofacial Implants*, **8**(2), 137–44.

Dumitrescu, A.L. (2010) *Etiology and Pathogenesis of Periodontal Disease*. Springer, Berlin.

Friberg, B., Ekestubbe, A., Mellstrm, D. & Sennerby, L. (2001) Brånemark implants and osteoporosis: a clinical exploratory study. *Clinical Implant Dentistry and Related Research*, **3**(1), 50–6.

Gondim, V., Aun, J., Fukuda, C., *et al.* (2013) Severe clinical attachment loss: an independent association with low hip bone mineral density in postmenopausal women. *Journal of Periodontology*, **84**(3), 352–9.

Huttner, E.A., Machado, D.C., De Oliveira, R.B., *et al.* (2009) Effects of human aging on periodontal tissues, *Special Care in Dentistry*, **29**(4), 149–55.

Koduganti, R., Gorthi, C., Reddy, P.V. & Sandeep, N. (2009) Osteoporosis: a risk factor for periodontitis. *Journal of Indian Society of Periodontology*, **13**(2), 90–6.

Listgarten, M.A., Schifter, C.C. & Laster, L. (1985) Three-year longitudinal study of the periodontal status of an adult population with gingivitis. *Journal of Clinical Periodontology*, **12**(3), 225–38.

Müller, T., Palluch, R. & Ackowski, J.J. (2011) Caries and periodontal disease in patients with Parkinson's disease. *Special Care in Dentistry*, **31**(5), 178–81.

Okamoto, N., Morikawa, M., Okamoto, K., *et al.* (2010) Relationship of tooth loss to mild memory impairment and cognitive impairment: findings from the Fujiwara-kyo study. *Behavioral and Brain Functions*, **6**, 77.

Shay, K. (2002) Infectious complications of dental and periodontal diseases in the elderly population. *Clinical Infectious Diseases*, **34**(9), 1215–23.

Siukosaari, P., Ajwani, S., Ainamo, A., *et al.* (2012) Periodontal health status in the elderly with different levels of education: a five-year follow-up study. *Gerodontology*, **29**(2), e170–8.

Stein, P., Desrosiers, M., Donegan, S., *et al.* (2007) Tooth loss, dementia and neuropathology in the Nun study. *The Journal of the American Dental Association*, **138**(10), 1314–22.

Vincent, G.K. & Velkoff, V.A. (2010) The next four decades: the older population in the United States: 2010 to 2050. Population estimates and projections. *Current Population Reports*. From https://www.census.gov/prod/2010pubs/p25-1138.pdf. Accessed March 26, 2014.

Van Dyke, T. & Sheilesh, D. (2005) Risk factors for periodontitis. *Journal of the International Academy of Periodontology*, **7**(1), 3–7.

Further reading

Dounis, G., Ditmyer, M., McClain, M., *et al.* (2010) Preparing the dental workforce for oral disease prevention in an aging population. *Journal of Dental Education*, **74**(10), 1086–94.

Friberg, B. (1994) Treatment with dental implants in patients with severe osteoporosis: a case report. *The International Journal of Periodontics Restorative Dentistry*, **14**(4), 348–53.

Haffajee, A.D. & Socransky, S.S. (1986) Attachment level changes in destructive periodontal diseases. *Journal of Clinical Periodontology*, **13**(5), 461–72.

Hellstein, J., Adler, R., Edwards, B., *et al.* (2011) Managing the care of patients receiving antiresorptive therapy for prevention and treatment of osteoporosis: executive summary of recommendations from the American Dental Association Council on Scientific Affairs. *The Journal of the American Dental Association*, **142**(11), 1243–51.

Redding, S. (2005) Cancer therapy-related oral mucositis. *Journal of Dental Education*, **69**(8), 919–29.

Research, Science, and Therapy Committee of The American Academy of Periodontology (1999) The pathogenesis of periodontal diseases. *Journal of Periodontology*, **70**(4), 457–70.

Sook-Bin Woo, Hellstein, J.W. & Kalmar, J.R. (2006) Systematic review: bisphosphonates and osteonecrosis of the jaws. *Annals of Internal Medicine*, **144**(10), 753–86.

Suzuki, K., Nomura, T., Sakurai, M., *et al.* (2005) Relationship between number of present teeth and nutritional intake in institutionalized elderly. *Bulletin of Tokyo Dental College*, **46**(4), 135–43.

Wright, W.E., Haller, J.M., Harlow, S.A. & Pizzo, P.A. (1985) An oral disease prevention program for patients receiving radiation and chemotherapy. *The Journal of the American Dental Association*, **110**(1), 43–7.

CHAPTER 12

Endodontic Management of the Aging Patient

Harold E. Goodis[1] and Bassam M. Kinaia[2]

[1] University of California School of Dentistry, San Francisco, CA, USA; Boston University Institute for Dental Research and Education, Dubai, UEA
[2] Department of Periodontology and Dental Hygiene, University of Detroit-Mercy School of Dentistry, Detroit, MI, USA

Introduction

At the turn of the 19th into the 20th century, life expectancy was to the mid 50s. In the 21st century, men can live into their late 70s with women's expectancy estimated to extend into the mid-80s. The aspect of living longer does not necessarily mean that people will live better. In dentistry, extension of life expectancy has led to the need for care of the oral cavity using new methods, materials, and technologies. In many instances, this presents clinicians with challenges of care modalities that were not expected (Centers for Disease Control and Prevention, 2012). The dental needs of the aging patient in the 21st century appear to be very different and more complex than those experienced by older patients in the mid to late 20th century (Chalmers, 2006a,b). As the population ages, people are taking more medications that may benefit their general health but not necessarily their dental or periodontal health (Ciancio, 1996). (See Chapter 11 for a discussion of periodontal disease.) Because we are living longer, more people suffer from chronic medical problems and diseases than those whose lives ended in earlier ages. As written in a newspaper opinion piece, treating today's aging patients many times appears as if dentists are attempting to relate to very young children, but without the "giggles and glee" (Fieler, 2012). The writer remembers his father saying that there were parallels between "… caring upward and caring downward on the family tree." Many middle-aged people are caring for their parents, in their own home or in a managed care facility. Emotionally, everything appears

to be backward "… taking care of someone who once took care of you." Mr. Fieler concluded with a profound statement, "… the lessons your children don't want to hear from you today are the same ones you don't want to hear from them later." That sentiment causes patients who are aging of attempting to understand the need for procedures that they don't expect nor understand. Therefore, the need for a root canal procedure can be daunting to them. Explaining not only the need for such a procedure but what it entails as far as what is done to a 70, 80, or even a 90-year-old patient may take up more time than one can imagine.

The need for dental care in aging patients is a multiphase situation and those needs grow yearly. Many of these patients will receive necessary care but many won't, primarily because of what occurs in teeth and oral soft tissues that many care providers have never treated. Therefore, this chapter will discuss the treatment regimens used in root canal therapy of older patients, compare, when applicable the form and function of the tooth, dental pulp, and dentin in young versus aging individuals, and the management of this treatment modality in an environment much different than that usually seen in private practice. The reader will find that, in many instances it is impossible to describe either clinical findings or step-by-step procedures. However, references to appropriate, published articles from refereed journals and textbooks will be suggested to supplement the information in this chapter. Thus, the following will be divided into a discussion of the structure of the inner and outer tissues of the tooth and the changes that occur over time, both physiologic and pathologic, that lead to a different

Geriatric Dentistry: Caring for Our Aging Population, First Edition. Edited by Paula K. Friedman.
© 2014 John Wiley & Sons, Inc. Published 2014 by John Wiley & Sons, Inc.
Companion website: www.wiley.com/go/friedman/geriatricdentistry

way of treating a large group of patients who need what can be considered primary care.

The dental pulp

The developing soft tissue of an adult and aging individual's tooth is a complex tissue surrounded by relatively hard tissues (Figs 12.1a,b & 12.2a,b). The dental pulp has several functions in a developing tooth, but in an adult tooth the pulp functions in a manner that is protective in nature. The protective mechanism, as in tissues throughout the body, warns us when something is wrong. In the pulp, the peripheral sensory nervous system composed of two types of pain fibers (neurons) and functions in a way that not only warns the individual that there is a problem but leads, in many instances, to proper diagnoses and treatment plans (Hargreaves *et al.*, 2012). These neurons are called the A delta and C fibers and, because they are located in different areas of the pulp, respond to different stimuli. The response is usually one of pain that may differ in length, severity, location, and stimulus (Hargreaves *et al.*, 2012).

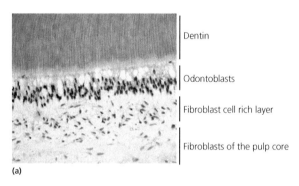

(a)

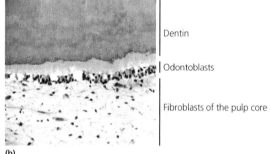

(b)

Figure 12.1 (a) Histologic section of the dental pulp complex of a young tooth (15 years old). Note the dense odontoblast and cell-rich zones. (b) Histologic section of the dental pulp complex of a 59-year-old patient. Note the lesser number of odontoblasts present. Figures courtesy of Dr. Peter Murray, Nova Southeastern University.

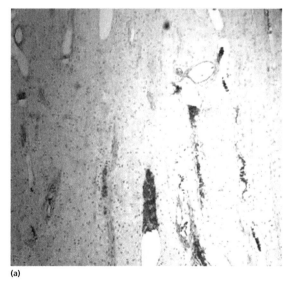

(a)

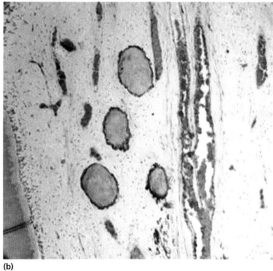

(b)

Figure 12.2 (a) Histologic section of the dental pulp complex of a young tooth (15 years old). Note the highly vascularized tissue. (b) Histologic section of the dental pulp complex of a second 59-year-old patient. Note the lesser number of odontoblasts present. Also note the calcifications found in the pulp tissue. Figures courtesy of Dr. Peter Murray, Nova Southeastern University.

The dental pulp has an infinite capacity to heal itself, not an unusual event in the body as many tissues do the same when injured. Pulp tissue submitted for histologic examination demonstrated the effects of multiple challenges to the tooth, including caries (initial and recurrent), marginal bacterial micro-leakage of restorations, direct trauma, and iatrogenic procedures such as cavity preparation (Bernick & Nedelman, 1975; Hillmann & Geurtsen, 1997; Nielsen, 1983; Stanley, 1961). All affect the pulp, causing an inflammatory response, which will initially be patho-logic, but can become physiologic, since the initial inflammatory response can lead to repair with possible regeneration of the pulpal tissue (Cooper *et al.*, 2010).

The dental pulp tissue is considered a low compli-ance tissue due to its location and the types of tissues surrounding it (Kim, 1985a). First, the pulp is a relatively large volume of tissue with a relatively small vascular supply. The largest artery to enter the pulp is the arteriole and the largest vessel to exit the pulp is the venule; therefore, the vascular system is referred to as a microcirculation. Second, the pulp is a terminal circulation with few, if any, vessel anastomoses. Multi-rooted molars have demonstrated anastomoses in the root portion of the tooth. Therefore, the ability to shunt blood from and to an inflamed area is not pos-sible and may compromise repair when injury occurs. Last, the pulp is surrounded by relatively hard, unyielding, dentin walls, which inhibits and, in many instances, completely suppresses the ability of the pulp to swell, as occurs in other soft tissues such as skin and muscle (Kim, 1985b). Taken together, the above mitigates toward an adverse ability to be protective in nature as it is designed to be. In sum, the potential for the dental pulp to repair itself is infinite. However, aging individuals have limitations for repair or regeneration of pulpal tissues due to limited blood supply, sensory deficits due to fewer neurons, and reduction of the pulp canal space resulting in less tissue available for repair to occur (Bernick & Nedelman, 1975). Therefore, the evidence points to the need for well-controlled root canal therapy to retain a tooth that may appear to be the easiest treatment rather than the best treatment (Trope, 2008). The potential of the dental pulp for healing is limitless. However, aging individuals have limitations for repair and regeneration. This is due to a limited blood supply, sensory deficits due to fewer neurons, and lesser amounts of pulp tissue due to continued mineralization of the tissue space (Trope, 2008).

Dentin and the odontoblasts

Normally the pulp of the developing and adult tooth, as described above, has the ability to form the matrix that becomes three types of dentin. Primary dentin is formed as the tooth develops with a structure that is tubular in nature. Secondary dentin begins to form as the tooth completes its form and erupts. It also con-tains a tubular structure with its tubules being contin-uous with those of primary dentin. The formation of

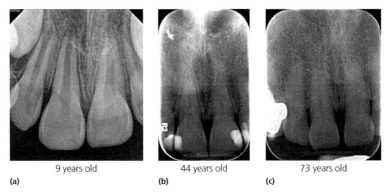

9 years old	44 years old	73 years old
(a)	(b)	(c)

Figure 12.3 (a) A 9-year-old patient with typically young incisors. Note the size of the root canal systems and the incomplete root end development of the three teeth pictured. (b) A 44-year-old patient with restored maxillary central incisors. Note the great change in the size of the root canal spaces, partially attributed to the mesial and distal deposition of tertiary dentin due to composite placement. (c) Maxillary right lateral incisor and central incisor of a 73-year-old patient. Note the absence of restorations with no history of trauma. When compared to Fig. 12.9, the physiologic deposition of secondary dentin is evident. Figures courtesy of Dr. Franklin Tay, Medical College of Georgia.

secondary dentin continues throughout the life of the tooth and is physiologic in nature, unless there is an injury or challenge to the pulp (Smith *et al.,* 1994, 1995) (Fig. 12.3a,b,c). Tertiary dentin generally occurs in teeth that have been injured in some manner (i.e., caries). It is not tubular in its formation but rather occurs as a solid kind of structure.

The importance of dentin cannot be overstressed. Therefore, it is the dentin that in fact may be considered as the partner to the pulp due to its location adjacent to the pulp (the pulp–dentin complex). Dentin's tubular structure contains pulpal fluid and the projecting arm of the odontoblast, the odontoblast process. The odontoblast is responsible for the initiation of dentin matrix formation that becomes mineralized over time and again acts as a protective mechanism (Holland *et al.,* 1985, 1994). The odontoblasts do not undergo mitosis nor they are replaced, unless the pulp is challenged, and continues to act as stated above. However, given the fact that humans are living longer, it is apparent that continued formation of secondary dentin may begin to narrow the root canal space as individuals age to a point that it may be difficult to perform a root canal procedure. Men will demonstrate narrowing of the root canal space in their 40s and it is not impossible that the entire upper and middle portions of the root canal system may be mineralized (Woo, 2001) (Fig. 12.4a,b,c). This event is a reminder that a completely physiologic process may become a pathologic process due to aging (Fig. 12.5a,b,c). Tertiary dentin is the last form of that hard tissue. It forms in response to an injury to the pulp caused by caries etc. Tertiary dentin is not physiologic but pathologic. Its matrix mineralizes as an atubular structure in response to placement of certain materials next to or over an exposed pulp. Tertiary dentin is of two types: reactionary where the dentin matrix is formed by surviving odontoblasts; and reparative dentin formed by a generation of new odontoblast-like cells, which are cells that may act differently than the original cells (Pääkkönen *et al.,* 2009). The formation of tertiary dentin in response to a stimulating type material, such as calcium hydroxide ($CaOH_2$), also narrows or closes the root canal space, but much more rapidly than secondary dentin. The new dentin formed also may lead to further closure of the root canal space and cause a nonresponse to temperature stimulation.

A normal dental pulp demonstrates its ability to survive throughout life. As mentioned above, the odontoblast, with its process extending into the dentinal tubules, is the cell responsible for formation of the dentin matrix. When caries are present (Stanley, 1977), and initially removed, the odontoblastic processes are cut, effectively causing the odontoblast to die. There are sufficient numbers of odontoblasts so that dentin continues to form. However, repeated placement or replacement of restorations, combined

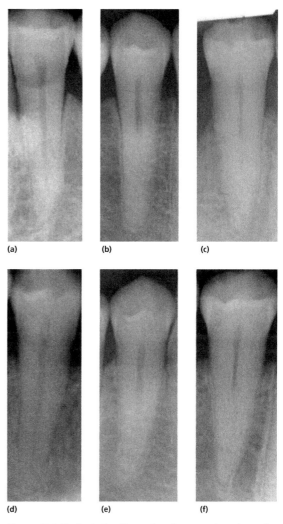

(a)   (b)   (c)

(d)   (e)   (f)

Figure 12.4 Periapical radiographs of a premolar taken of a male patient at three times over a 40-year period. (a) Mandibular first premolar at age 33. The root canal system can be seem to the apex of the tooth. (b) The same tooth at age 52. (c) The same tooth at age 73 years. The same pattern is seen in a second patient at the same time frames (d, e, f). Courtesy of Woo, 2001.

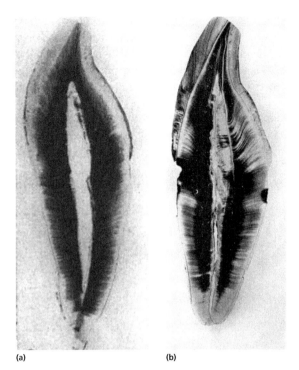

(a)   (b)

Figure 12.5 (a) Low power photomicrograph of an unstained root canal space (ground section) of an upper central incisor typical of a 26–30-year-old individual. Note the size of the root canal space (Original mag. ×20).
(b) Low power photomicrograph of an unstained root canal space (ground section) of an upper central incisor typical of a over 71-year-old individual. Secondary dentin fills the entire pulp chamber of the root canal space. Note that the secondary dentin formation is tubular as opposed to atubular dentin. Its formation is due to age and not to caries or placement of restorations. Courtesy of Philippas & Applebaum, 1966.

with marginal bacterial microleakage, may cause all odontoblasts in the area to die; therefore, the remainder of the tissue depends on formation of odontoblast-like cells to form a matrix that will result in tertiary dentin (About *et al.*, 2001; Couve & Schmachtenberg, 2011; Couve *et al.*, 2012; Murray *et al.*, 2000). Eventually, the remaining pulp tissue becomes overwhelmed and the remaining tissue becomes necrotic. In these cases, depending on the age of the patient, the patient's ability to sit for a period of time in the dental chair and the condition of the patient's teeth (caries, fractured cusps, lost restorations, periodontal status, and restorability), treatment choices may become overwhelming.

Sensory mechanisms

As mentioned above, the adult dental pulp attempts to function as a protective mechanism. As people age, the root canal space contracts, limiting the number of cells remaining in the pulp to be able react positively to an adverse stimulus. Therefore, aging also leads to decreases in the number of sensory (pain) nerves present in the pulp (Bernick 1962a, 1967a; Fried, 1992; Fried & Hildebrand, 1981; Matysiak *et al.*, 1986, 1988).

The presence of tertiary dentin may be capable of blocking peripheral pain fibers from being stimulated in a manner that will allow the patient to sense pain. Contracture of the pulp space limits the amount of pulp tissue present and can affect those remaining nerves in the body of the remaining pulp tissue, again limiting the ability to respond to an adverse stimulus. These events may compromise patient's responses to tooth testing, especially to applications of testing with cold or heat. The responses occur through stimulation of sensory neurons located in and around odontoblasts and within the body of the pulp. More recent studies appear to indicate that odontoblasts also may have a sensory function (El Karim *et al.*, 2011; Magloire *et al.*, 2010; Okumura *et al.*, 2005; Son *et al.*, 2009). This is an important finding since aging individuals have fewer odontoblasts and, if the pulp has been injured, the odontoblast-like cells may not function as did the original odontoblasts functioned. These studies have expanded the sensory ability of the dental pulp to respond to injury, and indicates that the dental pulp sensory pain mechanisms are much more complex that originally believed.

Since the tissue responds to injury to protect the remaining pulp by formation of odontoblast-like cells, the neural response in these situations may or may not be diagnostic. The formation of tertiary dentin may prevent contracture of dentinal fluid and movement into the pulp through what now may be obliterated tubules; hence, no or weak responses to cold. On the other hand, the atubular dentin may block the ability of a heat stimulus from reaching the body of the pulp to allow increase in temperatures to a level that patients will respond to heat (Zach & Cohen, 1962, 1967). The pulp has a greater tolerance in young people to decreases in temperature, therefore indicating that a coolant must be cold enough to elicit responses. The tissue is less tolerant to increases in pulp temperatures as responses generally occur with temperatures rising 5–7 degrees (Zach & Cohen, 1962, 1967). Ultimately, the main factor continues to be limitation of root canal space and decreases in the numbers of sensory neurons, lessening the patient's response being realistic.

Vascularity

The same limiting events occur with the vascular supply to the dental pulp. The microcirculation in normal pulp tissue maintains vitality. But as individuals age and the root canal system narrows due to continued secondary or tertiary dentin formation, fewer and smaller vessels are available to allow normal blood flow (Bernick, 1962b, 1967b, 1972). While the radicular vasculature is still effective, the gradual narrowing of the pulp volume indicates a diminished blood flow in the tissue (Domine & Holz, 1991). The metabolic ability of the dental pulp decreases gradually and the capillaries in the subodontoblasts become thinner with aging (Ma *et al.*, 1997). Interestingly, one could say that, of everything being equal, an individual living well into his or her 90s, who presents with what appears to be a completely calcified root canal system, would have been thought to have had a perfect root canal therapy without treatment. However, a remnant of pulp tissue remains apically but has no blood supply, and a lesion will be seen apically on a radiograph. Such a case would eventually require treatment, most often surgery. Unlike an event due to trauma, a 90-year-old patient's root canal closure would be due to a normal physiologic event of secondary dentin deposition throughout life. If that patient should require surgery, the situation and management changes and, depending on the health of the patient, treatment becomes more difficult (Eldarrat *et al.*, 2010; Kvaal *et al.*, 1994).

Management considerations

Diagnosis
Tooth testing
The need for a correct diagnosis in any treatment situation is a necessity. Tooth testing can be quite subtle or quite dramatic. The subtlety of endodontic

diagnosis is being able to understand pain responses to temperature changes and other stimuli to understand whether the patient presents with a reversible or irreversible pulpitis. For example, a response to a cold stimulus that disappears as soon as the stimulus is removed from the tooth is generally a reversible pulpitis. This indicates that the problem is something other than an irreversible pulpitis, as seen in fractured cusps, caries, or recurrent caries. The key to the diagnosis is that the symptom occurs because underlying dentin has been exposed. Covering the dentin with a new restoration after caries removal or removal of a fractured cusp tip ends the pain. On the other hand, a response to a heat stimulus that lingers for some time or beginning many seconds to a minute or two after removal of the stimulus is indicative of an irreversible pulpitis. In older patients, these responses can be quiet dramatic, with loud and painful responses and a look that will say that the patient believes he or she is in the wrong office.

As stated above, tissues change in the aging patient. While dentists are capable of making a correct diagnosis in older patients, they must remember to be more "patient" with their "patients" who are older. An axiom of tooth testing for pulpal and periradicular diseases, whatever the age of the patient, is to **listen to the patient!** So often, especially in a busy practice, practitioners think that they can take a radiograph and immediately form a diagnosis and treatment plan without patient input. Believe it or not, patients do have a clue as to which tooth is causing the problem. However, with older patients, especially those experiencing pain and with a history of several medical conditions, the dentist must understand the possible difficulty of getting to the "root" of the problem.

First, aging patients tend to be more anxious, thinking that everything touching a particular tooth causes pain. They will try to help by responding immediately to a temperature test when a cotton swab without a stimulant touches their tooth. When asked what they felt, they can't say. Therefore, each and every test used in the diagnostic process must be thoroughly explained to the patient. There have been many older patients who respond to a stimulant placed on the pontics of a fixed appliance. (A not uncommon event in the author's office [H.E.G.].) Second, they ask many questions, sometimes asking the same question several times, either because they don't understand or have a dementia and don't remember the answers. Older patients also have the need to attempt to dictate what type of treatment they require. It is, therefore, necessary to schedule more time with aging patients than normally would be required for a younger patient. Remember again that an aging patient's responses are not necessarily what a younger patient would report. With the root canal space compromised, either physiologically or pathologically, there may be no response to temperature-testing methods in what may ordinarily be a reversible pulpitis that turned into an irreversible pulpitis, because of recurrent caries or a fractured tooth structure present that can be treated without a root canal procedure. This may complicate the necessary treatment. A necrosis with a sinus tract and radiographic evidence of a lesion may be the easiest diagnosis to make and treat. The use of an electric vitalometer, especially after explaining how the device works, will sometimes frighten an older patient. Because of its limited ability, due to the need to be used only on tooth structure, in routine testing it should not be used for the aging patient. Older patients will always tell their friends how they were "electrocuted" in the dentist's office. A good rule to follow is to never test the suspected tooth first. Test the adjacent, opposing or contra-lateral tooth first, then the suspected tooth last. This not only demonstrates to aging patients that they will not be hurt, it will also be a baseline for the patient's responses.

Once the dental pulp becomes inflamed, the overriding symptom is the onset of pain. Since the volume of tissue in the root canal space of a young individual is relatively large, as opposed to older patients with much less tissue, diagnosis generally does not pose problems. Testing regimens are based on careful questioning of the patient to elicit as much history and information as possible. The input from the patient leads to the type of tooth testing that may be necessary to properly diagnose the problem. Since pain to temperature, either hot or cold, is a cardinal symptom of a pulpitis, this may be the best place to start. This, of course, occurs after a full intraoral and extraoral examination.

In many instances, symmetry of facial areas will have changed due to internal swelling in the mouth. Therefore, the testing begins with the easiest and most common tests prior to other, more complicated

tests. When a necrosis is suspected and the pain complaint comes from chewing hard food or swallowing, with normal occlusion, the use of a mirror handle to gently percuss teeth is enough to cause a response. Differentiating between pain when percussing in a vertical direction, for periradicular pain, and in a bucco-lingual direction helps in understanding the possibility of a periodontal problem rather than an endodontic problem. (Don't forget to take periodontal gingival sulcus readings.) Biting on a wet cotton roll, use of a Tooth Sleuth®, or percussing individual cusp tips may disclose the presence of a hard tooth structure fracture that certainly will change the diagnosis and may change the prognosis. The use of the ball of the index finger in the palpation test can pick up disease quickly and effortlessly; slight pressure in the cul-de-sac area is used to define sensitivity.

Since presence of vital tissue is necessary in the crown of the tooth for a response to temperature testing, a problem exists with a nonresponse in older patients. With gingival recession and closure of the root canal system, the remaining pulp tissue may be well below the cervical area of the tooth; hence, a possible nonresponse from an older patient. There is a possibility of periodontal recession that exposes dentinal tubules which curve down and then up to reach the pulp, the hot or cold stimulus may be placed somewhat lower towards the gingival crest of the tooth in an attempt to have a response. Care must be taken in these cases not to involve the soft tissue of the gingival crest which will result in a false positive. If radiographs disclose no periodontal ligament thickening or a radiolucent lesion and pain is the only symptom or sign, difficulties increase as to making a correct diagnosis. Keep in mind the difficulty of attempting to pulp test a child 3–5 years of age. That will make one understand the difficulty of testing that child's aging grandparents, who are brought to the dentist by the child's mother or father. A retrospective study concluded that general practitioners were able to detect radiographic changes when they are extensive, but they miss periodontal ligament widening and lamina dura changes (Sherwood, 2012). Remember that loss of restorations, secondary or recurrent caries, and fractured cusps, among other coronal conditions must be intercepted early enough to either prevent a pulpitis from occurring or from suffering the sequelae of a necrotic tooth.

Radiographs

The above is predicated on the fact that properly angled and exposed radiographs have been taken. This part of diagnosis is placed here as, while radiographs are incredibly important, too often dentists will take them first, glance at them when developed or if digital, and never look at them again. Hence, the placing of a radiographic discussion here after the discussion of tooth testing above is important. The dentist must return to view the radiograph after the information of listening to the patient, extraoral and intraoral examinations completed, with tooth testing having been generated. Ordinarily, the presence of a radiolucency at the apex of a tooth that doesn't respond to testing indicates a necrotic pulp with extension to the periradicular area. That is particularly true in a younger patient but not necessarily true in an aging patient. Being able to diagnose between a lesion of endodontic origin (LEO) and other pathologic entities can be delicate. Obviously, younger patients may present with a greater ability to represent their symptoms and dental history than an aging patient. Simply put, more than one radiograph needs to be taken at a different angle (mesio-distal) after the fully parallel position of the first film. If the lesion moves in the angled film, it's probably not a LEO. If the pulp tests are normal and there were no symptoms, the lesion will be a lesion other than a LEO; this is true in young and aging patients. Additionally, the angled film may better describe the number of roots present or dilacerations of roots not seen in the first film.

There is a very subtle situation that causes dentists to err in a diagnosis. It is referred to as a thickened periodontal ligament (PDL). Most dentists have never heard of or have forgotten that this entity exists. For example, a young patient will present with radiographic evidence of a thickened PDL. Confounding to the dentist – who believes that the symptoms indicate a pulpitis, which is confirmed by the tooth-testing results being positive to cold but with symptoms not lingering – an irreversible pulpitis is diagnosed and the dentist immediately begins a root canal procedure. As presented above, stimuli responses to cold are expressive of a reversible pulpitis, with exposure of dentin. To have this response in an older person with radiographic evidence of coronal closure of the root canal system may indicate that a deeper fracture is present that extends to the lower lever of the pulp

tissue. The subtly of a thickened PDL comes from knowing that it generally indicates a reversible pulpitis (find the exposed dentin, treat it), not an irreversible pulpitis. Remember that conventional radiographs used for diagnosis and management of endodontic problems result in limited information because of the two-dimensional nature of the images produced or the geometric distortion produced by the angulation. (Patel *et al.*, 2009) (The reader is referred to Berman & Hartwell, 2011, and other endodontic texts for a more detailed discussion of endodontic radiographs.)

Other methods of radiographic examination are presently being suggested to increase the ability of the dentist to make a correct diagnosis. Laser Doppler flowmetry (LDF) measures the presence or absence of blood flow in the pulp tissue. The device passes a laser beam through tooth structure that interacts with the red blood cells. The interaction causes a signal to bounce off of the blood cells, that are picked up by a receiver device. The resultant value is automatically converted to a number that indicates flow. The use of this device is limited as the laser beam will not go through metallic restorations and must be carried out in complete quiet with little or any type of airflow. In some instances, someone walking near the device will cause deviations in the values generated. The blood flow from gingival tissues also can cause marked deviations in the readings. However, when the environment is controlled, LDF can be used for research. One study tested 8–75-year-old participants' pulpal blood flow (PBF) at different ages. Resting PBF decreased with increasing age, indicating a smaller mass of tissue with fewer vessels. When cold was applied to the crown, all blood flow decreased with significance in aging patients (Ikawa, 2003; Jafazadh, 2009). Laser wavelengths also may become the method of choice for cleaning and shaping root canal systems, but the science still in not quite there. Lasers are suggested for treating sensitive dentin and other clinical methodology (Stabholtz *et al.*, 2004).

Cone beam computed tomography (CBCT) is presently being tested as having the ability to image oral structures (soft and hard tissue) three-dimensionally. Tests using extracted teeth or other models mimicking the mandible or maxilla with human teeth in place, demonstrated that ability (Gani & Visvisian, 1999; Hassan *et al.*, 2009; Ozer, 2010; Wang *et al.*, 2011). Patel and colleagues were able to detect periradicular pulpal disease before the disease process had perforated either cortical plates of bone when the lesion could not be seen by periradicular radiographs (Patel, 2009; Patel *et al.*, 2009). This has been increasingly utilized in the oral cavity (Agematsu *et al.*, 2010; Kaya *et al.*, 2011; Maret *et al.*,2011; Silva *et al.*, 2012). CBCT has not become standard of care in endodontics as the ability to see apices in most devices is not acceptable and it does not justify the extra expense. However, use of micro-CT devices in research (not clinically because of increased radiation and cost) demonstrated that decreases in interpulpal space due to secondary dentin in extracted teeth were higher in women than men. Space decreases occurred more often in older men in their 50s and 60s and in women in their 40s and 50s (Agematsu *et al.*, 2010). CBCT has greater utility for imaging maxillofacial areas (Maret *et al.*, 2011). Others suggest the use of CBCT to evaluate changes in root canal anatomy and morphology as individuals' age, which may allow more teeth in aging patients to be treated (Kaya *et al.*, 2011). *In vitro* studies compared the use of CBCT between periapical radiographs and CBCT in detection of artificial perforations in extracted teeth (Tyndall & Kohltfaber, 2012; Tyndall & Rathore, 2008). For the detection of periapical pathoses, Patel *et al.* (2012) found that CBCT demonstrated a lower healing rate for primary root canal therapy than that seen in periapical radiographs, particularly in molars. In teeth with existing preoperative periapical radiolucencies, CBCT images showed more failures (14%) compared with periapical radiographs (10.4%) (Patel *et al.* 2012).

Treatment methods

The late 20th century onwards has seen new treatment methods and materials brought to the market place. The advertising of these products implies that, if used as directed, time will be saved and procedures will be much easier, quicker, and better. This will allow the practitioner to see and treat more patients, earn a better income, and live the good life. While many of the products and devices (operating microscope, rotary instruments), when used correctly, may lower the stress levels of practitioners, they are not the new wonders of the modern world. Endodontists will say endodontics is labor intensive. The endodontist knows that he or she must sit at the chair, anesthetize a patient, and access,

clean and shape, and obdurate the root canal systems of the tooth to be treated. There are no short cuts. The new materials and devices certainly help, but each generation has its own new instruments and materials and endodontics remains a labor-intensive treatment modality. A successful root canal procedure connotes that diseased tissue has been removed from the root canal system and the tooth, with proper restoration, can be returned to original form and function (naturally, if it is periodontally sound or can be made so). This is a noble objective but not necessarily true, especially when treating aging patients on a regular basis. Goodis *et al.* (2001) surveyed Diplomates of the American Board of Endodontics in the changing demographics of their practices, with emphasis on the ages and numbers of the patients referred to their practices. Respondents reported that smaller root canal spaces more commonly occurred as the number of aging patients referred increased. The change in the size of the canals did not, however, compromise the success of their treatment (Figs 12.6a,b,c & 12.7a,b). Rather, it was the poor condition of the aging patient's teeth that caused the most problems. While acknowledgment was made to the greater difficulty in locating and treating smaller canal systems, most respondents spoke to the need of more studies that would lead to treating patients earlier using materials that would not cause closure of those same canal systems, and to the breakdown in dentitions and periodontal tissue breakdown that would require these procedures in aging individuals (Goodis *et al.*, 2001). The treatment of an aging patient in many instances may not necessarily be more difficult than treatment in a younger patient. It just may take more patience and time to complete treatment successfully.

As the US aging population has increased, other studies over the past 25 years have examined management considerations in this population (Galen, 1990). In the 19th century, and well into the 20th century, treatment consisted of removal of all the teeth that possibly could have been saved and their replacement with dentures. "If it was good enough for my father and mother, it's good enough for me." As reported by Walton (1997), the biologic and anatomic differences in the dental pulp and dentin between young and aging individuals must be understood and considered in the diagnosis, treatment planning, and actual treatment. Older patients are

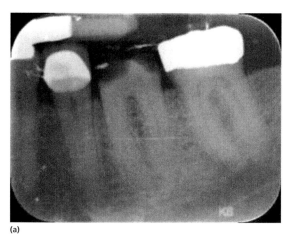
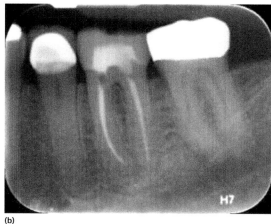

(a)   (b)

Figure 12.6 (a) Radiograph of a lower left first molar with little or any coronal structure remaining in a 67-year-old male patient. The patient's dentist suggests the tooth's removal and placement of a crown-restored implant. Note the thinness of the root canal systems, probably due to tertriary dentin formation. (b) Radiograph of the same tooth after endodontic therapy and placement of a crown. Courtesy of Dr. Franklin Tay, Medical College of Georgia.

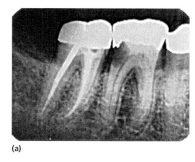
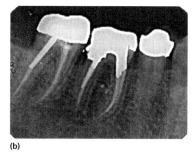

(a)   (b)

Figure 12.7 (a) Radiograph of a lower right first molar in a 71-year-old male patient. Note the large carious lesion at the distal gingival margin below the restoration with successful root canal therapy in the second molar. (b) The caries has been removed and packed with amalgam and the tooth has a second root canal treatment. This case was seen by a periodontist who told the patient that it could not be retained and a crown restored implant would be a better treatment.

more likely to have complex medical histories (strokes, heart disease, diabetes, dementias). This also is a product of living longer. One or another, by itself, may be daunting in successfully completing care (Qualtrough & Mannocci, 2011). The dentist today must be willing to vary how he or she treats the aging patient in relation to number of visits, different chair positions for the patients and the practitioner to accommodate physical disabilities, and working more closely with caregivers. It may be necessary to travel to homebound individuals to provide adequate care, which, in most instances, is the most difficult of conditions, requiring portable equipment, supplies, and room to deliver proper care.

Emphasis must be placed on the retention of teeth in order to maintain the ability of patients to properly chew for normal mastication. The knowledge that older patients' teeth may be badly broken down and/or heavily restored makes treatment extremely challenging (Allan & Whitworth, 2004; Qualtrough & Mannocci, 2011). The authors stress the need for strategic treatment planning and preservation of key teeth, even when diseased, to protect and retain natural teeth and associated soft tissue and bone. Age-related changes in the structure of dentin and pulp occur that require knowledge of new endodontic procedures and new instrumentation (Burke & Samarawickrama, 1995).

Endodontic therapy of aging patients

Appointments

Endodontics mostly has become a one-appointment discipline, with root canal system cleaning, shaping, and obturating the root canal space. Obviously, the time scheduled for an aging patient is dependent on the patients being able to sit in a normal dental chair and be reclined when required. If needed, more time can be scheduled, which may ease the patient's ability to sit for treatment. Aging patients will present with canes and wheelchairs, and offices must be designed to handle slower walking or walking-assisted patients. This includes the dental chair, ideally equipped with fold-down arms to allow ease of movement from a wheelchair or a walker to the dental chair.

Diagnosis

The first part of a diagnosis is listening to the patient. This is not actually a test, since all that is required is attention of the operator to what the patient is saying and the answers to questions asked by he or she. Listening to the patient applies both to young and aging patients. In most cases, absent senilities, the patient to be treated will have an idea as to where the problem is originating and what causes sensitivity.

Diagnosis involves the use of testing devices to elicit patient responses. Further, visualization of the surrounding soft tissue and underlying structure is required to locate pathoses. Devices to augment radiographs (digital films, CBCTs) will be useful in detecting radiolucent lesions associated with abscessed teeth. Accurately angled films are a must and their exposure is the second aspect of making a correct diagnosis.

Endodontic diagnosis depends both on external tooth testing devices applied to either natural tooth structure, or in many instances, to an artificial crown (metallic, ceramic, or combination). Use of percussion and palpation is an easy way to introduce an aging patient to tooth testing. The use of a mirror handle or the finger tip of the index finger is all that is needed. Percussion is a gentle tap to the crown of the tooth in an apical direction, keeping in mind to percuss each cusp of a posterior tooth. In many instances, sensitivity to the test will indicate a fracture, and a hard tap is not necessary (any tooth can be made to hurt if the stimulus is too strong). Biting on a wet cotton roll or on the Tooth Sleuth® also detects fractured cusps. Tapping in an apical direction and in a bucco-lingual direction distinguishes periradiular from periodontal disease and pain. Palpation is the easiest of tests as only the ball portion of the index finger is used. With the cheeks held away from the periodontium, the fingertip is moved anterior to posterior in the cul de sac above the apices of the teeth. Again, pressure applied should be very light. If slight swelling is present, the patient will indicate sensation much different than that on normal, not involved tissue. The use of a periodontal probe also may be used to differentiate between periapical and periodontal diseases.

Next in the testing hierarchy is the use of temperature testing. Contrary to some beliefs, natural tooth structure in not necessary to test for sensitivity to a stimulus in the environment of the oral cavity. Patients generally present for treatment complaining of pain. The pain is usually caused by temperature change to liquids or food, biting on various foods, or just swallowing, causing opposing teeth to occlude. Included in tooth testing, is the use of hot and cold applications whether an artificial or restored crown is present. If a patient presents with sensitivity to heat or cold while at home, that, in and of itself, tells the dentist that the pulp is involved. The temperature is transferred through the crown but if the tooth is already sensitive, that's the next test. In using temperature tooth testing stimuli, hold the stimulus on the middle third of the buccal surface, away from the gingival crest. The stimulus should be held for five seconds and the heat or cold should not be overly hot or cold. Do not use liquid nitrogen for cold testing nor overly hot, smoking gutta percha for heat testing.

A good rule to follow using these tests, is to test other teeth considered to be normal before testing the suspected tooth. Test adjacent, contralateral, or opposing teeth before testing the suspected tooth. Another test that can be used includes application of a dye to locate crown fractures. The reader is referred to Berman and Hartwell (2011) for a more complete discussion of tooth testing.

Since the radiographs or other visual aids were previously taken, now is a good time to revisit those films. The rule now is to coordinate all information generated, including radiographs. While periapical radiographs are the principle means of "looking inside" the soft tissue and bone, they can be augmented by use of three-dimensional imaging. The CBCT device or other such devices allow for a more complete diagnosis. Much as it has been used in periodontics, the three-dimensional micro-CT devices can be used in endodontics to find separated instruments, perforations, dilacerlations, and hidden root systems not easily demonstrated on peripical radiographs, especially from the standpoint of both bucco-lingual and mesio-distal views. Morse and colleagues (Morse, 1991; Morse *et al.*, 1993) detailed aging changes of the dental pulp and dentin, finding that normal teeth underwent root canal space loss as patients aged. While endodontists knew of these occurrences, not everyone remembered the process. A more recent study (Oginni *et al.*, 2009) found root canal space obliteration using the periapical index and radiographs helpful in developing a positive treatment plan for aging patients. Needless to say, older patients should respond to these tooth tests routinely everything else being equal. However, the reduction to canal space may not allow temperature changes to move fluid through the absent dentinal tubules (a delta response) or raise or lower temperatures in the core of the pulp (C-fibers) to evoke a response. The proper angulation of a radiograph with a second film at either a mesial or distal angulation is needed, including a bitewing to gauge the height of the pulp chamber in posterior teeth.

Medical history

There are common diseases in aging individuals that must be disclosed to the operator. If it appears that they are not complete, a telephone call to the patient's physician should clarify the medical history. The physical and mental problems may affect the success or failure of a particular treatment result. Borderline diabetes (type 2) in aging patients may not be understood nor have been diagnosed by the patient's physician. Inability to swallow from lack of saliva, pain in the left arm, radiating to the mandible, shortness of breath, pain in the chest, high blood pressure, and other conditions mirrored in a patient's face and mouth should be noted. There are many signs and symptoms of disease in other areas of the body that will be manifested in and around the oral cavity first, such as diabetes. A remark of an aging patient that he or she is always thirsty may trigger referral for a visit to their physician.

Diagnosis is built upon a series of questions, answers, examinations, testing, and past dental and medical histories. The drugs older patients are taking also may affect success or failure, especially in the case of senilities. Careful attention to the patient's ability to know what is being taken is as important as when it is to be taken. Failure to know or understand these and other conditions were, are or will be; may not cause just failure of oral treatment, but great harm to the aging patient.

Treatment plan

Simply put, proper diagnosis leads to a proper treatment plan. Not all patients can be treated endodontically successfully, especially older patients. However, the dentist should not consign a difficult endodontic procedure to the removal of a tooth just because of age. The treatment plan should be based on the relationship between the general dentist and the endodontist and with other specialists, if required. The advent of successful use of implants with osseous integration has changed the thinking of many practitioners, both generalists and specialists. Teeth that can be successfully treated endodontically may be removed because the dentist offers a dental implant instead. And teeth are treated that should be removed, again because the dentist doesn't know how to place implants. Managing the treatment of an older patient is not as simple as "just" doing a root canal procedure or removing a tooth. The treatment plan is a complex endeavor with any patient, no matter what age.

Endodontic treatment

Endodontists see a wide range of situations that may influence their ability to successfully complete a toot canal system procedure in older individuals. The first part of actual treatment is placement of a rubber dam. In optimum circumstances, placement of a rubber dam may be difficult (Fig. 12.6a,b). In an aging patient it may be close to impossible. The first rule is not to give in to older patients saying they won't be able to breathe or swallow with the dam in place. Older patients' tongues will wander more that younger patients and a dam in place will inhibit the tongue from being overly active. Without the dam, and the movement of the tongue, it will be easier to dislodge

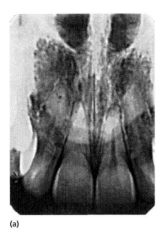 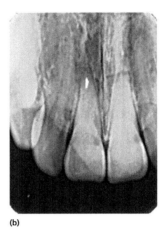

(a)   (b)

Figure 12.8 (a,b) Radiographs of a 73-year-old male patient. Note the almost complete calcification of the root canal systems of the maxillary second premolar and first and second molars. The premolar became sensitive to percussion and biting (Tooth Sleuth®). Endodontic surgery was carried out with placement of a reverse fill amalgam rather than remove the crown.

an instrument and swallow it. Again, it becomes a reversion of the patient to early childhood where the tongue is also very active. To ease breathing, cut the dam away from the nose. Four-handed assisting also aids in keeping the patient happy, and usind a saliva injector is necessary. Use a smaller rubber dam that only covers a quadrant with the mouth essentially clear. The use of the dam may be the most difficult aspect of treating aging patients endodontically. Successful root canal treatment depends on being able to isolate the tooth, as cotton rolls will not work,

There are a wide range of treatment modalities in enddontics, including the use of conventional (Fig. 12.6a,b & 12.7a,b), surgical (Fig. 12.8a,b), or combined treatments. Suffice it to say the success rates in endodontics are about 95% (Alley, 2011). The use of operating microscopes, micrometer instrumentation, rotary instruments, digital and three-dimensional radiographs, new materials to obturate root canal systems, as well as patience with the aging patients lead to such a high success rate and lead to greater numbers of teeth being retained by older individuals. Changes brought about with new instrumentation, improvements in vision enhancement, and new packing materials hasn't appreciably changed the face of endodontics. Success, either with conventional or surgical treatment is labor intensive. The

operator must sit at the chair and properly access, clean and shape, and obdurate conventionally or incise, expose, prepare, and fill root apices surgically. There are no shortcuts.

Access openings and cleaning and shaping

After the battle of rubber dam placement, access to the pulp chamber to develop straight line access is performed. Proper access should mirror the orifices of the root canal systems. However, the opening should only be as large as necessary to be able to manipulate the mouth mirror in a manner that each orifice is seen in its entirety and be accessed. Remember that all root canal systems have curves; therefore hand instruments can be curved for easier entry. Nickel–titanium (NiTi) instruments are softer than stainless steel hand instruments and they follow the curve of the system; therefore, they are not curved. They also are able to be centered in the canal system leading to a more round preparation, which is easier to obdurate. There is a tendency to under-shape systems with these instruments since they are not as sharp as hand instruments.

The objective remains that a preparation should be developed as a continuous, funnel-like, tapering preparation which can be packed three-dimensionally. Gates–Glidden burs may be used to augment the upper third of the preparation (Schilder, 1974) before other rotaries are introduced. Manufacturers claim that NiTi instrumentation is all that is needed in root canal system preparations. However, a hybrid methodology had been developed at the University of California School of Dentistry that uses NiTi files to within 3–4 mm of the apex with stainless steel hand instruments used to the radiographic orifice. The use of the stainless steel hand instruments ensures confinement of the apical portal of exit in its same position spatially. This results in a shape of the root canal system of the narrowest potion at is narrowest part of the canal at the apex and largest at the orifice of the orifice of the canal system. This is a great method that avoids over-enlargement of the apical portion of the system.

As with all cleaning and shaping regimens, irrigation after the use of each instrument is a major part of the protocol. Irrigation regimens and solutions generally disinfect the root canal system rather than sterilize it. Many studies have generated data that indicates that combinations of irrigants may result in sterilization within the root canal. Therefore, a method of irrigation should be used that will rid the system of debris, both inorganic and organic. The regimen recommended consists of the use of sodium hypochlorite (NaOCl at full strength: 6%) with ethylenediaminetetraacetic acid (EDTA: 17%). NaOCl dissolves organic debris while EDTA is used for inorganic debris (Siquiera et al., 1998). A smear layer is created during cleaning and shaping, and there is great controversy as to whether or not to remove it through use of irrigants. The recommended irrigants may be used in an alternating manner, with the last application being NaOCl. The use of these solutions is another good reason to apply a rubber dam, which will stop any leakage into the oral cavity (Bystrom & Sundqvist 1985; Lottanti et al., 2009; Rossi-Fedele et al., 2012; Siquiera et al., 2007; Zehnder, 2006).

A final word about the use of calcium hydroxide in an attempt to sterilize the canal systems. Many years ago, patients were treated over three appointments as endodontists believed that it was necessary to accomplish complete removal of microorganisms. The first appointment was for cleaning and shaping, the second to take a culture, and the third to obturate. If the second appointment culture was negative, the belief was that sterilization had occurred. The problem with this was that the wrong culture media was used and operators were culturing for aerobes instead of anaerobes and, thus, culturing was generally discarded. This eventually led to the elimination of multi-appointment procedures and one-appointment procedures became the treatment of choice for a great many practitioners. However, some studies used calcium hydroxide $(CaOH)_2$ placed in the root canal system after the first appointment, leaving it in place for at least a week if not two weeks. (Siquiera, et al. 2007). This regimen required multi-visit treatments and caused a great deal of discussion as to the need of at least two appointments and the value of sterilizing root canal systems. There has been no resolution of this issue. There is an old saying in endodontics that precedes completion of root canal therapy: "What is taken out of the root system is more important than what is put back into the system." The phrase is somewhat apocryphal but has been repeated many times over the years. It is certainly proper to take out the contents of the system as thoroughly as possible, but it may eventually lead to three-appointment endodontics and culturing before obturation.

Obturation

Over the years, many discussions in endodontics concerning the use of gutta percha (GP), spoke to its advantages and disadvantages as an obturation material. From the standpoint of cleaning and shaping, there appeared to be more disadvantages than advantages. This "dissonance" occurred due to how the material was used to end up with a very dense material. When used cold with spreaders, auxiliary cones were placed laterally around the master cone, the spreaders were inserted and the material distorted in an effort to completely pack the system space. The advent of warm GP changed the manner in how the material was packed (Langeland, 1974; Schilder, 1967). Studies found the removing increments of GP with warmed instruments softened the material ahead of the heated instruments and, when the removal reached 5 mm from the apical portal of exit, the remaining GP was now warm and could be pushed the last 0.5 mm to "cork" the apical opening. Flat surface pluggers engage the warmed GP and are able to move it apically in order to obtain a three-dimensional pack within the system. The ability move GP apically allowed the cleaning and shaping process to reach the radiographic apex.

Needless to say, examinations of well-prepared root canal systems demonstrated that the dentin surfaces were not entirely smooth. Therefore, together with GP, a sealer needed to be placed to fill any voids. The sealer also filled the many portals of exit (lateral or accessory canals) found in the apical 5 mm. The preferred sealer used with GP is a zinc oxide-eugenol (ZOE) -based sealer that is easily mixed and placed and allows sufficient working time. The use of Resilon® with a resin sealer can be used as GP and its sealer are used and give the operator another choice of a packing material. The material can be warmed and packed ad is GP.

The success of surgical operating microscopes increased the success of surgical procedures as their use disclosed more apical anatomy. They were first thought to increase the success rate of conventional treatments but seem to have somewhat less success than conventional treatments. The isthmus between mesio-buccal and mesio-lingual apical openings in lower molars and between MB 1 and MB 2 in upper molars also can be viewed (Del Fabbro et al., 2007; Hannahan & Eleazer, 2008; Naito, 2010; Ng et al., 2011; Seltzer et al., 2012).

Retreatment

Treatment modalities presently used in endodontics utilize methods that allow teeth once treated to be retreated conventionally. Retreatment has become the treatment of choice before surgical intervention in these situations and appears to be more successful than surgery (Barnes & Patel, 2011; Ng et al., 2011; Torabinejad, 2009; Wong, 2004). In aging patients, both retreatment and surgical options can be used to retain essential teeth.

Lastly, the introduction of dental implants offers another treatment option. However, their use should not become the be-all, end-all choice of a treatment modality. The easier route for these patients would be conventional and retreatment therapy. This can occur when the "team" approach to older patients is utilized. This allows the older patient to receive complete information as to the different treatment options, the better to make an educated decision. That approach also will prevent an endodontic procedure that will not succeed and prevent the loss of a tooth that can be successfully treated.

Vital pulp therapy

No discussion on endodontic treatments would be complete without consideration of vital pulp therapy. Most clinical investigations concerning direct or indirect pulp capping tend to be carried out in young to early middle-aged patient. (Bjorndal et al., 2010; Willershausen et al., 2011). A few studies have been classified as examining aging to elderly individuals 65–85 years of age or older. Therefore, the success or failure of pulp capping in aging patients has not thoroughly been examined. An early study evaluated the success of pulp capping in 148 patients aged 10–67 with a 3-year follow-up. The author found an 88% rate of clinical success with the older patients having a similar success rate (Weiss, 1966). A later study evaluated the success of pulp capping in 149 patients aged 8–74. There was a minimum 5–10 year follow-up. There was a similar success rate (Haskell et al., 1978). Barthel et al. (2000) found the same findings in a cohort of patients aged 10–70 when followed for 5–10 years. A slight trend towards failure was found when comparing patients over age 40 to those over 60 years of age (Matuso et al., 1996).

The above studies indicated that age as a prognostic factor didn't appear to play a decisive role in success or failure of pulp capping, However, there were no reports as to the extent of remaining pulp tissue in the root systems. In one retrospective study, authors reported that teeth pulp capped in 60-year-old patients showed significantly lower favorable outcomes (Dammasche et al., 2010). A second study found that the success rate in pulp capped teeth decreased as age increased (Auschill et al., 2003). Neither result is surprising due to the changes previously described as occurring in the dental pulp and dentin of aging patients.

Regenerative endodontics

The future of endodontics will embrace the field of soft tissue regeneration. Several studies have reported the formation of a new pulp-like tissue forming in adult teeth with incompletely formed apices. These cases include dens in dente, traumatized teeth, teeth with necrotic pulp tissue, and periradicular lesions (Banchs & Trope, 2004; Bose et al., 2009; Ding et al., 2009). The interest in regenerative endodontics began with the pulp capping procedures earlier in the 20th century. Today's research identifies a group of primitive cells (progenitor, stem cells) necessary to develop new odontoblast-like cells, dentin, periodontal ligament, and bone. However, studies to date have taken place in test tubes/plated laboratories and in animals. If, however, pulp capping procedures can succeed in some older patients, regenerative protocols also may be successful. With life expectancies continuing to increase, the field may lead to protocols that, rather than treat a tooth through a root canal procedure, a regenerative pulp procedure may be an approach that older patients would embrace as a treatment procedure that could be easier than a root canal or surgical procedure.

Periodontal considerations

Since periodontics and endodontics essentially treat the attachment apparatus of the tooth and may affect the success of procedures in the two specialties, a brief review is included of the effects of aging occurring in the adjacent periodontal tissue. The notion that age leads to periodontal disease progression has been a controversial topic over the past few decades. Early evidence shows increase in periodontal disease prevalence and severity with older age (Johnson et al., 1989; Van der Velden, 1984). Epidemiologic studies demonstrate that there is a significant increase in periodontal attachment loss, alveolar bone loss, and tooth loss with age. However, the effect of age on increase in periodontal probing depths appears to be nominal (Albandar, 2002). Although early studies demonstrated such effects of aging on the periodontium, age alone does not lead to severe periodontal attachment loss in elderly patients (Huttner, 2009). Therefore the notion that periodontitis is an expected outcome again has been questioned (Papapanou et al., 1991). Current evidence suggests that severe periodontal disease among elderly patients is not as common as thought of earlier (Burt & Eklund, 1999). Periodontal disease progression as seen in increase in attachment loss, increases with age in elderly patients. However, this is due to the time factor of successful aging rather than pathology (Locker et al., 1998). Thus, it is expected that changes in the oral cavity hard and soft tissue, such as the periodontium, will occur, but is due to the cumulative effect of time rather than the susceptibility of older patients to periodontal disease. This aspect of periodontal disease increase may occur due to inadequate manual dexterity to allow older patients to take care of their teeth and supporting oral structures.

Conclusion

This chapter has reviewed, as much as space permits, the tenets of endodontics in aging patients. A review of the biology of the dental pulp preceded a review of the treatment modalities. In most cases, older patients should be treated the same as younger patients, with the expectation of the same degree of success if correct treatment principles are followed before, during, and after treatment. But, as described in this chapter, in many instances the biology of older patients' pulp tissue and surrounding dentin undergoes changes that, if not recognized, will lead to mistreatment and loss of teeth. The changes that occur have been recognized for several years, yet the greater body of dentists will treat all their aging patients exactly as they treat their younger patients.

A final word: life expectancy appears to increase every decade. No one knows if these increases will continue or not. In any case, aging patients deserve the best care available, which means that dentists and endodontists must be aware of older patients' dental needs.

Case study 1

Mrs. Ethyl Smith is a new patient. She is 79 years old, walks with either a cane or a metal walker with wheels, has been diagnosed with type 2 diabetes, high blood pressure, osteoporosis and arthritis, and is somewhat frail. However, she appears to be mentally sharp with no history of a dementia. The patient is not capable of sitting upright for long periods of time. She is well-dressed, neat, and speaks to you quietly clearly. She admits to being nervous in a dental chair and is concerned that she will lose her teeth as she grows older.

Complaints

Pain on biting in the lower right quadrant and sensitivity to putting on her make-up at the outer lower right cheek area adjacent to the lower premolars and molars. All posterior teeth in her mouth have been restored with PBM crowns and the posterior areas appears to show calculus build-up. She presents with radiographs taken 4 months ago by another dentist. She claims that the other dentist frightened her with his treatment plan.

Case study questions: diagnosis and treatment planning

A Describe the methodology used to make the patient comfortable, both physically and mentally.
B What questions might you ask to put this patient at ease and comfortable in the chair? What questions might you ask concerning the patient's symptoms?
C List the diagnostic tests and the tooth testing needed to make a proper diagnosis. Discuss the rational of the tests used and what responses would possibly be forthcoming.
D What area of a tooth might you describe to the patient? What would you tell the patient to put her at ease during treatment?
(Up to this point the answers to each area above are rather generic. The dentist should now focus on the areas of treatment to be rendered based on his or her knowledge. Therefore, the review of these questions are based on specific knowledge known to the provider consistent with the answers to the following discussion questions.)

DISCUSSION QUESTIONS

1 Describe the tooth structures that normally protect the dental pulp.
2 Identify the various types of dentin in a tooth and the stimuli that causes them to form.
3 What is the role of the dental pulp in an adult tooth?
4 Describe the function of native odontoblasts.
5 What are the main reasons for older patients responding to tooth (pulp) testing?
6 What type dentin forms in response to caries reaching the pulp?
7 Why may treatment of an aging patient take take two or more appointments to complete treatment?
8 Discuss the treatment modalities used in contemporary endodontics and the materials used to complete treatment successfully.

References

About, I., Murray, P.E., Franquin, J.C., *et al.* (2001) The effect of cavity restoration variables on odontoblast cell numbers and dental repair. *Journal of Dentistry,* **29**(2), 109–17.

Agematsu, H., Someda, H., Hashimoto, M., *et al.* (2010) Three-dimensional observation of decrease in pulp cavity volume using micro-CT: age-related change. *Bulletin of the Tokyo Dental College,* **51**(1), 1–6.

Albandar, J.M. (2002). Global risk factors and risk indicators for periodontal diseases. *Periodontology 2000,* **29**, 177–206.

Allen, P.F. & Whitworth, J.M. (2004) Endodontic considerations in the elderly. *Gerodontology,* **21**(4), 185–94.

Alley, B.S. (2004) A comparison of survival of teeth following endodontic treatment performed by general dentists or by speicialists. *Oral Surgery Oral Medicine Oral Pathology Oral Radiology and Endodontics,* **98**(1), 115–18.

Auschill, T.M., Arweiler, N.B., Hellwig, E., *et al.* (2003) Success rate of direct pulp capping with calcium hydroxide. *Schweiz Monatsschr Zahnmed,* **113**(9) 946–52.

Banchs, F. & Trope, M. (2004) Revascualrization of immature permanent teeth with apical periodontitis: new treatment. *Journal of Endodontics,* **30**(4), 196–200.

Barnes, J.J. & Patel, S. (2011) Contemporary endodontics – part 1. *British Dental Journal,* **211**(10), 463–8.

Barthel C.R., Rosenkranz, B., Leuenberg, A. & Roulet, J.F. (2000) Pulp capping of carious exposures: treatment outcome after 5 and 10 years: a retrospective study. *Journal of Endodontics,* **26**(9), 525–8.

Berman, L.H. & Hartwell, G.R. (2011) Diagnosis. In: *Pathways of the Pulp* (eds. K.M. Hargreaves, S. Cohen & K. Keiser), 10th edn., pp. 2–39. Mosby, St. Louis.

Bernick, S. (1962a) Age changes in nerves of molar teeth of rats. *Anatomical Record,* **143**, 121–6.

Bernick, S. (1962b) Age changes in the blood supply to molar teeth of rats. *Anatomical Record,* **144**, 265–74.

Bernick, S. (1967a) Effect of aging on the nerve supply to human teeth. *Journal of Dental Research,* **46** (4), 694–9.

Bernick, S. (1967b) Age changes in the blood supply to human teeth. *Journal of Dental Research,* **46**(3), 544–50.

Bernick, S. (1972) Vascular and nerve changes associated with the healing of the human pulp. *Oral Surgery Oral Medicine oral Pathology Radiology Endodontics,* **33**(6), 983–1000.

Bernick, S. & Nedelman, C. (1975) Effect of aging on the human pulp. *Journal of Endodontics,* **1**(3), 88–94.

Bjorndal, L., Reit, C., Bruun, G., *et al.* (2010) Treatment of deep carious lesions in adults: randomized clinical trials comparing stepwise vs. direct complete excavation, and direct pulp capping vs. partial pulpotomy. *European Journal of Oral Sciences,* **118**(3), 290–7.

Bose, R., Nummikoski, P. & Hargreaves, K. (2009) A retrospective evaluation of radiographic outcomes in immature teeth with necrotic root canal systems treated with regenerative endodontic procedures. *Journal of Endodontics,* **35**(10), 1343–9.

Burke, F.M. & Samarawickrama, D.Y. (1995) Progressive chages in the pulpo-dentinal complex and their consequences. *Gerodontology,* **12**(12), 57–66.

Burt, B.A. & Eklund, S.A. (1999) *Dentistry, Dental Practice, and the Community.* Saunders, Philadelphia.

Bystrom, A. & Sundqvist, G. (1985) The antibacterial action of sodium hypochlorite and EDTA in 60 cases of endodontic therapy. *International Endodontic Journal,* **18**(1), 35–40.

Centers for Disease Control and Prevention (2012) *Health, United States 2012.* National Center for Health Statistics, Hyattsville, MD, pp. 106–7.

Chalmers, J.M. (2006a) Minimal intervention dentistry: part 1. Strategies for addressing the new caries challenge in older patients. *Journal of the Canadian Dental Association,* **72**(5), 427–33.

Chalmers, J.M. (2006b) Minimal intervention dentistry: part 2. Strategies for addressing restorative challenges in older patients. *Journal of the Canadian Dental Association,* **72**(5), 435–40.

Ciancio, S.G. (1996) Medications as risk factors for periodontal disease. *The Journal of Periodontology,* **67**, 1055–9.

Cooper, P.R., Takahashi, Y., Graham, L.W., *et al.* (2010) Inflammation–regeneration interplay in the dentine–pulp complex. *Journal of Dentistry,* **38**(9), 687–97.

Couve, E. & Schmachtenberg, O. (2011) Autophagic activity and aging in human odontoblasts. *Journal of Dental Research,* **90**(4), 523–8.

Couve, E., Osorio, R. & Schmachtenberg, O. (2012) Mitochondrial autophagy and lipofuscin accumulation in aging odontoblasts. *Journal of Dental Research,* **91**(7), 696–701.

Dammaschke, T., Leidinger, J., Schäfer, E. (2010) Long-term evalutation of direct pulp capping – treatment outcomes over and ave rage period of 6.1 years. *Clinical Oral Investigations,* **14**(5), 559–67.

Del Fabbro, M., Taschieri, S., Testori, T., *et al.* (2007) Surgical versus non-surgical endodontic re-treatment for periradicular lesions. *Cochrane Database and Systematic Reviews,* **18**(3), CD005511.

Ding, R.Y., Cheung, G.S., Chen, J. *et al.* (2009) Pulp revascularization of immature teeth with apical periodontitis: a clinical study. *Journal of Endodontics,* **35**(5), 745–9.

Domine, L., & Holz, J. (1991) The aging of the human pulp–dentin organ. *Schweizer Monatsschrift für Zahnmedizin,* **101**(6), 725–33.

Eldarrat, A.H., High, A.S. & Kale G.M. (2010) Age-related changes in AC-impedance spectroscopy studies of normal human dentine: further investigation. *Journal of Material Science and Materials in Medicine,* **21**(1), 45–51.

El Karim, I.A., Linden, G.J., Curtis, T.M., *et al.* (2011) Human odontoblasts express functional thermo-sensitive TRP channels: implications for dentin sensitivity. *Pain,* **152**(10), 2211–23.

Fieler, B. (2012) 'The father is child of the man'. *The New York Times,* July **29**, 2012.

Fried, K. (1992) Changes in pulpal nerves with aging. *Proceedings of the Finnish Dental Society,* **88** (Suppl 1), 517–28.

Fried, K. & Hildebrand, C. (1981) Pulpal axons in developing, mature, and aging feline permanent incisors. A study by electron microscopy. *Journal of Compendium Neurology,* **203**(1), 23–36.

Galen, D. (1990) Endodontics and the elderly patient – management considerations. *Journal of the Canadian Dental Association,* **56**(6), 483–7.

Gani, O. & Visvisian, C. (1999) Apical canal diameter in the first upper molar at various ages. *Journal of Endodontics,* **25**(10), 689–91.

Goodis, H.E., Rossall, J.C. & Kahn, A.J. (2001) Endodontic status in older US adults. Report of a survey. *Journal of the American Dental Association,* **132**(11), 525–30.

Hannahan, J.P. & Eleazer, P.D. (2008) Comparison of success of implants versus endodontically treated teeth. *Journal of Endodontics,* **34**(11), 1302–5.

Hargreaves, K.M., Goodis, H.E. & Tay, F.R. (2012) *Seltzer and Bender's Dental Pulp*, 2nd edn. Mosby Elsevier, St. Louis.

Haskell, E.W., Stanley, H.R., Chellemi, J. & Stringfellow, H. (1978) Direct pulp capping treatment: a long-term follow-up. *Journal of the American Dental Association*, **97**(4), 607–12.

Hassan, B., Metska, M.E., Ozok, A.R. *et al.* (2009) Detection of vertical root fractures in endodontically treated teeth by a cone beam computed tomography scan. *Journal of Endodontics*, **35**(5), 719–22.

Hillmann, G. & Geursten, W. (1997) Light-microscopic investigation of the distribution of extracellular matrix molecules and calcifications in human dental pulps of various ages. *Cell and Tissue Research*, **289**(1), 145–54.

Holland, G.R. (1985) The odontoblast process; form and function. *Journal of Dental Research*, **64**, 499–514.

Holland, G.R. (1994) Morphological features of dentine and pulp related to dentine sensitivity. *Archives of Oral Biology*, **39** (Suppl), 3S–11S.

Huttner, E.A., (2009) Effects of human aging on periodontal tissues. *Special Care in Dentistry*, **29**(4), 149–55.

Ikawa, M., Komatsu, H., Ikawa, K., *et al.* (2003) Age-related changes in the human pulpal blood flow measured by laser Doppler flowmetry. *Dental Traumatology*, **19**(1), 36–40.

Jafazadh, H. (2009) Laser Doppler flowmetry in endodontics: a review. *International Endodontic Journal*, **42**(6), 476–90.

Johnson, B.D., Mulligan, K, Kiyak, H.A. & Marder, M. (1989) Aging or disease? Periodontal changes and treatment considerations in the older dental patient. *Gerodontology*, **8**(4), 109–18

Kaya, S., Adiguzel, O., Yavuz, I., *et al.* (2011) Cone-beam dental computerized tomography for evaluating changes of aging in the dimensions central superior incisor root canals. *Medicina Oral Patologia Oral y Cirugia Bucal*, **16**(3), e463–6.

Kim, S. (1985a) Regulation of pulpal blood flow. *Journal of Dental Research*, **64**, 590–6.

Kim, S. (1985b) Microcirculation of the dental pulp in health and disease. *Journal of Endodontics*, **11**(11), 465–71.

Kvaal, S.I., Koppang, H.S. & Solheim, T. (1994) Relationship between age and deposit of peritubular dentine. *Gerodontology*, **11**(2), 93–8.

Langeland, D. (1974) Root canal sealers and pastes. *Dental Clinics of North America*, **18**(2), 309–27.

Locker, D., Slade, G.D. & Murray, H. (1998) Epidemiology of periodontal disease among older adults: a review. *Periodontology 2000*, **16**, 16–33.

Lottanti, S., Gautschi, H., Sener, B. & Zehnder, M. (2009) Effects of ethylenediaminetetracetic, etidronic and per-acetic acid irrigation on human root dentine and the smear layer. *International Endodontic Journal*, **42**(4), 335–43.

Ma, Q., Hu, X. & Yu, P. (1997) [Studies on aging enzyme activities of the human dental pulp blood vessels]. *Zhonghua Kou Qiang Yi Za Zhi*, **32**(2), 81–3.

Magloire, H., Maurin, J.C., Couble, M.L., *et al.* (2010) Topical review. Dental pain and odontoblasts: facts and hypotheses. *Journal of Oral Pain*, **24**, 335–49.

Maret, D., Peters, O.A., Dedouit, F., *et al.* (2011) Cone-beam computed tomography: a useful tool for dental age estimation? *Medical Hypotheses*, **76**(5), 700–2.

Matuso, T., Nakanishi, T., Shimizu, H. & Ebisu, S. (1996) A clinical study of direct pulp capping applied to carious-exposed pulps. *Journal of Endodontics*, **22**(10), 551–6.

Matysiak, M., Dubois, J.P., Ducastelle, T. & Hemet, J. (1986) Morphometric analysis of human pulp myelinated fibers during aging. *Journal de Biologie Buccale*, **14**(1), 69–79.

Matysiak, M., Dubois, J.P., Ducastelle, T. & Hemet, J. (1988) [Morphometric study of variations related to human aging in pulp unyelinated and myelinated axons]. *Journal de Biologie Buccale*, **16**(2), 59–68.

Morse, D.R. (1991) Age-related changes of the dental pulp complex in relationship to systemic aging. *Oral Surgery Oral Medicine Oral Pathology, Radiology and Endodontics*, **72**(6), 721–45.

Morse, D.R., Esposito, J.V., Schoor, R.S. (1993) A radiographic study of aging changes of the dental pulp and dentin in normal teeth. *Quintessence International*, **24**(5), 329–33.

Murray, P.E., About, I., Lumley, P.J., *et al.* (2000) Human odontoblast cell numbers after dental injury. *Journal of Dentistry*, **28**(4), 277–88.

Naito, T. (2010) Surgical or nonsurgical treatment for teeth with existing root filings? *Evidence Based Dentistry*, **11**(2), 54–5.

Ng, Y.L., Mann, V., Gulabivata, K. (2011) A prospective study of the factors affecting outcomes on non-surgical root canal treatment: part 1: periapical health. *International Endodontic Journal*, **44**(7), 583–609.

Ng, Y.L., Mann, V., Gulabivata, K. (2011) A prospective study of the factors affecting outcomes of non-surgical root canal treatment: part 2: tooth survival. *International Endodontic Journal*, **44**(7), 610–25.

Nielsen, C.J. (1983) Age-related changes in reducible cross-links of human dental pulp collagen. *Archieves of Oral Biology*, **28**(8), 759–64.

Oginni, A.O., Adekova-Sofowora, C.A. & Kolavole, K.A. (2009) Evaluation of radiographs, clinical signs and symptoms associated with pulp canal obliteration: an aid to treatment decision. *Dental Traumatology*, **25**(6), 620–5.

Okumura, R., Shima, K., Muramatsu, T., *et al.* (2005) The odontoblast as a sensory receptor cell? The expression of TRPV1 (VR-1) channels. *Archives of Histology and Cytology*, **68**, 251–7.

Ozer, S.Y. (2010) Detection of vertical fractures of different thicknesses in endodontically enlarged teeth by cone beam computed tomography versus digital radiography. *Journal of Endodontics*, **36**(7), 1245–9.

Pääkkönen, V., Bleicher, F., Carrouel, F., *et al.* (2009) General expression profiles of human native odontoblasts and pulp-derived cultured odontoblast-like cells are similar but reveal differential neuropeptide expression levels. *Archives of Oral Biology*, **54**(1), 55–62.

Papapanou, P.N., Lindhe, J., Sterrett, J.D. & Eneroth, L. (1991) Considerations on the contribution of ageing to loss of periodontal tissue support. *Journal of Clinical Periodontology*, **18**(8), 611–15.

Patel, S. (2009) New dimensions in endodontic imaging: part 2. Cone beam computed tomography. *International Endodontic Journal*, **42**(6), 463–75.

Patel, S., Dawood, A., Whaites, E. & Pitt Ford, T. (2009) New dimensions in endodontic imaging: part 1. Conventional and alternative radiographic systems. *International Endodontic Journal*, **42**(6), 447–62.

Patel, S., Wilson, R., Dawood, A., *et al.* (2012) The detection of periapical pathosis using digital periapical radiography and cone beam computed tomography – part 2: a 1 year post-treatment follow-up. *International Endodontic Journal*, **45**(8), 711–23.

Philippas, G.G. & Applebaum, E. (1966) Age factor in secondary dentin formation. *Journal of Dental Research*, **45**(3), 778–89.

Qualtrough, A.J. & Mannocci, F. (2011) Endodontics and the older patient. *Dental Update*, **38**(8), 559–62.

Rossi-Fedele, G., Doğramaci, E.J., Guastalli, A.R., *et al.* (2012) Antagonistic interactions between sodium hypochloride, Chlorhexidine, EDTA, and citric acid. *Journal of Endodontics*, **38**(4), 426–31.

Schilder, H. (1967) Filling root canal in three dimensions. *Dental Clinics of North America*, **4**, 723–44.

Schilder, H. (1974) Cleaning and shaping the root canal. *Dental Clinics of North America*, **18**(2), 269–96.

Seltzer, F.C., Kohli, M.R., Shah, S.B., *et al.* (2012) Outcome of endodontic surgery: a meta-analysis of the literature – part 2: comparison of endodontic microsurgical techniques with and without the use of higher magnification. *Journal of Endodontics*, **38**(1), 1–10.

Sherwood, I.A. (2012) Pre-operative diagnostic radiograph interpretation by general dental practitioners for root canal treatment. *Dentomaxillofacial Radiology*, **41**(1), 43–54.

Silva, J.A., de Alencar, A.H., da Rocha, S.S. *et al.* (2012) Three-dimensional image contribution for evaluation of operative procedural errors in endodontic therapy and dental implants. *Brazilian Dental Journal*, **23**(2), 127–34.

Siqiera, J.F., Jr., Batista, M.M., Fraga, R.C. & de Uzeda M. (1998) Antibacterial effects of endodontic irrigants on black-pigmented gram-negative anaerobes and facultative bacteria. *Journal of Endodontics*, **24**(6), 414–16.

Siqiera, J.F., Jr., Guimarães-Pinto, T., Rôças, I.N. (2007) Effects of chemomechanical preparation winth 2.5% sodium hypochlorite and intracanal medication with calcium hydroxide on cultivable bacteria in infected root canals. *Journal of Endodontics*, **33**(7), 800–5.

Smith, A.J., Tobias, R.S., Cassidy, N., *et al.* (1994) Odontoblast stimulation in ferrets by dentine matrix components. *Archieves of Oral Biology*, **39**(1), 13–22.

Smith, A.J., Cassidy, N., Perry, H., *et al.* (1995) Reactionary dentinogenesis. *International Journal of Developmental Biology*, **39**(1), 273–80.

Son, A.R., Yang, Y.M., Hong, J.H., *et al.* (2009) Odontoblasts TRP channel and thermo/mechanical transmission. *Journal of Dental Research*, **88**(11), 1014–19.

Stabholz, A., Sahar-Helft, S. & Moshonov, J. (2004) Lasers in endodontics. *Dental Clinics of North America*, **48**(4), 809–32.

Stanley, H.R. (1961) Traumatic capacity of high-speed and ultrasonic dental instrumentation. *Journal of the American Dental Association*, **63**, 749–66.

Stanley, H.R. (1977) Management of the aging patient and the aging pulp. *Journal of the California Dental Association*, **5**(5), 62–4.

Torabinejad, M. (2009) Outcomes of nonsurgical retreatment and endodontic surgery: a systematic review. *Journal of Endodontics*, **35**(7), 930–7.

Trope, M. (2008) Regenerative potential of dental pulp. *Journal of Endodontics*, **34**(7 Suppl), S13–17.

Tyndall, D.A. & Kohltfarber, H. (2012) Application of cone beam volumetric tomography in endodontics. *Australian Dental Journal*, **57**(Suppl 1), 72–81.

Tyndall, D.A. & Rathore, S. (2008) Cone-beam CT diagnostic applications: caries, periodontal bone assessment, and endodontic applications. *Dental Clinics of North America*, **52**(4), 825–41.

Van der Velden, U. (1984). Effect of age on the periodontium. *Journal of Clinical Periodontology*, **11**(5), 281–94.

Walton, R.E. (1997) Endodontic considerations in the geriatric patient. *Dental Clinics of North America*, **41**(4), 795–816.

Wang, P., Yan, X.B., Lui, D.G., *et al.* (2011) Detection of dental root fractures by using cone-beam computed tomography. *Dentomaxillofacial Radiology*, **40**(5), 290–8.

Weiss, M. (1966) Pulp capping in older patients. *New York State Dental Journal*, **32**(10), 451–7.

Willershausen, B., Willershausen, I., Ross, A., *et al.* (2011) Retrospective study on direct pulp capping with calcium hydroxide. *Quintessence International*, **42**(2), 165–71.

Wong, R. (2004) Conventional endodontic failure and retreatment. *Dental Clinics of North America*, **48**, 265–89.

Woo, S.P. (2001) *Secondary dentin formation and root canal occlusion in middle-aged to elderly men in a VA dental logitudinal study.* Master of Science thesis, University of California, School of Dentistry, CA, USA.

Zach, L. & Cohen, G. (1962) Thermogenesis in operative techniques. *Journal of Prosthetic Dentistry*, **12**, 977–84.

Zach, L. & Cohen, G. (1967) Pulp response to externally applied heat. *Oral Surgery Oral Medicine Oral Pathology Radiology and Endodontics*, **19**, 515–30.

Further reading

Alian, A., McNally, M.E., Fure, S. & Birkhed, D. (2006) Assessment of caries risk in elderly patients using the car-iogram model. *Journal of the Canadian Dental Association,* **72**(5), 459–63.

American Association of Endodontists; American Academy of Oral and Maxillofacial Radiology (2011) Use of cone-beam computed tomography in endodontics. Joint Position Statement of the American Association of Endodontists and the American Academy of Oral and Maxillofacial Radiology. *Oral Surgery Oral Medicine Oral Pathology Radiology and Endodontics,* **111**(2), 234–7.

Cooper, P.R., McLachlan, J.L., Simon, S., *et al.* (2011) Mediators of inflammation and regeneration. *Advances in Dental Research,* **23**(3), 290–5.

CHAPTER 13

Oral Mucosal Lesions

Miriam R. Robbins

Department of Oral and Maxillofacial Pathology, Radiology, and Medicine, New York University College of Dentistry, New York, NY, USA

Introduction

The intent of this chapter is to identify some of the most common oral lesions in the older adult and present the information in an easily accessible format. Clinical photos are presented with each condition to facilitate identification and diagnosis.

The oral mucosa is a common site for a wide variety of lesions, including ulcerative, vesiculobullous, desquamative, lichenoid, infectious, and malignant. Both normal changes associated with aging and pathologic factors can contribute to the presence of oral pathoses. As people age, the mucosa becomes atrophic resulting in thinner and less elastic tissue. This change in cellular structure combined with a decline in the immunologic responsiveness also associated with aging, results in an increased susceptibility to infection and trauma. Other contributing factors are the increases in incidence of systemic diseases and the use of multiple medications, especially those that result in xerostomia (discussed in Chapter 14).

Any mucosal lesion that does not respond as expected within an appropriate period of time or that persists despite all attempts to resolve any underlying etiology should be biopsied to determine the diagnosis. All patients, even if edentulous, should have an annual head and neck exam with a through intraoral soft tissue examination to evaluate the presence of any lesions and to intervene at an early stage with appropriate treatment.

Each of the conditions presented will be discussed according to the following format:

1 Etiology
2 Clinical presentation
3 Diagnosis
4 Treatment.

Burning mouth syndrome

Burning mouth syndrome (BMS) is characterized by a continuous burning sensation of the oral mucosa and/or tongue, usually without accompanying clinical and laboratory findings (Patton *et al.*, 2007). It is more common in middle-aged or older women with increasing prevalence associated with increasing age (Bergdahl & Bergdahl, 1999), and is often accompanied by subjective complaints of dysgeusia and xerostomia.

Etiology

The most common etiology of BMS is idiopathic, although it may represent a chronic neuropathic condition that may be exacerbated by psychogenic factors. Other conditions including lichen planus, candidiasis, menopause and other hormone imbalances, nutritional or vitamin deficiencies, xerostomia, gastrointestinal disorders, diabetes, thyroid disorders, nerve injuries, or medication side effects may need to be considered (Patton *et al.*, 2007).

Clinical presentation

BMS is characterized by the absence of clinical signs. Candidiasis and salivary hypofunction may be concurrent findings.

Diagnosis

The diagnosis is established after all possible etiologic factors have been eliminated based on history, physical evaluation and laboratory studies. Baseline

Geriatric Dentistry: Caring for Our Aging Population, First Edition. Edited by Paula K. Friedman.

© 2014 John Wiley & Sons, Inc. Published 2014 by John Wiley & Sons, Inc.

Companion website: www.wiley.com/go/friedman/geriatricdentistry

complete blood count (CBC) with differential, fasting glucose, vitamin B12, folic acid, iron, ferritin, and thyroid levels should be obtained.

Treatment

There is no definitive cure. Patients should be reassured that this is not an infectious or malignant condition, but should be counseled that this is a chronic pain condition. Approximately 50% of patients with BMS show improvement of symptoms after 6–7 years (Sardella *et al.*, 2006). Treatment is aimed at relieving discomfort and should be individualized based on symptoms. A variety of topical and systemic treatments have been proposed with variable evidence to support their use (Patton *et al.*, 2007). There is some evidence to support cognitive behavioral therapy as an adjunct to pharmacologic therapies (Sardella *et al.*, 2006).

Topical treatments include clonazepam-dissolvable wafers (0.5 mg twice daily) or mouth rinse (1 mg/5 ml), oral capsaicin, doxepin solution (10 mg/ml), viscous lidocaine, and diphenhydramine elixir (12.5 mg/5 ml).

Systemic treatments include alpha-lipoic acid (600 mg daily), low doses of selective serotonin reuptake inhibitors (SSRIs), tricyclic antidepressants, benzodiazepines, anticonvulsants, clonazepam (0.5 mg tablets 3 times a day) or alprazolam (0.25 mg tablets 3 times a day). Dosages need to be adjusted according to the individual response and the presence/severity of side effects. Older patients taking central nervous system depressants should not be prescribed these medications without consultation with the patient's physician. In fact, systemic treatments may best be managed the patient's physician or by an appropriate dental specialist due to the prolonged nature and potential side effects (including addiction/dependency) of these therapies.

Candidiasis (see also Chapter 2)

Etiology

Oral candidiasis is an opportunistic infection most commonly caused by *Candida albicans* overgrowth, although there are other *Candida* species that can also cause this condition. In adults, oral yeast infections become more common with increased age,

especially among denture wearers (Darwazeh *et al.*, 1990). Other risk factors include antibiotic therapy, xerostomia, uncontrolled diabetes mellitus, immunosuppression, corticosteroids (both systemic and inhaled), and poor oral hygiene (Peterson, 1992).

Clinical presentation

Pseudomembraneous candidiasis (Fig. 13.1)
- Most common form.
- Soft-white elevated plaques present on mucosal membranes.
- Easily wiped away, leaving an erythematous base.
- Anywhere in mouth, but hard palate, tongue, and buccal mucosa common sites.
- May extend into oropharynx.

Erythematous (atrophic) candidiasis (Fig. 13.2)
- Erythematous sensitive patches that look "raw."

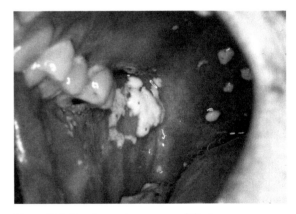

Figure 13.1 Pseudomembranous candidiasis.

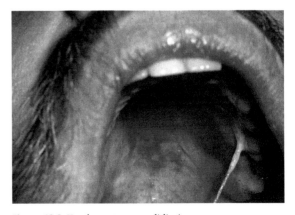

Figure 13.2 Erythematous candidiasis.

- Several forms characterized by cause and location:
  - Acute atrophic (antibiotic sore mouth):
    - Commonly caused by broad spectrum antibiotics.
    - Atrophic dorsal surface of tongue.
    - Complaint of burning sensation.
  - Chronic atrophic (denture stomatitis) (Fig. 13.3):
    - Commonly seen in patients who wear poorly fitting removable prostheses for extended periods of time (i.e., do not remove at night).
    - Well-demarcated erythematous mucosa present under denture base (usually maxilla).
    - Patients usually asymptomatic.
  - Angular chelitis (Fig. 13.4):
    - Erythema and fissuring of commissures of lips (usually bilaterally).
    - Often caused by a combination of fungal and bacteria infection.

- Median rhomboid glossitis (central papillary atrophy) (Fig. 13.5):
  - Well-demarcated rhomboid area seen in the midline of the tongue anterior to the circumvallate papillae.
  - "Kissing" lesion frequently seen on hard palate.

Hyperplastic candidiasis (candida leukoplakia) (Fig. 13.6)

- Well-defined confluent white patches that can not be wiped off.
- Common on buccal mucosa near commissures, but can be seen on hard palate and lateral tongue.
- May be leukoplakia that is colonized by *Candida*.
- Biopsy is warranted if no resolution following antifungal treatment or if there are focal areas of erythema associated with white patches.

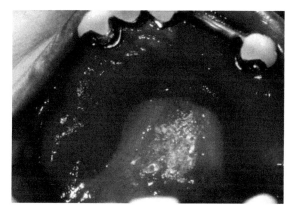

Figure 13.3 Denture stomatitis.

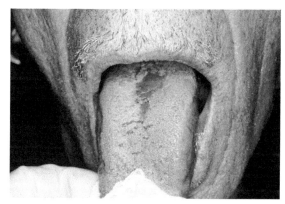

Figure 13.5 Median rhomboid glossitis.

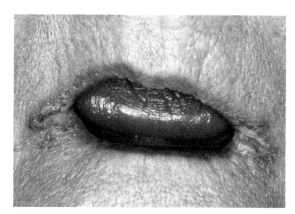

Figure 13.4 Angular chelitis.

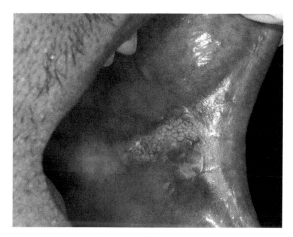

Figure 13.6 Hyperplastic candidiasis.

Diagnosis

The diagnosis of oral candidiasis is often made based on the clinical signs and symptoms and is treated empirically with antifungal medications. Additional adjunctive methods for the diagnosis of oral candidiasis include exfoliative cytology, biopsy, and culture.

Treatment

Oral candidiasis may be treated with topical or systemic antifungal therapy (Tables 13.1 & 13.2). Chronic candidiasis often requires a prolonged period of therapy. Topical applications of various forms of antifungal medications are commonly used to treat acute cases. Rinses tend to be less effective than other topical forms because the duration of tissue contact is suboptimal. Topical troches/pastilles prolong the contact of the medication with oral mucosa and are generally safe to use because of poor systemic absorption. They may not be appropriate for patients with xerostomia due to decreased ability to dissolve this form. These forms are often high in sugar and need to be used with care in diabetic patients. Oral hygiene should be emphasized to decrease the development of caries. Patients who wear dentures should be instructed to remove them prior to using a rinse, troche, or pastille (Giannin *et al.*, 2011).

Azole antifungals (the most common type of systemic medications) are potent inhibitors of cytochrome P450 system and therefore have many drug–drug interactions with other commonly prescribed medications (e.g., statins, tricyclic antidepressants, oral hypoglycemic, and warfarin) (Gubbin & Heldenbrand, 2010). Prolonged use can also lead to hepatotoxicity and liver function tests should be performed if the medication is used for more than 3 weeks.

All medications, whether topical or systemic, should be continued for several days after resolution of clinical signs. Recurrence is common while underlying etiologic factors exist. For patients with denture stomatitis, a topical antifungal can be applied to the mucosa and denture base prior to insertion (Webb *et al.*, 2005). Additionally, all removable prostheses must also be treated with antifungals to prevent a potential source of reinfection. Patients should be advised to remove and clean dentures every night. Following brushing the dentures, they can be soaked in a dilute bleach solution (1 part bleach to 10 parts water) tissue side down

Table 13.1 Topical antifungal agents

Agents	Dose/unit	Daily dosage
Nystatin topical cream, powder, ointment	100 000 U/g	Apply thin layer to affected area 3 times daily (can be applied to inner surface of denture as well)
Nystatin oral suspension	100 000 U/ml	400 000–600 000 U po; swish and swallow 4–5 times a day
Nystatin pastilles	200 000 U	200 000–400 000 U po 4–5 times a day
Nystatin vaginal suppositories (OTC)	100 000 U	100 000 U po, dissolve in mouth 4 times a day
Clotrimazole troche	10 mg	10 mg dissolved po 5 times a day for 2 weeks
Clortrimazole vaginal cream (OTC)	1%	Apply thin layer to tissue side of denture and/or affected area of mouth 4 times a day
Miconazole nitrate vaginal cream (OTC)	2%	Apply thin layer to tissue side of denture and/or affected area of mouth 4 times a day
Miconazole vaginal suppository	100 or 200 mg	Dissolve one suppository in mouth 4 times a day
Miconazole (Oravig®) buccal tablet	50 mg	Place one tab on buccal mucosa in morning for 14 days. Allow to dissolve, do not chew
Ketoconazole cream	2%	Apply thin layer to tissue side of denture and/or affected area of mouth 4 times a day
Amphotericin B suspension	100 mg/ml	100–200 mg po; swish and swallow 4 times a day
Nystatin–tramcinolone acetonide ointment	15 g tube	Apply to corners of mouth after meals and at bedtime for 2 weeks

OTC, over the counter; po, by mouth.

Table 13.2 Systemic antifungal agents

Agents	Form	Dosage
Fluconazole (Diflucan®)	Capsules	100 mg qd
Ketoconazole (Nizoral®)	Tablets	200 or 400 mg qd
Miconazole (Daktarin®)	Tablets	50 mg qd
Itraconazole (Sporanox®)	Capsules	100 mg qd

qd, once a day.

for 10 minutes. Angular chelitis generally respond well to combination therapy containing both an antifungal and steroid.

Epulis fissuratum (inflammatory fibrous hyperplasia, denture-induced fibrous hyperplasia, denture granuloma)

Epulis is a nonspecific term used for tumor-like masses of the gingiva. Epulis fissuratum occurs as a result of trauma from an ill-fitting or over-extended denture. It appears to occur more frequently in women (Zhang *et al.*, 2007).

Etiology
As alveolar bone resorbs, the denture flange become overextended and traumatizes the sulcular tissue resulting in an overgrowth of fibrous connective tissue.

Clinical presentation
Epulis presents as a single or multiple folds of hyperplastic granulation tissue surrounding the denture flange, usually in the anterior maxillary and mandibular vestibule. The tissue can become ulcerated and painful.

Diagnosis
Diagnosis is based on clinical appearance and presence of removable prostheses. Any ulcerated area that does not heal once the etiology has been resolved should be biopsied to rule out squamous cell carcinoma.

Treatment
Surgical resection of tissue is usually necessary followed by fabrication of new prostheses with reduced flange.

Geographic tongue (benign migratory glossitis)

This is a relatively common chronic condition that is usually asymptomatic.

Etiology
It is suggested, but not confirmed, that this condition may be related to psoriasis or to a hypersensitivity reaction. Some patients report exacerbation during times of stress, eating certain foods, or using certain oral hygiene products.

Clinical appearance
The dorsum of the tongue is the most common site; however, it can be found on the buccal mucosa or lip (erythema migrans). It is characterized by a migrating pattern of irregularly shaped erythematous, atrophic patches surrounded by a raised yellowish-white hyperkeratotic border (Fig. 13.7). Lesions may completely resolve and then reappear in a different pattern later. Patients are usually asymptomatic, although there may be some sensitivity to acidic or spicy foods

Diagnosis
Typical lesions can be diagnosed clinically. It may be confused with lichen planus or candidiasis with more atypical presentation.

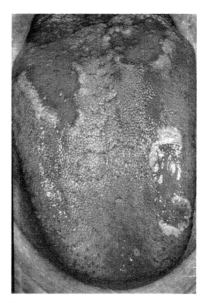

Figure 13.7 Geographic tongue.

Treatment

Since most lesions are asymptomatic, no treatment is needed. Topical steroids can be used to treat symptomatic lesions. Candidal infection should be considered in persistently symptomatic cases.

Hairy tongue

Etiology

Hairy tongue is caused by overproduction of keratin by the filiform papillae. Antibiotics, tobacco, poor oral hygiene, chronic use of hydrogen peroxide or chlorohexadine, systemic corticosteroids, xerostomia, and oral candidiasis have all been implicated in contributing to the condition. The hyperkeratinized papillae can become colored by a variety of exogenous factors such as coffee, tobacco, and chromogenic bacteria.

Clinical presentation

Elongation and pigmentation of the filiform papillae located in the posterior center of the tongue giving the dorsum of the tongue a hairy appearance (Fig. 13.8). Colors can range from white to green to brown to black.

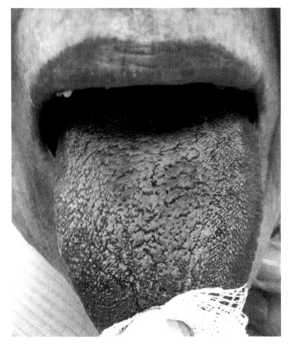

Figure 13.8 Hairy tongue.

Treatment

Elimination of possible etiologic factors and improved oral hygiene, including routine brushing and/or scraping of the tongue. Podophyllum resin (1% solution) can be painted over the affected area 3–5 times daily to help reduce the overgrowth. Immediately after application, the oral cavity must be thoroughly rinsed and the rinse expectorated due to systemic side effects of ingested podophyllum. Treatment with antifungals is indicated in those cases where fungal infection is suspected.

Herpes simplex (recurrent)

Etiology

Primary oral herpes transmission is by physical contact with the virus and is often subclinical although some individuals may have systemic symptoms including headache, fever, and vesicular eruption of the oral and perioral tissues. Following the primary occurrence, the herpes virus remains in a latent state in the trigeminal ganglion. When reactivated, the virus travels down the nerve to the site of the initial infection, most commonly the lip (herpes labialis) and causes localized vesicles and ulceration. Reactivation triggers can include exposure to sunlight or cold, trauma, stress, or immunosuppression.

Clinical presentation

Secondary or recurrent herpes infection usually affects the vermillion border of the lip and surrounding skin. Intraorally, it usually occurs on keratinized tissue (such as the hard palate or gingiva) in immunocompetent hosts (Fig. 13.9). Patients with suppressed immune systems can have lesions on any mucosal site. Patients often experience a prodrome of tingling, burning, or itching prior to the development of multiple vesicles. These vesicles quickly break and become ulcers that coalesce. The process is usually self-limiting and lesions heal in 1–2 weeks without treatment.

Diagnosis

Diagnosis is usually made based on clinical presentation. It can be differentiated from aphthous ulcers in most cases by the different regional distribution.

Treatment

Use of antivirals such as acyclovir and valacyclovir can shorten the clinical course of the lesions especially if started during the prodromal phase (Table 13.3).

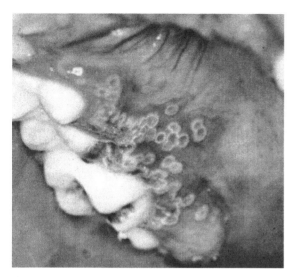

Figure 13.9 Recurrent intraoral herpes.

Topical application of penciclovir topical (Denavir®) can be used for herpes labialis. Topical analgesics (Table 13.4) can be used to alleviate pain but patients should be cautioned to use with care prior to eating due to the increased potential for aspiration secondary to reduced gag reflex. Viscous lidocaine should be used with care for patients with impaired cardiovascular function, bradycardia, or altered ability to expectorate without swallowing the medication.

Herpes zoster (shingles)

Etiology

Reactivation of herpes varicella virus (chickenpox) often precipitated by thermal or mechanical trauma or immunosuppression. It is more common in elderly patients.

Table 13.3 Medications used to treat recurrent herpetic infections

Medication	Form	Treatment
Penciclovir cream 1%	2 g tube	Dab on lesion every 2 h during waking hours for 4 days. Begin treatment at first sign of symptoms
Valacyclovir 500 mg or 1000 mg	8 caps	**Episode dose:** Take 2000 mg at first sign of symptoms and then 2000 mg 12 h later **Suppressive dose:** 500 mg every day, reassess need at 4 months **Zoster dose:** 1000 mg every 8 h for 7 days, begin treatment within 48 h of symptom onset
Acyclovir 400 mg	15 capsules	Take one capsule 3 times a day for 5 days

Table 13.4 Topical analgesics

Analgesics	Form	Treatment
2% Viscous lidocaine hydrochloride (HCL) (20 mg/ml)	250 ml	Swish 5 ml for 2 min and spit before meals and at bedtime or apply with cotton swab (Use with care in patients with impaired cardiovascular function or bradycardia)
Lidocaine/prilocaine 5% cream	30 g tube	Apply to lesions as needed
Diphyenhydramine 12.5 mg/5 ml elixir and magnesium hydroxide (Maalox®) or kaolin and pectate (Kaopectate®)	4 oz of each mixed 1 : 1	Rinse with 5–10 ml for 2 min and spit before meals and at bedtime
Diphyenhydramine 12.5 mg/5 ml elixir, Maalox® or Kaopectate®/viscous lidocaine	4 oz of each mixed 1 : 1	Rinse with 5–10 ml for 2 min and spit before meals and at bedtime
Sucralfate 1 g/10 ml suspension	420 ml	Rinse with 5–10 ml for 2 min and spit before meals and at bedtime

Clinical presentation

Herpes zoster presents as a painful unilateral vesicular eruption along the distribution of a sensory nerve that rupture to form multiple, shallow ulcerations. Patients aged over 60 are prone to develop post-herpetic neuralgia, which can be a persistent and debilitating sequela of shingles.

Diagnosis

Diagnosis is usually made on clinical presentation based on distribution of lesions. Sometimes the appearance of lesions can be preceded by neuropathic pain that can mimic odontogenic pain in cases where the trigeminal nerve is involved.

Treatment

Antiviral therapy should be initiated as soon as possible to reduce the duration of the lesions. Short-term, high dose corticosteroids may be prescribed to decrease the development of post-herpetic neuralgia.

Irritation fibroma

Etiology

The etiology is repeated trauma to the oral mucosa.

Clinical presentation

Irritation fibroma presents as a dome-shaped, immovable solitary soft tissue mass, frequently found on the buccal mucosa, lower lip, and lateral tongue surface (Fig. 13.10). It is generally moderately firm and

the surface coloration is usually similar to or slightly paler than the surrounding mucosa. Ulceration may be present from recurring trauma. Patients generally report the lesion being present for a long period time with little change.

Diagnosis

Clinical appearance and patient history is generally sufficient. Histopathologic examination is needed for definitive diagnosis from other soft tissue growths.

Treatment

Treatment is by excisional biopsy.

Leukoplakia

Leukoplakia is a clinical term to describe a white, nonremovable patch present on any oral mucosal surface that cannot be attributed to any other clinically diagnostic condition. A small percentage may show premalignant or malignant epithelial changes that may eventually become a malignancy.

Etiology

Leukoplakia may be idiopathic or the result of chronic irritation due to trauma from ill-fitting dentures, broken teeth, or restorations; smoking or excessive alcohol use.

Clinical presentation

This lesion typically occurs in older adults. It is most commonly found on the buccal mucosa and lateral border of the tongue (Fig. 13.11). The floor of the

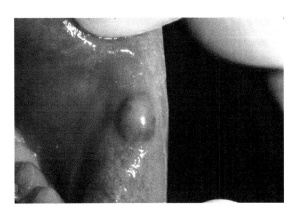

Figure 13.10 Irritation fibroma.

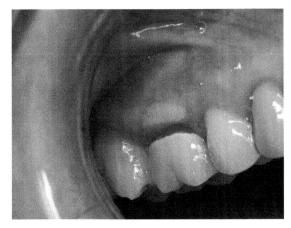

Figure 13.11 Leukoplakia.

mouth is considered a higher risk site. (Rethman *et al.*, 2010) The degree of opacity (slight to dense) and surface texture (smooth to corrugated) may vary depending on the amount of keratin produced.

Diagnosis
Biopsy is indicated due to potential for malignancy.

Treatment
Treatment depends on the histologic finding. Treatment for those lesions showing simple hyperkeratosis includes removing the source of irritation if present. Complete surgical excision of lesions showing moderate or more severe dysplastic changes by scalpel or laser is indicated. Other treatments include topical retinoids, bleomycin, photodynamic light therapy, and cryotherapy although no treatment has proved to be effective in preventing malignant transformation in high-risk lesions (Lodi *et al.*, 2002). Careful monitoring with routine intraoral soft tissue examination is important even after surgical removal.

Lichen planus

Lichen planus is a relatively common disease that can affect the skin and/or mucous membranes. In its erosive form, it appears as chronic, multiple oral mucosal ulcers.

Etiology
Oral lichen planus is a chronic inflammatory condition that has exacerbations and remissions. Although the etiology is uncertain, current data suggest that it is an autoimmune process that involves T-cell infiltration of the oral mucosal tissues (Sugerman, 2002). It generally occurs in patients over 50 years of age with a female to male ratio of 1.4 : 1.0.

Clinical presentation
The reticular form of the disease presents with asymptomatic lacy white lines (Wickham's striae, frequently found bilaterally on the buccal mucosa as well as the lateral border of the tongue and the gingiva) (Fig. 13.12a). Oral erosive lichen planus can have a variety of appearances. Most commonly, it manifests as painful eroded ulcerated areas surrounded by peripheral white radiating striae or as erythema and ulceration of the gingiva (desquamative gingivitis) (Fig. 13.12b).

Diagnosis
While cases of reticular lichen planus with classic lesions may be diagnosed clinically, a biopsy is required to definitely differentiate between oral lichen planus and other white or chronic ulcerative lesions or to exclude malignancy.

Treatment
There is no known cure. The condition is chronic and lesions frequently recur once treatment is stopped. Asymptomatic patients with reticular lesions do not need to be treated. Topical analgesics can be useful in patients with symptomatic lesions (Table 13.4). High-potency topical corticosteroids can be used to control the inflammation and reduce pain (Table 13.5).

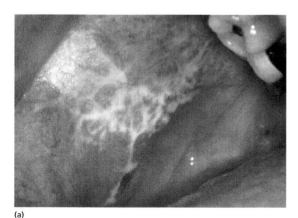
(a)

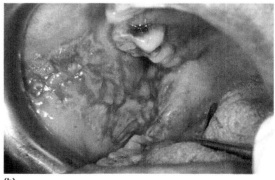
(b)

Figure 13.12 (a) Reticular lichen planus. (b) Erosive lichen planus.

Table 13.5 Medications (in order of increasing potency) for treatment of ulcerative lesions

Agent	Dose/unit	Dosage
Amlexanox 5% oral paste	5 g tube	Apply to ulcer after meals and before bedtime
Topical steroids		
Steroids are listed in order of increasing potency. Mixing topical steroid with equal parts of Orabase® B helps with adhesion to lesion. Prolonged use >2 weeks is discouraged		
Triamcinolone acetonide 1%	5 g tube	Apply to ulcer after meals and before bedtime
Fluocinonide 0.05% cream or ointment	30 g tube	Apply to ulcer after meals and before bedtime
Dexamethasone elixir	0.5 mg/5 ml 100 ml bottle	Rinse with 5 ml for 2 min and spit after meals and before bedtime. Do not eat or drink for 30 min after rinsing
Clobetasol propionate 0.05% cream or ointment	30 g tube	Apply to ulcer after meals and before bedtime
Systemic steroids and immunosuppressants for severe cases		
Dexamethasone elixir 0.5 mg/5 ml	320 ml	Rinse for 2 min after meals and before bedtime. Do not eat or drink for 30 min after rinsing: • For 3 days, rinse with 15 ml 4 times daily and swallow • For 3 days, rinse with 5 ml 4 times daily and swallow • For 3 days, rinse with 5 ml 4 times daily and swallow every other time • For 3 days, rinse with 5 ml 4 times daily and spit out all
Methylprednisolone 4 mg/tablet	Medrol® Dosepak	Follow instructions on pack for initial dose and gradual taper
Prednisone 10 mg	26 tablets	Take 4 tablets in morning for 5 days and then decrease by 1 tablet on each successive day until finished
Tacrolimus 0.03% ointment	30 g tube	Apply to affected region 2 times per day

Systemic therapy may be necessary to fully control the disease if the lesions prove to be refractory to topical therapy (Al-Hashimi *et al.*, 2007).

There is controversy about whether lichen planus is associated with an increased risk of oral cancer (Eisen, 2002), so regular exams to monitor for potentially malignant changes are indicated for all diagnosed patients. Any persistent or refractory erosive lesion should be biopsied to rule out a malignancy.

Mucous membrane pemphigoid (cicatricial pemphigoid)

This is a disease of older adults, especially women. Any area of the mucosa can be affected, but lesions most commonly present on the gingiva.

Etiology
Autoantibodies are produced against the hemidesmosomes in the basement membrane.

Clinical presentation
Patients present with patchy ulceration that are sometimes preceded by blisters that may be blood filled. Any mucosal surface can be affected, but many patients only have gingival lesions that may appear as red, nonulcerated desquamative gingivitis. The lesions are persistent, with periods of remission and exacerbation. The ulcerations are frequently painful. Conjunctival lesions are also common and can lead to blindness due to scarring.

Diagnosis
Biopsy is needed and reveals subepithelial clefting. Direct immunofluorescence shows linear deposits along the basement membrane.

Treatment
Topical high potency and systemic corticosteroids are usually the first line agents for this condition (Table 13.5). For patients with lesions limited to the palate and gingiva, custom trays may be used to help

hold topical steroids against the tissue. Excellent oral hygiene can help reduce local inflammation. Patients with ocular lesions need immediate referral to an ophthalmologist.

Papillary hyperplasia

This lesion is one of many reactive hyperplasias seen in oral mucosal membranes

Etiology
Generally found on the hard palate under ill-fitting complete or partial denture, it is thought to be the result of a combination of negative pressure, poor hygiene, and *C. albicans* overgrowth.

Clinical presentation
Clinically, multiple small papillary lesions give the mucosa of the anterior hard palate a pebbly or cobblestone appearance (Fig. 13.13). The tissue is generally erythematous due to increased inflammation.

Diagnosis
Diagnosis is based on clinical presentation and the presence of a prostheses.

Treatment
Tissue conditioner, improved oral hygiene, and topical antifungal therapy may reduce the problem in mild cases. Surgical removal of tissue with fabrication of new denture is necessary in more severe cases.

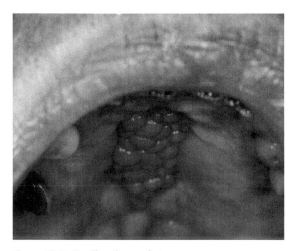

Figure 13.13 Papillary hyperplasia.

Pemphigus

An autoimmune, mucocutaneous disease that results in multiple bullae that quickly become large, shallow ulcerations. Dental prostheses can exacerbate formation because rubbing of the appliances on the mucosal membranes produces blister formation (Nickolsky's sign) although this is not pathognomonic.

Etiology
Circulating autoantibodies directed against desmoglein 3 (an epithelial desmosomal protein) results in the loss of cell-to-cell adhesion.

Clinical presentation
Oral lesions often precede skin lesions. More than one mucosal region is affected at a time. Large, shallow ulcers result from the rupture of short-lived bullae.

Diagnosis
Biopsy is needed and reveals intraepithelial separation. Direct immunofluorescence reveals fluorescent uptake in the intracellular layer.

Treatment
Prednisone is usually the first agent used. Immunosuppressants and immunomodulators such as azathioprine, dapsone, mycophenolate mofetil, cyclosporine, and methotrexate are also used for more extensive lesions but have the potential for serious side effects and need careful monitoring.

Recurrent aphthous ulcers

Recurrent aphthous ulcers (or canker sores) are the most commonly occurring nontraumatic ulcerations in the oral cavity, affecting anywhere from 20% to 60% of the population (Chavan *et al.*, 2012).

Etiology
Aphthous ulcers are recurrent painful mucosal lesions of unknown cause. They are usually self-limiting. Potential causes include focal immune dysfunction, deficiencies in vitamin B12, folic acid, and/or iron, hormonal changes, trauma, stress, and food allergies. The most commonly used medications

associated with intraoral aphthous-like ulcerations are nonsteroidal anti-inflammatory drugs (Chavan *et al.*, 2012).

Clinical presentation

Aphthous stomatitis occurs as recurring painful ulcerations usually involving movable nonkeratinized mucosa (such as the labial and buccal mucosa, the ventral surface of the tongue, and the floor of the mouth). Classification is based on the size and number of ulcers present. Minor aphthae (canker sores) are the most common form and presents as single or multiple oval ulcers less than 0.5 cm in dimension that heal within 10–14 days without scarring. They are covered with grayish-white pseudomembrane and surrounded by an erythematous halo (Fig. 13.14a). Prodromal symptoms of tingling or burning may precede the ulceration. Major aphthae are >0.5 cm in dimension and last several weeks to months (Fig. 13.14b). They generally heal with mucosal scarring. Herpetiform aphthae are multiple, very small (0.1–0.2 cm) crops of ulcers that often coalesce into a single larger ulcer (Scully, 2006). While they resemble intraoral herpes simplex infection, they are found on movable nonkeratinized tissue and there is no initial vesicle or blister associated with them (Figure 13.14c).

Diagnosis

Diagnosis is generally based on history of similar lesions, clinical presentation, and distribution of lesions. A CBC with differential and iron/vitamin B12 levels may be indicated in some patients.

Treatment

Most patients with minor aphthae generally heal without treatment. Over-the-counter barrier agents (like amlexanox 5% paste) and topical analgesics (Table 13.4) can provide palliative relief. For more severe cases or prolonged lesions, therapy includes topical or systemic corticosteroids (Table 13.5). Mixing topical steroid ointments with equal parts of Orabase® B paste (Colgate Oral Pharmaceuticals, Inc.) allows for prolonged contact of the medication with the lesions (Siegel *et al.*, 2006). Low dose doxycycline administered as a topical gel or minocycline rinses (0.2%) have shown some efficacy (Preshaw *et al.*, 2007; Skulason *et al.*, 2009). In patients with

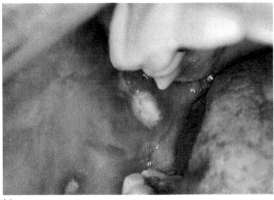
(a)

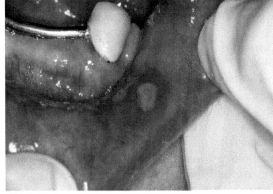
(b)

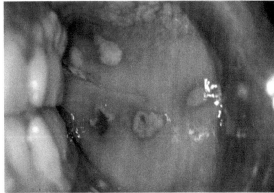
(c)

Figure 13.14 (a) Minor aphthous ulcers; (b) Major aphthous ulcers; (c) Herpetiform aphthous ulcers.

severe persistent recurring aphthae, systemic therapy with medication such as mycophenolate mofetil, pentoxifylline, colchicine, or thalidomide has been used (Gonsaves *et al.*, 2007; Ship, 1996), but close collaboration with the patient's physician is advised because of increased chance of adverse side effects.

Traumatic ulcerations

Ulcers are among the most common lesions seen in oral mucous membranes. There are many causes of oral ulcers. Most ulcers seen are the result of trauma, especially in patients wearing dental prostheses.

Etiology
Secondary to trauma from biting, improper tooth brushing, broken restorations or teeth, improperly fitting removable prostheses, alterations in motor control, excessive heat or chemical burns.

Clinical presentation
Traumatic ulcers usually present as painful ulcerations with a yellow fibrinous base and erythematous halo that can be found on any intraoral tissue. Size and shape can vary depending on source of trauma.

Diagnosis
Diagnosis is usually based on patient history and clinical appearance.

Treatment
Recurrent sources of irritation such as ill-fitting prostheses or broken teeth/restorations should be removed. Topical anesthetics and over-the-counter barrier medications may be used for pain relief in larger lesions (Table 13.4). Lesions may take longer to heal in elderly patients. If no resolution occurs in 3–4 weeks, biopsy is indicated.

Varices (varix)

Varices (or varicosities) are dilated tortuous veins that cause an elevation of the overlying mucosa. They are rarely seen before the age of 40 but more than two-thirds of adults aged over 60 will have at least one.

Etiology
Their development may be related to age-related weakening of connective tissue in the wall of superficial veins, resulting in dilatation. Sun exposure may be responsible for their presence on the vermillion border of the lip.

Clinical presentation
Varices appear as red, blue, or deep purple elevated lesions that are compressible and blanch upon pressure, unless they have thrombosed. The term "caviar tongue" is used to describe small, multiple, soft, well-circumscribed bluish-purple papules found on the ventral tongue. Solitary varix are more commonly found on the lips and buccal mucosa, and are usually larger and firmer due to thrombus formation secondary to sluggish vascular flow. The term venous lake is used to describe solitary lesions located on the vermillion border of the lips.

Diagnosis
Diagnosis is usually based on clinical appearance and the age of the patient.

Treatment
If they do not interfere with function or are not a cosmetic concern, varices do not need to be treated. Treatment includes surgical excision, cryotherapy, or laser ablation.

Case study

Mrs. Gilbert is an 83-year-old female who is frail with mild cognitive impairment. She lives with her 85-year-old husband at home. She has diabetes, hypertension, mild congestive heart failure, and osteoarthritis affecting both hands. Her chief complaint is "My mouth feels like I have cotton balls in it and the roof of my mouth and tongue are burning".
Her medications include metformin, nifedipine, hydrochlorothiazide, ramipril, donepezil, lorazepam, trazodone, tolterodine, and acetaminophen. On extraoral exam, there is fissuring and erythema present at the commissures of the mouth (Fig. 13.15a). Intraorally, there is poor oral hygiene with debris present (Fig. 13.15b). Her gingival tissues appear inflamed. Her saliva appears thick and ropy. When you remove her upper partial denture, there is erythema present on the palate in the outline of the denture base (Fig. 13.15c).

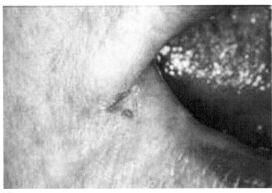

(a)

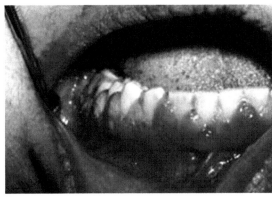

(b)

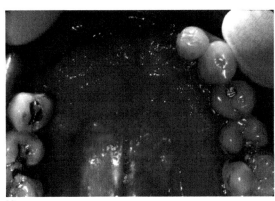

(c)

Figure 13.15 (a) Angular chelitis; (b) poor oral hygiene with debris present; (c) denture stomatitis. See case study for further details.

References

Al-Hashimi, I., Schifter, M., Lockhart, P.B., *et al.* (2007) Oral lichen planus and oral lichenoid lesions: diagnostic and therapeutic considerations. *Oral Surgery, Oral Medicine,*

Oral Pathology, Oral Radiology, and Endodontics, **103** (Suppl 1), S25–31.

Bergdahl, M. & Bergdahl, J. (1999) Burning mouth syndrome: prevalence and associated factors. *Journal of Oral Pathology & Medicine,* **28**(8), 350–4.

Chavan, M., Jain, H., Diwan, N., *et al.* (2012), Recurrent aphthous stomatitis: a review. *Journal of Oral Pathology & Medicine,* **41**(3), 201–6.

Darwazeh, A., Lamey, P., Samaranayake, L., *et al.* (1990) The relationship between colonisation, secretor status and in-vitro adhesion of *Candida albicans* to buccal epithelial cells from diabetics. *Journal of Medical Microbiology,* **33**(1), 43–9.

Eisen, D. (2002) The clinical features, malignant potential and systemic associations of oral lichen planus: a study of 723 patients. *Journal of the American Academy of Dermatology,* **46**, 207–14.

Giannin, P.J. & Shetty, K.V. (2011) Diagnosis and management of oral candidiasis. *Otolaryngologic Clinics of North America,* **44**(1), 231–40.

Gonsaves, W.C., Chi, A.C. & Neville, B.W. (2007) Common oral lesions: part 1. *American Family Physician,* **75**(4), 501–7.

Gubbins, P.O. & Heldenbrand, S. (2010) Clinically relevant drug interactions of current antifungal agents. *Mycoses,* **53**(2), 95–113.

Lodi, G., Sardella, A., Bez, C., *et al.* (2002) Systematic review of randomized trials for the treatment of oral leukoplakia *Journal of Dental Education,* **66**, 896–902.

Patton, L.L., Siegel, M.A., Benoliel, R. & De Laat, A. (2007) Management of burning mouth syndrome: systematic review and management recommendations. *Oral Surgery, Oral Medicine, and Oral Pathology,* **103** (Suppl), S39.e1–13.

Peterson, D.E. (1992) Oral candidiasis. *Clinics in Geriatric Medicine,* **8**(3), 513–27.

Preshaw, P.M., Grainger, P., Bradshaw, M.H., *et al.* (2007) Subantimicrobial dose doxycycline in the treatment of recurrent oral aphthous ulceration: a pilot study. *Journal of Oral Pathology & Medicine,* **36**, 236–40.

Rethman, M.P., Carpenter, W., Cohen, E.E., *et al.* (2010) Evidence-based clinical recommendations regarding screening for oral squamous cell carcinomas. *Journal of the American Dental Association,* **141**(5), 509–20.

Sardella, A., Lodi, G., Demarosi, F., *et al.* (2006) Burning mouth syndrome: a retrospective study investigating spontaneous remission and response to treatments. *Oral Diseases,* **12**(2), 152–5.

Scully, C. (2006) Clinical practice: aphthous ulceration. *New England Journal of Medicine,* **355**(2), 165–72.

Ship, J.A. (1996) Recurrent aphthous stomatitis. *Oral Surgery, Oral Medicine, Oral Pathololgy, Oral Radiology,* **81**, 141–7.

Siegel, M.A., Silverman, S. Jr. & Sollecito, T.P. (eds.) (2006) *Clinician's Guide to Treatment of Common Oral Conditions,* 6th edn. BC Decker, Lewiston, NY, pp. 49–50.

Skulason, S., Holbrook, W.P. & Kristmundsdottir, T. (2009) Clinical assessment of the effect of a matrix metalloproteinase inhibitor on aphthous ulcers. *Acta Odontologica Scandinavica*, **67**, 25–9.

Sugerman, P.B., Savage, N.W., Walsh, L.J., *et al.* (2002) The pathogenesis of oral lichen planus. *Critical Reviews in Oral Biology and Medicine*, **13**(4), 350–65.

Webb, B.C., Thomas, C.J. & Whittle, T. (2005) A 2-year study of *Candida*-associated denture stomatitis treatment in aged care subjects. *Gerodontology*, **22**(3), 168–76.

Zhang, W., Chen, Y., An, Z., *et al.* (2007) Reactive gingival lesions: a retrospective study of 2439 cases. *Quintessence*, **38**, 103–10.

CHAPTER 14

Xerostomia

Jadwiga Hjertstedt

Department of Clinical Services, Marquette University School of Dentistry, Milwaukee, WI, USA

Introduction

Xerostomia (dry mouth) is a subjective sensation of oral dryness and it may be associated with salivary gland hypofunction (SGH), and changes in salivary composition. It is a very common complaint among older adults but it is not a normal part of the aging process (Heft & Baum, 1984). Dry mouth is often neglected or unrecognized by some practitioners due to a variety of reasons such as diverse symptom presentation, patients not reporting due to an unawareness of its consequences to oral health, and practitioners being more focused on restorative needs of their patients considering these as more urgent or important. Nonetheless, clinicians need to have a good understanding of this condition and recognize its etiology, signs, and symptoms in order to recommend the most effective treatment to prevent oral health complications and improve their patients' overall well-being and quality of life.

Role of saliva and functions of salivary components

An adequate amount of saliva is vital for maintaining oral health and for overall well-being. Saliva with its components (over 300 proteins, peptides, and electrolytes) plays an essential role in the maintenance of healthy soft and hard oral tissues as well as overall oral comfort (Dawes, 2008). The unpleasant symptoms reported by patients who experience xerostomia are the best evidence of how important saliva is to

quality of life and serve as reminders of saliva's important and versatile properties. Saliva has several protective functions affecting the oral mucosa and teeth. The salivary mucins lubricate and protect mucous membranes by coating and enhancing elasticity. Several proteins such as lysozyme, lactoferrin, histatins, cystatins, and secretory immunoglobulins have broad antimicrobial activity with the overlapping defensive systems. Together they prevent oral microorganisms' aggregation and adherence; the proteins also inhibit microbial growth. Additionally, the bicarbonate/carbonate buffer system stabilizes intraoral pH by neutralizing acids which, in combination with certain proteins coating tooth enamel, is essential in the remineralization process thus protecting the dentition from dental caries (van Nieuw Amerongen *et al.*, 2004). In addition, saliva facilitates speech and has several food intake-related functions. It assists with chewing activities, bolus formation, and digestion of starches (amylase) and fats (lipase), as well as aids in swallowing and taste mediation (Kaplan & Baum 1993).

Xerostomia has been called the "invisible" oral disease. Both patients and clinicians take saliva for granted and usually recognize the importance of its presence by the sequellae of its absence; therefore, it is important to recognize clinical signs and symptoms of xerostomia and/or SGH and to elucidate its cause. By doing so, clinicians may offer the patient recommendations and interventions that will prevent deleterious effects of hyposalivation, alleviate discomfort, and enhance a person's quality of life.

Geriatric Dentistry: Caring for Our Aging Population, First Edition. Edited by Paula K. Friedman.

© 2014 John Wiley & Sons, Inc. Published 2014 by John Wiley & Sons, Inc.

Companion website: www.wiley.com/go/friedman/geriatricdentistry

Defining and recognizing xerostomia and SGH

Although xerostomia and SGH share common causes and seem to be interrelated, they refer to two separate entities. Xerostomia is the subjective sensation of dry mouth; therefore, patients themselves are its best "diagnosticians." It should be differentiated from SGH or hyposalivation, which is an objective finding determined by measuring salivary gland output. The accepted reference values for hyposalivation are <0.1 ml/minute for unstimulated whole saliva (UWS) and <0.5 ml/min for stimulated whole saliva (SWS) (Dawes, 1996). These cut-off flow rates, however, do not account for variations based on factors that may affect salivary output such as degree of hydration, gender, circadian rhythms, gland size, medications, and age, among others.

Patients with xerostomia and/or SGH experience a variety of oral and nonoral symptoms (Närhi, 1994; Sreebny *et al.*, 1989;) which may vary somewhat in nature, duration, and intensity among individuals. Common oral complaints associated with xerostomia include the sensation of a dry sticky mouth and tongue, thick saliva, mouth soreness, altered taste, increased thirst, and difficulty with speaking, eating, and swallowing (Table 14.1). Diets consisting of dry and spicy foods exacerbate problematic swallowing. Additionally, the need to drink in order to swallow when eating particularly dry foods is common, and it is known as the *cracker sign*, associated with the experience of eating dry crackers. Patients with xerostomia who wear removable prosthesis report several problems related to dry mouth including impaired denture retention, mouth soreness, and fungal infections (Turner *et al.*, 2008).

Table 14.1 Subjective symptoms and clinical findings associated with xerostomia and/or salivary gland hypofunction

Oral symptoms	Nonoral symptoms
• Dry mouth that feels sticky • Dry lips • Thick saliva that feels like glue • Mouth soreness • Sores at the corners of the lips • Burning mouth and/or tongue sensation • Difficulty speaking (dysphonia) • Difficulty eating, especially dry and spicy foods • Difficulty swallowing (dysphagia) • Increased thirst and need to sip water frequently • Need to drink water to be able to swallow, especially dry foods • Altered taste (dysgeusia) • Halitosis • Difficulty wearing dentures • Lipstick may stick to front teeth (for women)	• Dry skin (xeroderma) • Dry, sore throat and hoarseness • Dry eyes, feeling of sand or gravel in the eyes; blurred vision, need to use tear substitutes • Enlarged/swollen major salivary glands especially in patients with Sjögren's syndrome, sarcoidosis, and HIV infection (usually firm and nontender upon palpation) • Dry nasal passages • Vaginal dryness and itching • Constipation

Clinical findings and consequences of salivary gland hypofunction
• Dry lips that can be chapped or cracked
• Dry oral mucous membranes that stick to the glove, dental mirror, or tongue blade
• Thick, viscous saliva
• Dry tongue that appears reddened, depapillated, and fissured
• Oral mucosa appears pale and dull
• Little or no pooling of saliva on the floor of the mouth
• Viscous and thick, or no saliva expressed from the duct orifices of the major salivary glands (Stensen's or Wharton's)
• Increased prevalence of dental caries: cervical and root surface and on atypical sites, i.e., incisal edges of mandibular anterior teeth or on cusps
• Oral candidiasis with erythematous patches on the palate, or dorsal surface of the tongue
• Angular cheilitis
• Increased plaque accumulation and calculus

These oral-related symptoms may lead to changes in eating habits including selection and avoidance of certain foods. For older adults social interaction with friends and family is a major aspect of their overall well-being. Since food plays an important role in the feeling of connecting with relatives, friends, and culture, xerostomia-associated oral symptoms may be very upsetting and frustrating, and ultimately may adversely affect their quality of life and contribute to social isolation. In addition, avoidance of certain foods may compromise the nutritional status in the geriatric population (Rhodus & Brown, 1990). Patients with xerostomia and SGH may also present with several nonoral symptoms such as dry skin and throat; dry, itching eyes and blurred vision; as well as vaginal itching and fungal infections (Table 14.1).

Dry mouth is a difficult and complex issue, with many questions still unanswered. The reasons for the complexity surrounding xerostomia will be discussed in this chapter. While xerostomia is most commonly linked to SGH, not all patients complaining of oral dryness have abnormally low salivary flow rates (Sreebny & Valdini, 1988; Thomson *et al.*, 1999). Similarly, not all patients with SGH complain of dry mouth sensation. This may possibly be explained by the fact that patients first begin to experience symptoms of dry mouth when their unstimulated salivary volume has decreased by approximately 40–50% (Dawes, 1987).

Because hyposalivation has the potential to lead to significant deterioration of oral health including rapidly developing cervical and root caries, erosion, mucosal lesions, and opportunistic infections to name a few, it is imperative to properly identify patients with suspected SGH. The clinician should elicit responses to follow-up questions about their symptoms from those patients who complain of continual oral dryness. Positive responses to questions such as those listed below have been shown to be predictive in identifying patients with hyposalivation (Fox, 1996):

1 Do you sip liquids to aid in swallowing dry foods?
2 Does your mouth feel dry when eating a meal?
3 Do you have difficulties swallowing any foods?
4 Does the amount of the saliva in your mouth seem to be too little, too much, or you don't notice it?

Additionally, several extraoral and intraoral findings identified during oral examination should alert the astute clinician to consider SGH in a differential diagnosis (with or without xerostomia) (Table 14.1). Extraoral signs frequently include: dry, cracked lips

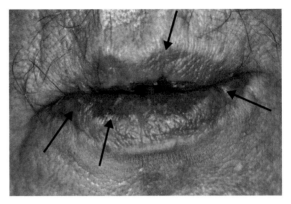

Figure 14.1 Dry, cracked (arrows) lips in an elderly patient with medication-induced xerostomia. Courtesy of Dr. Ralph H. Saunders, URMC, Rochester, NY.

(Fig. 14.1) often with redness in the corners of the mouth suggesting angular cheilitis. Some patients (including those with Sjögren's syndrome, sarcoidosis or viral infections) may have unilateral- or bilaterally enlarged parotid or submandibular glands that may or may not be tender on palpation. In some instances, salivary gland palpation will yield very little or no saliva. The expressed secretion may be more viscous than watery. Intraoral findings through visual inspection may reveal: dry, pale mucous membranes; reddened, fissured, and often a depapillated tongue (Fig. 14.2); and decreased or absent pooling of saliva on the floor of the mouth. One simple objective method to identify patients with SGH is whether the examiner's gloved finger, a dental mirror, or a tongue blade sticks to the cheek during retraction.

The most deleterious consequence of hyposalivation (with or without xerostomia) is the increased risk of rapidly progressive dental caries. Patients with severe SGH often present with rampant new or recurrent caries lesions that are often present on atypical surfaces such as cervical margins or incisal edges of the mandibular anterior teeth. Older adults with remaining teeth are a particularly vulnerable group. They are at significant risk for root caries (Fig. 14.3) because of exposed root surfaces from gingival recession as well as their compromised ability (i.e., impaired manual dexterity, sensory and cognitive deficits) to maintain good oral hygiene.

Other common intraoral findings with SGH in older adults include increased plaque accumulation

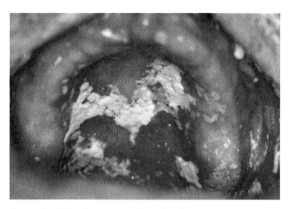

Figure 14.4 Erythematous, dry palatal mucosa (mucositis) with white plaques indicative of an opportunistic fungal infection caused by *Candida albicans*. Courtesy of Dr. Ralph H. Saunders, URMC Rochester, NY.

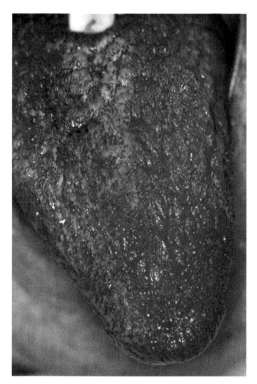

Figure 14.2 Dry, red and depapillated, fissured tongue. Courtesy of Dr. Ralph H. Saunders, URMC, Rochester, NY.

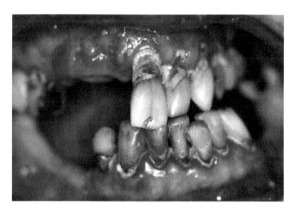

Figure 14.3 Root caries, plaque accumulation and dry erythematous oral mucosa due to medication-induced dry mouth. Courtesy of Dr. Ralph H. Saunders, URMC, Rochester, NY.

and frequent oral mucosal yeast infections primarily resulting from *Candida albicans* (Fig. 14.4). Together these extraoral and intraoral findings are valid indicators of hyposalivation (Navazesh *et al.*, 1992)

and stand as evidence to the importance of saliva for healthy soft and hard oral structures.

Prevalence

Dry mouth is a common patient complaint, particularly among the elderly. Reviews of studies on the prevalence of xerostomia show that approximately 20% of the general adult population and 30% of those aged 65 and older report symptoms of oral dryness (Orellana *et al.*, 2006; Ship *et al.*, 2002). The reported estimates from studies on xerostomia prevalence have shown rates ranging from 0.9 to 64.8% with generally higher rates for women and for those in nursing homes (Handelman *et al.*, 1989; Locker, 1995). The considerable variability in prevalence rates may be explained by lack of uniform methodology to measure and collect data. For example, inconsistent definition of xerostomia, varying content, and number of questions asked in the questionnaires, and use of small convenience study samples may affect reported prevalence rates (Orellana *et al.*, 2006; Thomson, 2005). Understandably, nearly all patients with Sjögren's syndrome and those who received radiotherapy for head and neck cancers report xerostomia (Chambers *et al.*, 2007; Fox *et al.*, 2000).

Similarly, studies conducted on prevalence of the SGH have shown significant variability, mainly due to the inconsistent measurement standards such as cut-off measurement values used for defining hyposalivation (Nederfors, 2000). Studies investigating concurrent prevalence of xerostomia and SGH within the same sample found much lower rates (ranging from 2 to 5.7%) of both conditions compared to rates reported separately (Bergdahl, 2000; Hochberg *et al.*, 1998; Thomson *et al.*, 1999). This finding supports the notion that these are two discrete conditions and further research is needed to explain the complex relationship between xerostomia and SGH.

Effect of aging on salivary glands and flow rates

There are significant age-related structural changes affecting all major and minor salivary glands. The reported histologic changes include significant acinar atrophy, with the acinar cells being replaced by fat, connective tissue, and duct-like epithelial structures (Scott *et al.*, 1987; Waterhouse *et al.*, 1973). These changes affect men and women similarly (Azevedo *et al.*, 2005).

In the past it was the general belief that dry mouth is a natural part of aging. This notion was based on the fact that early studies found age-related changes in salivary glands and lower salivary flow rates among older adults when compared to younger individuals. These studies, however, had methodologic flaws, such as cross-sectional designs, and did not control for medication use nor health status (Becks & Wainwright, 1943; Bertram, 1967; Gutman & Ben-Aryeh, 1974).

Contrary to the past assumption that xerostomia is a normal part of aging, more recent data on changes in salivary glands function indicate that they retain their secretory capacity with aging. Prospective longitudinal studies conducted on healthy older adults consistently demonstrated no age-related changes in both unstimulated and stimulated secretions from parotid glands (Heft & Baum, 1984; Ship *et al.*, 1995). Reports from studies on the flow rates from submandibular/sublingual and minor salivary glands provide conflicting results of reduced secretions (Pedersen *et al.*, 1985) or no changes in salivary output with aging (Ship *et al.*, 1995; Tylenda *et al.*, 1988).

The retained overall functional capacity, despite age-related acinar atrophy, has been explained by the remaining adequate secretory reserve in salivary glands to compensate for some losses without causing dry mouth symptoms in healthy unmedicated older adults (Ghezzi & Ship, 2003). Therefore, complaints

of dry mouth and/or SGH in older adults are likely to be caused by factors other than aging.

Etiology of xerostomia and/or SGH

Patients who present with complaints of dry mouth or clinical evidence of reduced salivary flow require careful assessment for possible etiologic factors in order to select appropriate interventions to prevent oral complications. Xerostomia and/or SGH have been linked to several different origins such as medications, radiation therapy to the head and neck, underlying systemic disease, and behavioral as well as other local factors. These factors will be discussed in the sections that follow.

Medication use

The predominant cause of dry mouth is the use of medications; both prescription and nonprescription. Older adults are the primary consumers of medications and this may explain why dry mouth complaints are far more common among them than among younger individuals. More than 500 commonly prescribed and over-the-counter drugs are associated with xerostomia or reduced salivary flow (Sreebny & Swartz, 1997). The agents that are most frequently implicated in dry mouth symptoms and reduced salivary output have anticholinergic properties that reduce the volume of serous saliva or have a sympathomimetic mechanism of action that makes saliva more viscous. Table 14.2 lists examples of common xerogenic drugs and their classes that include: antihistamines, anticholinergics, antidepressants, anxiolytics, antipsychotics, antihypertensive agents, and diuretics among others. It is worth noting that certain drugs such as loop diuretics and inhaled medications may cause xerostomia without any adverse effects on salivary secretion (Atkinson *et al.*, 1989). The prevalence and severity of dry mouth symptoms have been linked to the duration of use and the number of medications that an individual is taking. Polypharmacy, or the use of multiple medications, and the interaction between these medications has been shown to increase the incidence of xerostomia and SGH in the elderly because of the cumulative effects of combining drug therapies in an individual with multiple systemic problems (Thomson *et al.*, 2000, 2006). Increased number of medications has also been associated with reduction in stimulated and unstimulated saliva flow

Table 14.2 Examples of frequently used medications causing xerostomia

Classification (by therapeutic/ pharmacologic category)	Generic name	Brand name
Analgesics (opioids and nonopioids)	Hydrocodone/acetaminophen	Anexia®; Dolacet®; Hydrocet®; Hydrogesic®; Vicodin®
	Propoxyphene	Darvon®
Analgesics (NSAIDS)	Ibuprofen	Advil®, Excedrin IB®, Ibuprin®, Motrin®, Nuprin®
Antianginals (nitrates)	Isosorbide	Isordil®
Antianxiety/ sedative/ hypnotics		
Benzodiazepines (sedatives)	Alprazolam	Xanax®
	Diazepam	Valium®
	Clonazapam	Klonopin®
	Lorazepam	Ativan®
	Oxazepam	Serax®
Benzodiazepines (hypnotics)	Temazepam	Restoril®
Anticonvulsants	Gabapentin	Neurontin®
Antidepressants		
Tricyclic	Amitriptyline	Elavil®
	Doxepin	Sinequan®
Tetracyclic	Maprotiline HCL	Ludiomil®
Selective serotonin reuptake inhibitors (SSRIs)	Paroxetine	Paxil®
	Sertraline	Zoloft®
	Escitalopram	Lexapro®
Atypical	Fluoxetine	Prozac®
	Trazodone HCL	Desyrel®
Antiarrhythmics	Procainamide	Pronestyl®
	Disopyramide	Norpace®
Antihistamines	Cetirizine HCL	Zyrtec®
	Diphenhydramine	Benadryl®
	Fexofenadine HCL	Allegra®
	Loratadine	Claritin®
Antihypertensives		
Beta-adrenergic antagonists	Atenolol	Tenormin®
	Metoprolol succinate	Toprol-XL®; Lopressor®
Angiotensin-converting enzyme inhibitors	Lisinopril	Prinivil®; Zestril®
Calcium channel blockers	Amlodipine besylate	Norvasc®
Antiparkinsonian drugs	Benztropine	Cogentin®
	Trihexyphenidyl HCL	Artane®
Antipsychotics	Haloperidol	Haldol®
(butyrophenones and phenothiazines)	Chlorpromazine	Thorazine®
	Clozapine	Clozaril®
	Quetiapine fumarate	Seroquel XR®
	Risperidone	Risperdal®
	Olanzapine	Zyprexa®
Antispasmodics	Oxybutynin	Ditropan®
Bronchodilators	Albuterol	Airet®; Proventil®; Rotocaps®; Ventolin®; Ventomax®
Diuretics	Furosemide	Lasix®
	Hydrochlorothiazide	Dyazide®; Maxzide®
Gastrointestinal drugs (gastric acid secretion inhibitor)	Lansoprazole	Prevacid®
Sedative – hypnotics	Zolpidem	Ambien®
Skeletal muscle relaxants	Cyclobenzaprine	Flexeril®

rates (Wu & Ship 1993). Moreover, older adults who take multiple medications report more severe and longer-lasting symptoms of xerostomia than do younger individuals (Patel *et al.*, 2001).

Radiotherapy to head and neck

Another major cause of xerostomia is associated with fractionated radiation for treatment of malignant tumors of head and neck (Chambers *et al.*, 2007). In the USA more than 50,000 individuals are annually diagnosed with head and neck cancers, which account for 3–5% of all cancers. A majority of these patients are older than 50 years of age (Jemal *et al.*, 2010). Standard treatment is usually 5–7 weeks of radiotherapy for oral cancers with a dose of up to 70 Gy. This can have a profound and a long-lasting adverse effect on the function of salivary glands within the field of radiation. Loss of function is total dose, time, and gland dependent. Serous cells are more radiosensitive than mucous cells and parotid glands' serous cells are more sensitive than the acinar cells in other glands. Patients receiving radiation begin to experience a significant decrease in salivary flow, increase in saliva viscosity, and xerostomia within the first week after initiation of therapy or when doses exceed 10 Gy. Doses exceeding 60 Gy cause permanent damage consisting of the loss of acinar cells, glandular fibrosis, and fatty degeneration of the gland parenchyma (Henriksson *et al.*, 1994). The multiple symptoms resulting from salivary gland destruction and hyposalivation persist indefinitely, adversely affecting the patients' quality of life.

Systemic disorders

Xerostomia in patients not taking any medications may be an indication of underlying systemic disease requiring further evaluation. The coexistence of multiple chronic diseases is very common among older adults. Many of these conditions adversely affect salivary gland function and are associated with hyposalivation.

Sjögren's syndrome (SS) is the most common autoimmune disease affecting exocrine glands predominantly in middle-aged women. The characteristic histopathologic features of affected salivary glands in SS include lymphocytic infiltration, sialadenitis, acinar atrophy, and ductal hyperplasia leading to the formation of epithelial foci called epimyoepithelial islands. These are irreversible and destructive changes of salivary and lacrimal glands' parenchyma resulting in decreased secretions leading to the symptoms of dry

mouth and dry eyes. Many patients may also present with enlarged major salivary glands. The exocrinopathy is termed *primary SS* when it presents as a "sicca complex" with dry eyes (xerophthalmia) and dry mouth only. When xerophthalmia and xerostomia symptoms occur in combination with another autoimmune rheumatic disease, most commonly rheumatoid arthritis, systemic lupus erythematosus, or scleroderma, the term *secondary SS* is used. The coexistence and involvement of these connective tissue diseases in affected individuals may lead to fatigue, malaise, and several extraglandular systemic abnormalities including peripheral neuropathies, cutaneous vasculitis, dry skin, disorders of thyroid gland function, pulmonary diseases, nephritis, and gastrointestinal tract dysfunction.

Other conditions that may cause complaints of xerostomia and/or SGH include diabetes mellitus, psychogenic disorders such as depression, chronic anxiety and emotional stress, rheumatoid arthritis, sarcoidosis, hepatitis C virus infection, Parkinson's disease, and infection with human immunodeficiency virus/acquired immunodeficiency syndrome (AIDS). Individuals with graft-versus-host disease or those undergoing hemodialysis that have insufficient fluid intake may experience xerostomia because of dehydration. Various genetic diseases as well as conditions that cause metabolic changes (e.g., nutritional deficiencies, eating disorders, and dehydration) are associated with SGH (von Bültzingslöwen *et al.*, 2007). Patients with Alzheimer's dementia or stroke may complain of dry mouth despite normal salivary flow because of perception changes (Gupta *et al.*, 2006). Symptoms of dry mouth, regardless of cause, may be increased by smoking, tobacco chewing, and mouth breathing. Lastly, certain local obstructive factors such as sialoliths, cysts, viral, and bacterial infections affecting salivary glands may cause short-term decreased salivary flow.

Treatment modalities

Currently, there is no cure or single treatment approach that is effective for all patients with symptoms of dry mouth and/or salivary hypofunction. The practitioner's decision is most often based on past experience when treating patients with these conditions as well as information available in professional journals and from peers. Nevertheless, the management for the majority of these patients is primarily symptomatic with goals to: (i) prevent deleterious consequences of decreased or insufficient amount of saliva; (ii) attempt to stimulate salivary flow; and (iii) alleviate symptoms in order to improve the patient's quality of life. The treatment of any disease begins with an accurate diagnosis which in this context is a question of xerostomia or SGH, or both. Therefore, the starting point for the practitioner begins with an accurate medical and dental history, a careful clinical examination, and assessment of salivary flow rates. These essential elements of the diagnostic process can be rather complicated to perform when treating elderly patients. They often present with several chronic health conditions, take multiple medications, and the health information they provide may be incomplete or inaccurate. In patients with compromised decision-making capacity, it may be prudent to confirm the information with a family member or other caregiver. Additionally, a consultation with the patient's physician may be warranted to ensure not only the accuracy of the information provided by the patient in regards to health status but also to discuss the patient's medications. Since drug-induced SGH may be a reversible condition, it is certainly worthwhile to discuss with the physician the possibility of modifying the dosage or changing the medication to an agent with less adverse effects on saliva. Further, a review of medications may result in shortening the list of prescribed medications. Oftentimes, however, the benefits of medications to the patient's general health outweigh the adverse effects on salivary flow. As a result, the only alternative will be a palliative easing of the patient's dry mouth symptoms along with the initiation of aggressive caries preventive interventions in dentate patients. Prevention modalities and palliative strategies will be discussed in the following sections.

Preventing dental caries and mucosal diseases

Based on the established diagnosis (xerostomia, SGH, or both) the clinician can develop an individualized comprehensive program to prevent or minimize the risk of developing dental caries, and oral mucosal diseases.

The recommendations to patients with SGH, regardless of the cause, should emphasize: dietary modifications that limit sugar intake only to meals, elimination or decrease of between meal snacking,

maintenance of meticulous oral hygiene, and the use of patient- and professionally-applied topical fluorides (rinses, gels, and varnishes) (Beltrán-Aguilar et al., 2000). For caries control, patients can rinse twice daily with a nonprescription 0.05% sodium fluoride mouthrinse. Patients may benefit further from the daily use of prescription products with higher concentration of fluoride (i.e., 1.1% sodium fluoride or 0.4% stannous fluoride) that can be applied either as a brush-on gel preparation or delivered in custom-made acrylic fluoride trays. Moreover, in patients with clinical signs of severe salivary hypofunction, professionally applied fluoride varnish may help to prevent rapid development of dental caries. These patients will also require more frequent dental visits, so the clinician can monitor any changes in the patient's oral health status, oral-hygiene efforts, and apply, when necessary, high concentration fluorides. While all these efforts individually have some benefit in preventing dental caries, the combination of all of them has been shown to be most effective (Dreizen el al., 1977). As an adjunct, patients with the highest risk of caries and older patients unable to brush and floss could benefit from periodically rinsing with alcohol-free 0.12% chlorhexidine gluconate (1 minute daily for 2 weeks), to lower the number of *mutans streptococci* in the oral microflora. The above preventive interventions can be effective only if the patient (and his/her caregiver) understands the importance of regular dental visits and is motivated to participate actively in the process by consistently following the practitioner's recommendations. Noncompliance can result in deterioration of dentition and, potentially, tooth loss.

Patients with SGH also are more susceptible to oral mucosal infections. Candidiasis, a fungal infection, is particularly prevalent in geriatric patients. When clinical signs are suggestive of oral candidiasis, topical antifungal drugs should be prescribed (Table 14.3). It should be noted that many oral antifungal medications contain high amounts of sucrose and are cariogenic. Therefore, high caries-risk patients should use nystatin vaginal tablets, which are less cariogenic because they contain lactose instead, by dissolving them orally. (These tablets may be used in high caries-risk patients of both genders.) Patients who wear complete or partial dentures and have oral candidiasis should be reminded to wear their prosthesis only in the daytime, clean them with a denture toothbrush and disinfect them by soaking overnight in a nystatin suspension or 0.12%

Table **14.3** Antifungal agents for treatment of oral candidiasis

Topical oral suspensions

Rx: Nystatin oral suspension 100 000 units/ml (Mycostatin®, Nilstat®, Nystex®)
Disp: 240 ml
Sig: Use one teaspoonful (5 ml) 4–5 times per day for 14 days. Swish for 1 min and expectorate or swallow. Do not eat or drink for 30 min after using this medication
Patients with pharyngeal candidiasis should be directed to "swish and swallow"
Note: Products contain sucrose

Rx: Clotrimazole 10 mg/ml oral suspension (Lotrimin®)
Disp: 60 ml (14-day supply)
Sig: Swab 1–2 ml the affected area PC (after meals) and HS (at bedtime). Do not eat or drink for 30 min after using this medication.

Rx: Itraconazole oral solution 10 mg/ml (Sporanox®)
Disp: 280 ml (14-day supply)
Sig: Vigorously swish with two tsp (10 ml) for several seconds and expectorate twice daily (BID)

Lozenges

Rx: Clotrimazole 10 mg oral troches (Mycelex®)
Disp: 50 troches
Sig: Dissolve slowly in the mouth one tablet 3–5 times a day for 14 days

Rx: Miconazole 50 mg buccal tablets (Oravig®)
Disp: 15 tablets
Sig: Once daily for 14 days. Place one tablet against your upper gum near back teeth and press gently against the side of cheek for 30 seconds to make sure the tablet stays in place. Leave the tablet until next morning. Switch the sides of your mouth each morning using a new tablet

Rx: Nystatin vaginal tablets 100 000 U
Disp: 30 tablets
Sig: Slowly dissolve one tablet in the mouth, then swallow twice daily (BID) for 14 days

Rx: Clotrimazole 100 mg vaginal tablets (Gyne-Lotrimin®, generic)
Disp: 9 tablets
Sig: Dissolve slowly ½ tablet in mouth, then swallow twice daily (BID) for 14 days; Do not eat or drink for 1 hour following application

Ointment/cream

Rx: Nystatin ointment 100 000 units/g (Mycostatin®, Nilstat®, generic)
Disp: 15 g tube
Sig: Apply thin coat to affected areas in the corners of mouth (angular cheilitis) or inner surface of denture (denture-associated *Candida*) after each meal and before bedtime.

Rx: Clotrimazole 1% cream (Lotrimin®)
Disp: 15 g tube
Sig: Apply thin coat to affected areas in the corners of mouth (angular cheilitis) or inner surface of denture (denture-associated *Candida*) after each meal and before bedtime.
Available over the counter (OTC) as Lotrimin® AF, but labeled for athlete's foot and jock itch

Rx: Ketoconazole 2% cream (Nizoral®)
Disp: 15 g tube
Sig: Apply thin coat to affected area in the corners of mouth and inner surface of denture after each meal and before bedtime for 2 weeks

Systemic

Rx: Fluconazole 100 mg tablets (Diflucan®)
Disp: 15 tablets
Sig: Take two tablets as initial dose, one tablet daily thereafter for 14 days.

Rx: Ketoconazole 200 mg tablets (Nizoral®)
Disp: 10 tablets
Sig: Take one tablet daily for 10 days

chlorhexidine gluconate. The prosthesis must be thoroughly rinsed before reinserting into the mouth. To prevent reinoculation and recurrence of the infection, patients should be reminded to use a new denture brush that is not contaminated with the *Candida* yeast when the infection has been successfully resolved. In cases where the patient has concurrent angular cheilitis, nystatin or clotrimazole cream may be prescribed as concomitant therapy.

Interventions to stimulate salivary flow

Management of SGH and xerostomia can be achieved by saliva stimulation and/or by saliva replacement. In patients with some remaining functional gland tissue, salivary output can be enhanced through several local and systemic interventions (Fox, 2004; von Bültzingslöwen *et al.*, 2007). Salivary flow may be increased by mechanical and gustatory stimulation. Sucking on sugar-free (to minimize a cariogenic environment) hard candy, mints, or lozenges, as well as chewing sugar-free gum can provide temporary relief of oral dryness. Many of these products have additional benefits. Those sweetened with xylitol (e.g., Xylifresh®, Trident®, Xponent®, Smint®), in addition to stimulating salivary flow, possess antimicrobial properties. Xylitol has been shown to inhibit plaque adhesion to the tooth and growth of *streptococci mutans*, the main pathologic organism found in dental caries. Moreover, Biotene® dry mouth therapy products contain antimicrobial enzymes, such as lactoperoxidase, lysozyme, lactoferrin with bacteriostatic or bactericidal activity, that mimic the naturally present human salivary defense system. Patients should be informed that mints or hard candy containing citric acid, although effective in stimulating salivary flow, can pose a risk of enamel erosion (Ram *et al.*, 2011).

Systemic saliva stimulants

There are several pharmacologic salivary stimulants available for patients with dry mouth and SGH, however, pilocarpine and cevimeline are the ones that have been most extensively studied (Fox, 2004; von Bültzingslöwen *et al.*, 2007). Currently, they are the only two drugs approved by the US Food and Drug Administration (FDA) for relief of oral dryness symptoms and/or salivary hypofunction caused by SS (pilocarpine and cevimeline) or radiotherapy for head and neck cancer (pilocarpine). These are both cholinergic, parasympathomimetic agents acting primarily via muscarinic receptors; thus they increase salivary flow and reduce sensation of oral dryness in individuals with remaining viable gland tissue. Their effects are dose-related and temporary, however. Both pilocarpine and cevimeline are available only by prescription. The recommended initial dose for pilocarpine (Salagen®, MGI Pharma Inc., Bloomington, MN, USA) is 5 mg to be taken orally 3–4 times a day. The cevimeline hydrochloride (Evoxac®, Daiichi Pharmaceuticals, Tokyo, Japan) recommended oral dose is 30 mg three times daily.

Both pilocarpine and cevimeline are relatively safe with rare serious adverse effects. Excessive sweating, nausea, dizziness, and rhinitis are the most frequently observed adverse reactions. Both drugs are contraindicated in patients with narrow-angle glaucoma, uncontrolled asthma, and acute iritis. Also, it is advisable to consult with the patient's physician before prescribing either drug to a geriatric patient who may have cardiovascular or pulmonary disease as well as decreased renal and/or hepatic function.

Other lesser-known medications and interventions used to enhance salivary output include: low dose human interferon-alpha lozenges (Shiozawa *et al.*, 1998), acupuncture (Blom *et al.*, 1992), and electrostimulation (Weiss *et al.*, 1986).

Saliva substitutes

Patients who do not respond to mechanical local or systemic saliva stimulation may benefit from a variety of saliva substitutes or artificial saliva products available over-the-counter (Table 14.4). These products do not enhance saliva flow. Their intended use is mainly palliative to replace saliva's lubricating and moisturizing capacity. Topical, alcohol-free moisturizers are available as mouthwashes, sprays, gels, or lozenges (e.g., Biotene®, Oralube®, Moi-Stir®, Oasis®, Orajel®, MouthKote®), and can be used when needed to provide transient relief of oral dryness symptoms. The most common thickening agents used to boost the viscosity of saliva substitutes are carboxylmethyl cellulose (CMC), hydroxyethylcellulose, polyacrylic acid, xantham gum, and animal mucin. All of these act to aid to lubrication of the oral mucosa.

It is difficult for clinicians to recommend specific salivary substitutes to their patients as product performance is affected by patient's particular circumstances and clinical presentation. Individual

Table 14.4 Examples of saliva replacement products (salivary substitutes) commercially available

Product name	Manufacturer/distributor
A.S. Saliva Orthana Moisturizing spray Moisturizing lozenges Mucin-based	A.S. Pharmaceuticals, Andover, Hampshire, UK web: www.aspharma.co.uk
Aquoral®spray Citrus flavor Prescription only	Bi-Coastal Pharmaceuticals Corp., Red Bank, NJ, USA web: www.bicoastalpharm.com
Biotene® Moisturizing mouth spray PBF oral rinse Oral balance liquid Oral balance moisturizing gel	GlaxoSmithKline Moon Township, PA, USA web: us.gsk.com; www.biotene.com
BioXtra Moisturizing gel Moisturizing spray gel Contains xylitol	Lighthouse Health Products Inc. Cambridge, ON, Canada web: www.bioxtra.ca
GC America dry mouth gel Five flavors: raspberry, fruit salad, mint, lemon and orange	GC America, Inc. Alsip, IL, USA web: www.gcamerica.com
Moi-Stir® oral spray	Kingswood Laboratories, Inc. Indianapolis, IN, USA web: www.Kingswood-labs.com
Mouth Kote® dry mouth spray Contains xylitol	Parnell Pharmaceuticals Inc. San Rafael, CA, USA www.parnellpharm.com
Numoisyn® Lozenges Liquid Rx only	Align Pharmaceuticals, LLC Berkeley Heights, NJ, USA web: www.alignpharma.com
Oasis® Mouth spray Mouthwash Contains xylitol Two flavors: peppermint and spearmint	Gebauer Consumer Healthcare Cleveland, OH, USA web: www.oasisdrymouth.com
Orajel® dry mouth moisturizing gel	Church and Dwight Co., Inc. Princeton, NJ, USA web: www.orajel.com
Oralube® spray Lemon flavor	Orion Laboratories Pty, Ltd Balcatta, Western Australia web: www.orion.net.au
OraMoist® dry mouth patch Contains xylitol	Quantum, Inc. Eugene, OR, USA web: www.oramoist.com
Salese® soft lozenges Contains xylitol Three flavors: peppermint, wintergreen, and mild lemon	Nuvora Inc. Salta Clara, CA, USA web: www.nuvorainc.com
SalivaSure® lozenges Contains xylitol Citrus flavor	Scandinavian Formulas, Inc. Sellersville, PA, USA web: www.scandinavianformulas.com

parameters such as salivary flow rates are unique to each patient. Therefore, patients should try each product individually for few weeks to determine which is most effective in relieving their symptoms.

Other general recommendations for patients with xerostomia should include: (i) avoiding anything that could exacerbate dryness, such as: caffeinated or alcoholic beverages; alcohol containing mouthwashes and rinses (contributes to dehydration), and dry or spicy foods that can irritate oral mucous membranes; (ii) sipping water frequently or sucking on ice chips to maintain hydration; (iii) using a cold air humidifiers, especially at night for mouth breathers when their symptoms are exacerbated; (iv) using water- or lanolin-based moisturizers on the lips and under dentures to prevent cracking, and mucosal soreness; (v) using powered toothbrushes which have been shown to improve salivary flow (Hargitai *et al.*, 2005); and (vi) avoiding products and toothpaste containing sodium lauryl sulfate since in some individuals it can trigger the occurrence of aphthous ulcers (canker sores). Smokers should also be encouraged to quit smoking cigarettes for obvious medical reasons and because cigarettes promote oral dryness.

Future directions

Ongoing research efforts on interventions for SGH focus on several promising areas. These include the investigation of adult stem cells grafting which may show potential in replacing nonfunctioning salivary glands (Coppes & Stokman, 2011), gene therapy to replace and/or supplement nonfunctional genes controlling salivary secretion with healthy ones (Zheng *et al.*, 2011), development of artificial salivary glands for those who have lost all salivary glands function, and the development of new therapeutic biologic agents (Chen *et al.*, 2009; Tran *et al.*, 2005). In the future, the application of nanotechnology to pharmacology may yield new drugs that provide long-lasting palliative effects, have fewer adverse effects, and target-specific salivary glands.

Case study 1

A 64-year-old white female is seen for the first time in your office. She presents with a chief complaint of "My teeth are falling apart and are kind of cracked." In addition, she complains of dry mouth. Her medical history is significant for myocardial infarction 10 years ago, followed by placement of a defibrillator and stents. The stents have been replaced 6 months ago. Patient has also Crohn's disease and hypertension that is controlled by medications. She reports allergy to metronidazole (Flagyl®). The patient is a former smoker. She quit 10 years ago but smoked one pack/day for 30 years. In regards to her oral hygiene habits, she flosses and brushes twice daily with over-the-counter fluoride toothpaste. Her drinking water contains fluoride. To ease the sensation of oral dryness she drinks sweetened beverages and eats candy multiple times between meals to moisten her mouth.

The patient takes the following medications: metaproponol (beta-blocker), enalapril (ACE-inhibitor), hydrochlorothizide (diuretic), aspirin, clopidogrel (antiplatelet), simvastatin (cholesterol-lowering medication), loperamide (an opioid-receptor agonist for Crohn's disease), and L-methylfolate (nutritional supplement). Her vital signs are normal with a blood pressure of 130/76 mmHg, a pulse rate of 74 beats per minute, a respiration rate of 18 breaths per minute, and temperature 96.4° F.

Oral examination

Extraoral examination was within normal limits, with no lymphadenopathy. Intraoral examination revealed dry buccal mucous membranes and dry, depapillated tongue. There was very small amount of saliva on the floor of the mouth. Soft and hard palate appeared normal. The patient has most of her natural dentition. Radiographs and clinical examination reveals multiple teeth with both primary and recurrent caries (Figs 14.5a,b, 14.6 & 14.7). Other clinical findings include: fractured teeth, missing teeth, and defective restorations.

Case study questions

1 What is the most likely cause of patient's symptoms of dry mouth and why?
2 What findings in the history and oral examination are of interest?
3 What dietary counseling would you provide for this patient?
4 What would be the next most appropriate step to do?
5 What palliative treatment interventions would you suggest to the patient to alleviate her symptoms of dry mouth?
6 What caries preventive strategies could you recommend?

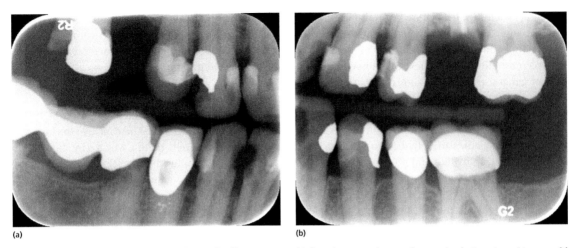

(a) (b)

Figure 14.5 (a,b) Posterior bitewing radiographs illustrating multiple primary and secondary caries lesions in a 64-year-old woman with dry mouth and hyposalivation.

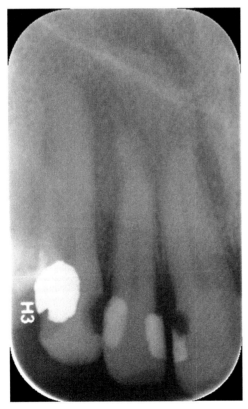

Figure 14.6 Maxillary periapical radiograph illustrating multiple interproximal recurrent caries on anterior teeth in a 64-year-old woman with dry mouth and hyposalivation.

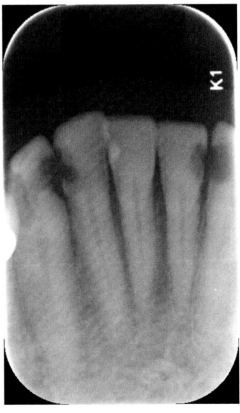

Figure 14.7 Mandibular periapical radiograph illustrating multiple recurrent caries lesions on anterior teeth in a 64-year-old woman with dry mouth and hyposalivation.

Case study 2

A 59-year-old white male presents to your office with a chief complaint of "I broke some teeth off and I need repairs to my partial." He has been your patient for the past 3 years (Fig. 14.8). About 1.5 years ago, following extraction of multiple teeth due to caries, the patient received a maxillary full denture and a mandibular removable distal extension partial denture (Fig. 14.9, remaining teeth after treatment). The patient wished to retain as many natural teeth as possible. It was recommended to the patient to brush his remaining teeth with *PreviDent® 5000 Plus* to lower the risk of new caries to the remaining dentition. Two months after delivery of his dentures, the patient was diagnosed with squamous cell carcinoma (SCC) of the inferior left lateral border of the tongue and anterior tonsillar pillar. He and was treated with radiation and chemotherapy with a total dose of less than 50 Gy. The radiation treatment was completed 3 months after the diagnosis.

Other significant medical history findings include: arthritis (severe lower back pain), depression and anxiety, anemia (post-chemotherapy), and blood transfusions, hypothyroidism (following radiation). He is also a former smoker who quit 4 years prior being diagnosed with SCC of the tongue and throat.

Patient takes the following medications: gabapentin (for neuropathic back pain), baclofen (muscle relaxant), bupropion (antidepressant), ziprasidone (antipsychotic), fentanyl (for pain), oxycodone (analgesic opioid), naproxen (NSAID), levothyroxine (thyroid hormone), atorvastatin (cholesterol lowering). His vital signs are blood pressure 110/70 mmHg, a pulse rate of 88 beats per minute, and a respiration rate of 12 breaths per minute.

Oral examination

Extraoral examination was within normal limits (WNL). On intraoral examination the mucous membranes appear dry and slightly erythematous. There is very small amount of viscous saliva on the floor of the mouth. The tongue appears red and depapillated with white plaques that can be scraped off. The palatal mucosa is dry and slightly erythematous with localized petechiae (Fig. 14.10). Teeth nos. 23–26 are fractured at the gumline with retained root tips (Fig. 14.11). These mucosal findings are indicative of a possible candidiasis. The remaining mandibular teeth: nos. 21, 22, and 27 have root and coronal caries (Fig. 14.12). Teeth nos. 21, 22, and 27 have moderate periodontitis with gingival recession, no mobility. The maxillary full denture is ill-fitting due to weight loss of 50 lbs following radiation and chemotherapy.

Case study questions

1 What else in addition to radiotherapy could exacerbate this patient's symptoms of xerostomia and hyposalivation?

2 What preventive techniques are available to prevent post-radiation caries?
3 What methods to stimulate saliva would you suggest to the patient if there is remaining viable salivary tissue?
4 What palliative treatment strategies would you suggest to alleviate this patient's symptoms of dry mouth?
5 What treatment modalities would you recommend to treat oral candidiasis infection?
6 What instructions would you provide the patient regarding the handling and storing of his dentures to prevent recurrence of his *Candida* infection?

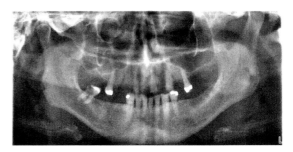

Figure 14.8 Panoramic radiograph demonstrating the status of dentition at the initial visit.

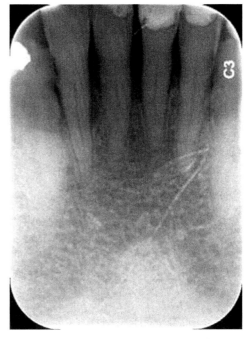

Figure 14.9 Mandibular periapical radiograph illustrating the anterior teeth after delivery of dentures and prior to radiotherapy for head and neck cancer.

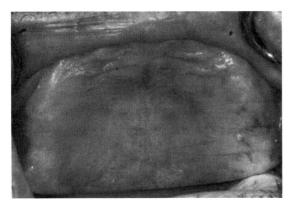

Figure 14.10 Dry palatal mucosa with localized erythema and soreness secondary to radiation and medication-induced xerostomia. Courtesy of Dr. Brandon Jones.

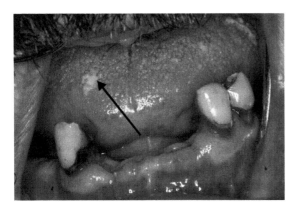

Figure 14.11 Mandibular periapical radiograph illustrating gross caries and retained root tips of anterior teeth in a 59-year-old man with radiation and medication-induced xerostomia. Patient received radiation for treatment of SCCA of the tongue and throat a year ago. Note white plaques on the tongue that are indicative of candidiasis (arrow).

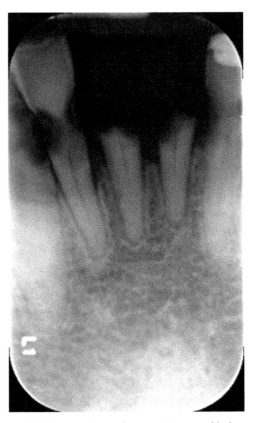

Figure 14.12 Root caries on the remaining mandibular teeth in a 59-year-old man who a year ago received radiation therapy for oral cancer. The teeth were caries free prior to radiotherapy. Courtesy of Dr. Brandon Jones.

Case study 3

A 53-year-old female presents to your office complaining that her mouth is falling apart despite the fact that she has been brushing twice daily. In addition, she complains of dry mouth and some difficulty speaking. She noticed these symptoms started about 10 months ago but they were not as severe and were intermittent in duration. In the past 2 months, however, the symptoms became more frequent and bothersome. Her last dental visit was about 3 years ago due to lack of dental insurance. She is a social worker and during the course of her work she talks to several clients, so having difficulty speaking is really problematic and frustrating to her. In addition she started to have problems sleeping at night and feels constantly tired. To help relieve the sensation of dry mouth she eats hard candy and drinks a variety of beverages (coffee, water, juice, soda, etc.) several times a day. She also notices that she needs to drink water to help in the swallowing of meat and dry foods such as bread, crackers, and cookies. She has had no pain on swallowing, has a good appetite and did not lose any weight (despite periodic upset stomach).

Her medical history is significant for an appendectomy when she was 18 years old and a cholecystectomy at the age of 43. Except for recent years' general joint soreness and stiffness in the morning that she attributes to getting older, she has no other complaints. The patient is on no prescribed medications but takes over-the-counter antihistamines and decongestants to help with her seasonal allergies that recently got worse. She drinks minimal alcohol (2–3 glasses of wine

(Continued)

a week) and smokes 5–10 cigarettes a day. There is no lymphadenopathy. However, the patient recalls that sometime in the past her submandibular glands were swollen but not painful and this resolved after a week or so. Her blood pressure is 110/70 mmHg and her radial pulse is 70 beats per minute.

Oral examination

Extraoral examination is as follows: the patient looks generally tired and her eyes are slightly red. Intraoral examination reveals dry and pale buccal mucous membranes (Fig. 14.13), little saliva on the floor of the mouth, moderate amounts of plaque, and multiple primary and recurrent caries (Figs 14.14 & 14.15). Her remaining dentition is heavily restored.

Case study questions

1 What syndrome are patient's oral and systemic findings suggestive of?
2 How would you confirm the diagnosis?
3 What treatment recommendations would you make to help this patient prevent dental caries?
4 What systemic pharmacologic agents could you recommend to increase salivary flow for this patient?
5 What other therapeutic agents and interventions may be recommended to this patient to alleviate the discomfort associated with her xerostomia?

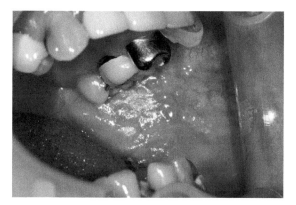

Figure 14.13 Dry, pale mucosa in a patient with xerostomia and hyposalivation. Courtesy of Dr. Sarah Chambers.

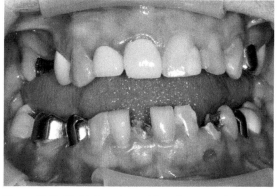

Figure 14.15 Multiple caries and heavily restored dentition in a patient with xerostomia and hyposalivation. Courtesy of Dr. Sarah Chambers.

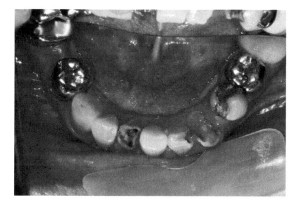

Figure 14.14 Gross coronal caries on mandibular anterior teeth in a patient with xerostomia and hyposalivation. Courtesy of Dr. Sarah Chambers.

MULTIPLE CHOICE QUESTIONS

Answers are found at the end of the book.
1 Xerostomia is a normal part of aging resulting from age-related acinar atrophy. Complaints of dry mouth in older adults are caused by factors other than aging.
   A The first statement is true, the second statement is false
   B The first statement is false, the second statement is true
   C Both statements are true
   D Both statements are false

2 Which of the following statements regarding xerostomia is TRUE?
  A Xerostomia is always consistent with diminished salivary gland function
  B Salivary gland hypofunction is always associated with xerostomia
  C Xerostomia is diagnosed by measuring salivary flow rates
  D Xerostomia may be an indication of underlying systemic disease

3 A 70-year-old man presents to your office with complaints of dry mouth and occasionally difficulty when swallowing dry foods. The most appropriate next step is to:
  A Refer for blood tests for Sjögren's syndrome markers
  B Measure salivary flow rates
  C Perform oral examination with palpation of major salivary glands
  D Review medical history and medications

4 The most common cause of dry mouth in the elderly is:
  A Dehydration
  B High blood pressure
  C Use of medications
  D Age-related changes in salivary glands

5 Which clinical findings are consistent with hyposalivation?
  1 Increased risk for fungal infections such as oral candidiasis
  2 Increased risk for severe periodontitis
  3 Increased risk for dental caries
  4 Increased risk for oral cancer
  A 1 and 2
  B 1 and 3
  C 2 and 3
  D All of the above

6 All of the systemic diseases/conditions listed below may be a cause for xerostomia in older adults except for one. Which one is the EXCEPTION?
  A Hyperlipidemia
  B Chronic depression
  C Sjögren's syndrome
  D Diabetes mellitus

7 Which of the following statements regarding Sjögren's syndrome is TRUE?
  A Patients with Sjögren's syndrome are more likely to develop non-Hodgkin's lymphoma
  B The hallmark symptoms of Sjögren's syndrome are dental caries and joint pain
  C Sjögren's syndrome is a disorder which affects equally older men and women
  D Sjögren's syndrome is diagnosed by serum rheumatoid factor assay

8 Which salivary glands are most sensitive to radiation?
  A Submandibular and sublingual glands
  B Minor salivary glands
  C Parotid glands
  D All glands are equally sensitive to radiation

9 Symptoms of radiation-induced xerostomia are transient and improve with time after the treatment is competed. Total dose of radiation exceeding 60 Gy results in permanent damage to salivary gland tissue.
  A The first statement is true, the second statement is false
  B The first statement is false, the second statement is true
  C Both statements are true
  D Both statements are false

10 The treatment goal/s for xerostomia and salivary gland hypofunction include:
  A Improve salivary gland function
  B Alleviate oral discomfort
  C Prevent dental caries
  D Prevent oral candidiasis
  E All of the above

11 General recommendations for patients with xerostomia and/or hyposalivation include:
  A Dietary counseling (such as avoiding frequent snacking especially sugary and dry foods as well as caffeine and alcohol containing drinks)
  B Reinforcing the importance of meticulous oral hygiene
  C Recommending more frequent check-ups with professional cleanings and fluoride applications (when the natural dentition is present)
  D All of the above

References

Atkinson, J.C., Shiroky, J.B., Macynski, A., *et al.* (1989) Effects of furosemide on the oral cavity. *Gerodontology*, **8**(1), 23–6.

Azevedo, L.R., Damante, J.H., Lara, V.S., *et al.* (2005) Age-related changes in human sublingual glands: a post mortem study. *Archives of Oral Biology*, **50**(6), 565–74.

Becks, H. & Wainwright, W.W. (1943) Human saliva. XIII. Rate of flow of resting saliva of healthy individuals. *Journal of Dental Research*, **22**, 391–6, 408–14.

Beltrán-Aguilar, E.D., Goldstein, J.W. & Lockwood, S.A. (2000) Fluoride varnishes. A review of their clinical use, cariostatic mechanism, efficacy and safety. *Journal of the American Dental Association*, **131**(5), 589–96.

Berghahl, M. (2000) Salivary flow and oral complaints in adults dental patients. *Community Dentistry and Oral Epidemiology*, **28**, 59–66.

Bertram, U. (1967) Xerostomia: studies of salivary secretion (thesis). *Acta Odontologica Scandinavica*, **25** (Suppl 49), 12–59.

Blom, M., Dawidson, I. & Angmar-Månsson, B. (1992) The effect of acupuncture on salivary flow rates in patients with xerostomia. *Oral Surgery, Oral Medicine, and Oral Pathology*, **73**(3), 293–8.

Chambers, M.S., Rosenthal, D.I. & Weber, R.S. (2007) Radiation induced xerostomia. *Head & Neck*, **29**(1), 58–63.

Chen, M.H., Chen, Y.J., Liao, C.C., *et al.* (2009) Formation of salivary acinar cell spheroids in vitro above a polyvinyl alcohol-coated surface. *Journal of Biomedical Materials Research*, **90**(4), 1066–72.

Coppes, R.P. & Stokman, M.A. (2011) Stem cells and the repair of radiation-induced salivary gland damage. *Oral Diseases*, **17**(2), 143–53.

Dawes, C. (1987) Physiological factors affecting salivary flow rate, oral sugar clearance, and the sensation of dry mouth in man. *Journal of Dental Research*, **66**, 648–53.

Dawes, C. (1996) Factors influencing salivary flow rate and composition. In: *Saliva and Oral Health*, 2nd edn (eds. W.M. Edgar & D.M. O'Mullane), pp. 27–41. British Dental Association, London.

Dawes, C. (2008) Salivary flow patterns and the health of hard and soft oral tissues. *Journal of the American Dental Association*, **139** (Suppl), 18–24.

Dreizen, S., Brown, L.R., Daly, T.E., *et al.* (1977) Prevention of xerostomia-related dental caries in irradiated cancer patients. *Journal of Dental Research*, **56**(2), 99–104.

Fox, P.C. (1996) Differentiation of dry mouth etiology. *Advances in Dental Research*, **10**(1), 13–16.

Fox, P.C. (2004) Salivary enhancement therapies. *Caries Research*, **38**(3), 241–6.

Fox, R.I., Stern, M., & Michelson, P. (2000) Update in Sjögren syndrome. *Current Opinion in Rheumatology*, **12**, 391–8.

Ghezzi, E.M. & Ship, J.A. (2003) Aging and secretory reserve capacity of major salivary glands. *Journal of Dental Research*, **82**(10), 844–8.

Gupta, A., Epstein, J.B, & Sroussi, H. (2006) Hyposalivation in elderly patients. *Journal of the California Dental Association*, **72**(9), 841–6.

Gutman, D. & Ben-Aryeh, H. (1974) The influence of age on salivary content and rate of flow. *International Journal of Oral Surgery*, **3**, 314–17.

Handelman, S.L., Baric, J.M., Saunders, R.H., *et al.* (1989) Hyposalivatory drug use, whole stimulated salivary flow, and mouth dryness in older, long-term care residents. *Special Care in Dentistry*, **9**(1), 12–18.

Hargitai, I.A., Sherman, R.G., & Strother, J.M. (2005) The effects of electrostimulation on parotid saliva flow: a pilot study. *Oral Surgery, Oral Medicine, Oral Pathology, Oral Radiology, and Endodontics*, **99**(3), 316–20.

Heft, M.W. & Baum, B.J. (1984) Unstimulated and stimulated salivary flow rate in different age groups. *Journal of Dental Research*, **63**, 1182–5.

Henriksson, R., Frojd, O., Gustafsson, H., *et al.* (1994) Increase in mast cells and hyaluronic acid correlates to radiation-induced damage and loss of serous acinar cells in salivary glands: the parotid and submandibular glands differ in radiation sensitivity. *British Journal of Cancer*, **69**(2), 320–6.

Hochberg, M.C., Tielsch, J., Munoz, B., *et al.* (1998) Prevalence of symptoms of dry mouth and their relationship to saliva production in community dwelling elderly: the SEE project (Salisbury Eye Evaluation). *Journal of Rheumatology*, **25**(3), 486–91.

Jemal, A., Siegel, R., Xu, J., *et al.* (2010) Cancer statistics 2010, *CA: A Cancer Journal for Clinicians*, **60**(5), 277–300.

Kaplan, M.D. & Baum, B.J. (1993) The functions of saliva. *Dysphagia*, **8**, 225–9.

Locker, D. (1995) Xerostomia in older adults: a longitudinal study. *Gerodontology*, **12**(1), 18–25.

Närhi, T.O. (1994) Prevalence of subjective feelings of dry mouth in the elderly. *Journal of Dental Research*, **73**(1), 20–5.

Navazesh, M., Christensen, C., & Brightman, V. (1992) Clinical criteria for the diagnosis of salivary gland hypofunction. *Journal of Dental Research*, **71**(7), 1363–9.

Nederfors, T. (2000) Xerostomia and hyposalivation. *Advances in Dental Research*, **14**, 48–56.

Orellana, M.F., Lagravere, M.O., Boychuk, D.G., *et al.* (2006) Prevalence of xerostomia in population-based samples: a systematic review. *Journal of Public Health Dentistry*, **66**(2), 152–8.

Patel, P.S., Ghezzi, E.M., & Ship, J.A. (2001) Xerostomic complaints induced by an anti-sialogogue in healthy young vs. older adults. *Special Care Dentistry*, **21**, 176–81.

Pedersen, W., Schubert, M., Izutsu, K., *et al.* (1985) Age-dependent decreases in human submandibular gland flow rates as measured under resting and post-stimulation conditions. *Journal of Dental Research*, **64**(5), 822–5.

Ram, S., Kumar, S., & Navazesh, M. (2011) Management of xerostomia and salivary gland hypofunction. *Journal of the California Dental Association*, **39**(9), 656–9.

Rhodus, N.L. & Brown, J. (1990) The association of xerostomia and inadequate intake in older adults. *Journal of the American Dietetic Association*, **90**(12), 1688–92.

Scott, J., Flower, E.A., & Burns, J. (1987) A quantitative study of histological changes in the human parotid gland occurring with adult age. *Journal of Oral Pathology*, **16**(10), 505–10.

Shiozawa, S., Tanaka, Y., & Shiozawa, K. (1998) Single-blinded controlled trial of low-dose oral IFN-alpha for the treatment of xerostomia in patients with Sjögren's syndrome. *Journal of Interferon & Cytokine Research,* **18**(4), 255–62.

Ship, J.A., Nolan, N.E., & Puckett, S.A. (1995) Longitudinal analysis of parotid and submandibular salivary flow rates in healthy, different-aged adults. The Journals of Gerontology. *Series A, Biological Sciences and Medical Sciences,* **50**(5), M285–9.

Ship, J.A., Pillemer, S.R., & Baum, B.J. (2002) Xerostomia and the geriatric patient. *Journal of the American Geriatrics Society,* **50**, 535–43.

Sreebny, L.M. & Schwartz, S.S. (1997) A reference guide to drugs and dry mouth – 2nd edition. *Gerodontology,* **14**(1), 33–47.

Sreebny, L.M. & Valdini, A. (1988) Xerostomia. Part I: relationship to other oral symptoms and salivary gland hypofunction. *Oral Surgery, Oral Medicine, and Oral Pathology,* **66**(4), 451–8.

Sreebny, L.M., Valdini, A., & Yu, A. (1989) Xerostomia. Part II: relationship to non-oral symptoms, drugs, and diseases. *Oral Surgery, Oral Medicine, and Oral Pathology,* **68**(4), 419–27.

Thomson, W.M. (2005) Issues in the epidemiological investigation of dry mouth. *Gerodontology,* **22**, 65–76.

Thomson, W.M., Chalmers, J.M., Spencer, A.J. *et al.* (1999) The Xerostomia Inventory: a multi-item approach to measuring dry mouth. *Community Dental Health,* **16**, 12–17.

Thomson, W.M., Chalmers, J.M., Spencer, A.J., *et al.* (2000) Medication and dry mouth: findings from a cohort study of older people. *Journal of Public Health Dentistry,* **60**(1), 12–20.

Thomson, W.M., Chalmers, J.M., Spencer, A.J., *et al.* (2006) A longitudinal study of medication exposure and xerostomia among older people. *Gerodontology,* **3**, 205–13.

Tran, S.D., Wang, J., Bandyopadhyay, B.C., *et al.* (2005) Primary culture of polarized human salivary epithelial cells for use in developing an artificial salivary gland. *Tissue Engineering,* **11**(1–2), 172–81.

Turner, M., Jahangiri, L., & Ship, J.A. (2008) Hyposalivation, xerostomia and the complete denture. *Journal of the American Dental Association,* **139**, 146–50.

Tylenda, C.A., Ship, J.A., Fox, P.C., *et al.* (1988) Evaluation of submandibular salivary flow rate in different age groups. *Journal of Dental Research,* **67**(9), 1225–8.

van Nieuw Amerongen, A., Bolscher, J.G.M., & Veerman, E.C. (2004) Salivary proteins: protective and diagnostic value in cariology? *Caries Research,* **38**, 247–53.

von Bültzingslöwen, I., Sollecito, T.P., Fox, P.C., *et al.* (2007) Salivary dysfunction associated with systemic diseases: systematic review and clinical management. *Oral Surgery, Oral Medicine, Oral Pathology, Oral Radiology, and Endodontics,* **103** (Suppl 1), S57,e1–15.

Waterhouse, J.P., Chisholm, D.M., Winter, R.B., *et al.* (1973) Replacement of functional parenchymal cells by fat and connective tissue in human submandibular salivary glands. *An age-related study. Journal of Oral Pathology,* **2**, 16–27.

Weiss, W.W. Jr, Brenman, H.S., Katz, P., *et al.* (1986) Use of an electronic stimulator for the treatment of dry mouth. *Journal of Oral and Maxillofacial Surgery,* **44**(11), 845–50.

Wu, A.J. & Ship, J.A. (1993) A characterization of major salivary gland flow rates in the presence of medications and systemic diseases. *Oral Surgery, Oral Medicine, Oral Pathology,* **76**(3), 301–6.

Zheng, C., Cotrim, A.P., Rowzee, A., *et al.* (2011) Prevention of radiation-induced salivary hypofunction following hKGF gene delivery to murine submandibular glands. *Clinical Cancer Research,* **17**(9), 2842–51.

CHAPTER 15

Prosthetic Considerations for Frail and Functionally Dependent Older Adults

Ronald L. Ettinger

Department of Prosthodontics, Dows Institute for Dental Research, University of Iowa College of Dentistry, Iowa City, IA, USA

Introduction

Earlier chapters have dealt with the demographic imperative and the decline in edentulousness, which has changed the treatment needs of the older population from noninvasive replacement of dentures to the complex needs of the dentate.

There is no such person as a typical older adult because they are extremely heterogeneous, ranging from the healthy to the frail, from the highly educated to the illiterate, from the affluent to the poor (Ettinger, 1993). This heterogeneity results from the fact that each person is influenced by their heredity, their diet, exercise, various diseases accidents, and lifestyle (Chalmers & Ettinger, 2008). The variance among older adults also influences their health literacy, with varying levels of knowledge and motivation regarding health and oral health (Shelley *et al.*, 2008).

In the past, the primary focus of prosthodontics for older adults was how to deliver complete dentures to the population (Eklund, 1999). The retention of teeth and the influence of aging, wear and tear, as well as iatrogenic issues, means that the dental needs of older adults have now become much more complex when compared to younger persons. The need for tooth/teeth replacement, which is the area of dentistry known as prosthodontics, has increased significantly in this population and the younger cohorts of older adults will no longer accept the simple solutions of the past, that is, the extraction of remaining teeth and the construction of complete dentures (Berkey *et al.*, 1996).

The aging population

The elderly have been defined as a cohort of persons aged 65 years and older. The utilization of only a chronological criterion is not particularly useful in dentistry because, as previously discussed, there is a great variation in the population. These older adults have experienced differences in physical health, medical issues and mental conditions as well as different life experiences. Thus, from an oral health perspective, a functional definition is much more useful. Ettinger and Beck (1984) separated the older population into three broad functional categories to reflect their ability to seek dental services:

- *Functionally independent older adults:* These adults live in the community unassisted and comprise about 70% of the population over age 65 years. Many of these persons may have some chronic medical problems such as, hypertension, type 2 diabetes (DM2), or osteoarthritis for which they are taking a variety of medications. Assuming the dental practitioner understands his or her patients' medical issues and the effects of their medications, treatment will depend on their perception of need and the amount they are prepared to pay for it. These older adults can access dental care independently using their own vehicles or public transportation, if it exists. Their prosthodontic treatment has been well-described by Budtz-Jorgensen (1999) in his textbook *"Prosthodontics for the Elderly."*

Geriatric Dentistry: Caring for Our Aging Population, First Edition. Edited by Paula K. Friedman.
© 2014 John Wiley & Sons, Inc. Published 2014 by John Wiley & Sons, Inc.
Companion website: www.wiley.com/go/friedman/geriatricdentistry

- *Frail older adults:* These are those persons who have lost some of their independence, but still live in the community with the help of family and friends or who are using professional support services such as Meals on Wheels, visiting nurses, home health aides, etc. They make up about 20% of the population over age 65 years. These older adults can no longer access dental services without the help of others. Their oral health needs require a greater understanding of medicine and pharmacology and a careful evaluation of their ability to maintain daily oral hygiene. The prosthodontic decision making for this segment of the population is the primary focus of this chapter.
- *Functionally dependent older adults:* These are those persons who are no longer able to live in the community independently and are either home-bound (about 5% of population over 65) or living in institutions (another 5% of population over 65). These older adults can only access dental services if they are transported to a dentist's office and many may use wheelchairs so the offices should be wheelchair accessible. If they cannot be transported, then the services need to be brought to them through mobile programs. This means that dental offices need to be wheelchair-accessible, the dental professional needs mobile equipment to visit the patient, or the institution in which the older adult resides must have a dental facility. This chapter does not deal in detail with the prosthodontic care of this group of older adults. (See Chapters 17 and 18 for alternative dental care delivery models.)

Decision making in prosthodontics

The knowledge base required to manage the oral problems of frail older adults does not depend on the development of new technical skills but rather on the following:

1. An understanding of normal aging;
2. An understanding of pathologic aging;
3. An understanding of older adults' medical problems and recognizing the oral implications of their systemic diseases;
4. A knowledge of pharmacology and drug-induced dental diseases;
5. The interpersonal skills needed to communicate with the patient, his or her family, and his or her other healthcare providers;
6. Knowing special communication techniques with older persons who have sensory deficits;
7. Having practical experience in clinical decision-making for frail and functionally dependent older adults.

The bulk of dental care for frail older adults still remains reconstructive, that is, the restoration of teeth and the restoration of function of the stomatognathic system with fixed and removable partial dentures (Douglass & Watson, 2002). The clinical techniques are usually similar to those needed for treating younger persons; however, more problems are encountered. For example, in recurrent caries the margins of interproximal restorations will need to be placed subgingivally with all the associated problems due to bleeding, marginal adaptation of restorative materials, and finishing (Bader *et al.*, 1991).

Deciding what constitutes appropriate care may vary for an older cohort of individuals because those decisions must include the consideration of a variety of age-related and age-associated psychologic, sociologic, biologic, and pathologic changes. Therefore, it is essential to identify modifying factors before a comprehensive treatment plan is formulated, as illustrated by the the following case study of a functionally independent older adult (Case study 1).

Case study 1

Functionally independent older adult

Mr. Arthur Z. is 75 years old. He is married and is a retired cabinet maker and lives about 20 miles away. His chief complaint is that he is having problems chewing his food and that his dentures no longer fit. His wife who came with him does not like the way his mouth looks. He has a history of hypertension which was diagnosed 10 years ago for which he is taking hydrochlorothiazide 25 mg twice daily. He has a history of cardiac arrhythmia which was diagnosed 6 years ago, for which he is taking disopyramide 100 mg per day. He has had arthritis in his hands for the last 15 years and has been taking ibuprofen 400 mg twice daily. He is very hard of hearing and wears a hearing aid.

An oral examination reveals an ill-fitting complete maxillary denture and severe resorption of the anterior segment of the maxillary ridge with a prominent nasal spine (Figs 15.1 & 15.2).

The remaining mandibular teeth are heavily worn, probably due to the porcelain teeth of the maxillary denture. The mandibular teeth all test vital except for no. 25, which has been root treated but has a periapical lesion (Fig. 15.3). He has bilateral large mandibular tori. He has not worn his mandibular cast removable prosthesis (RPD) because it no longer fits well. Due to the wear of the denture teeth and his natural teeth he is clearly overclosed. His oral hygiene is very good and none of the teeth have periodontal pockets deeper than 3 mm.

What are the impacts of the following medical problems on treatment?

a) **Hypertension.** His blood pressure was 135/80 mmHg and his pulse rate was 68 beats per minute. We will need to monitor his blood pressure at the beginning of each appointment, especially if we are going to use local anesthesia. It would be best to see him at mid-morning or early afternoon when he is rested. We would want to limit epinephrine to 0.036 mg, which is approximately two 1.7 ccs cartridges of lidocaine with 1 : 100 000 epinephrine and reduce stress whenever possible.

b) **Arrhythmia.** His arrhythmia has been stable and is not causing him any problems. He has had no episodes in the last 2 years and the problem seems to be controlled by his medications. We would want to reduce stress during his appointments and limit the use of epinephrine.

c) **Arthritis.** It is mainly in his hands and fingers. His oral hygiene is very good but a simple electric toothbrush might be a useful aid.

d) **Hearing.** We need to remind him to make sure his hearing aid is turned on and to remember to talk to him face to face so that, if necessary, he can lip read. Also, it is important to provide written post-appointment instructions to make sure that the information has been communicated and received.

Dental treatment

He was not in pain so no immediate treatment was necessary. Impressions were made and records taken for diagnostic casts and a diagnostic wax-up were done to develop several treatment plans, which were presented to the patient at a subsequent appointment. What treatment alternatives would you suggest? Some alternative treatment plans you can offer and the rationale for each are outlined below.

Treatment plan no. 1

Maxilla   Bone graft in the anterior, two implants on each side connected by a bar with Hader clips to support a complete overdenture.

Mandible   Surgical removal of the tori. Fixed partial denture (FPD) no. 20–22, crowns on nos 27, 28, 29, root canal treatment (RCT) nos. 23–26, post and core and crowns and one implant on each side for a molar unit.

Comment   This treatment plan is the most expensive and sophisticated, and the most stressful.

Treatment plan no. 2

Maxilla   New complete denture.

Mandible   Surgical removal of the tori FPD nos. 20–22, crown no. 27–29, RCT nos. 23–26 with post and core and crowns, distal extension RPD.

Comment   This treatment plan stabilizes the mandibular arch, is less stressful, but is time-consuming and expensive.

Treatment plan no. 3

Maxilla   New complete denture.

Mandible   Surgical removal of the tori extract nos. 20, 23, 24, 25, 26, 28, 29; cut down nos. 22 and 27 as vital overdenture, abutments for a complete overdenture. Wait 6 weeks before constructing dentures.

Comment   This treatment plan is the least expensive and least stressful and provides the patient with a functional dentition

After presentation of these treatment plans, a modified final treatment plan was developed with the patient and his wife that was within their budget and was aesthetic and functional (Fig. 15.4a–d).

Maxilla   New complete denture.

Mandible   Surgical removal of the tori. FPD nos. 20–22, crowns nos. 27–29, RCT no. 25, Teeth nos. 23–26 cut down as vital overdenture abutments for a cast partial distal extension overdenture. He was prescribed PreviDent® 5000 gel to be used in his RPD on a daily basis after breakfast and after cleaning.

Evaluation of treatment

This dental treatment did solve the patient's chewing and eating problems and improved the quality of his life. His wife approved of the change in his appearance due to the increase in the vertical dimension of occlusion. The problem of the wear of his denture was resolved by a combination of fixed prosthodontics and a removal partial denture. The continuing wear of his teeth was halted by the use of acrylic resin teeth on his complete maxillary denture and his removable partial overdenture. The patient was asked to return in 3 months for evaluation.

Key: FPD = fixed partial denture;   RPD = removable partial denture;   RCT = root canal treatment.

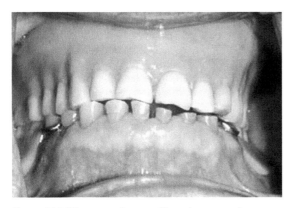

Figure 15.1 Worn complete maxillary denture and worn mandibular teeth with ill fitting removable prosthesis (RPD) (see Case study 1 for more details).

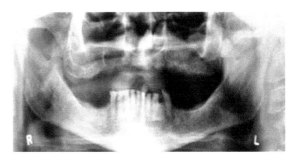

Figure 15.2 Orthopantomograph showing resorbed anterior maxilla and worn mandibular teeth (see Case study 1 for more details).

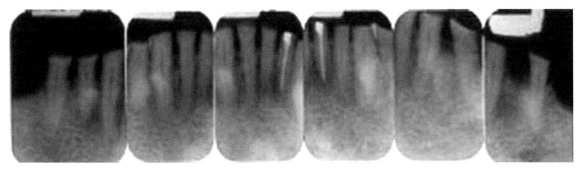

Figure 15.3 Periapical radiographs showing worn dentition and periapical lesion on no. 25 (see Case study 1 for more details).

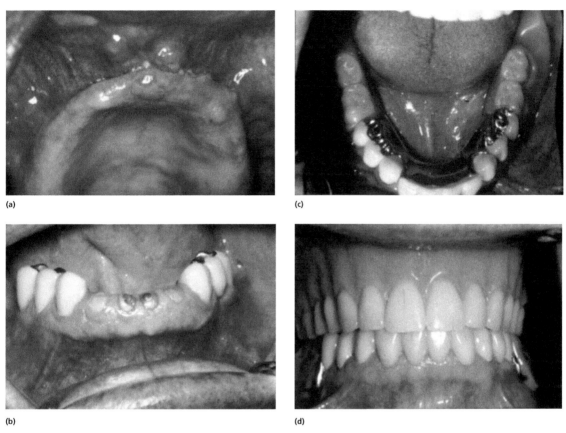

Figure 15.4 (a–d) The restored dentition (see Case study 1 for more details).

Sociodemographic information

To understand the prosthodontic needs of a patient, one must understand the environment in which the patient functions and how oral health care fits into their life style. It is not sufficient to gather a lot of data on age, gender, occupation, and education without understanding how these factors influence the needs and expectations of a patient. Life experiences such as the Depression of the 1930s, the World War of the 1940s, the Korean War of the 1950s, and the Vietnam War of the 1960s influence attitudes, values, and beliefs. The value of a dentition depends on the attitude of the patient, his or her family, or caregivers, which impacts treatment. The question is, does this person utilize health care or dental care only in response to some symptoms such as pain and discomfort? If so, how can the dentist influence and educate the patient to change these behaviors? Is this a patient who is educated about health issues and who would appreciate the presentation of several treatment plans of varying costs, which would allow the patient to choose one which best fits their expectations and lifestyle? If not, how can we help to educate the patient to increase oral health literacy?

Health history

As a population ages, there is a higher risk for chronic diseases and the patient is more likely to take medications, some of which have the potential to affect the oral tissues (Jainkittivong *et al.*, 2004). The most common side effect of many of the drugs used by this population is hyposalivation, which may induce xerostomia and increase the risk of caries and periodontal disease (Guggenheimer, 2002; Shinozaki *et al.*, 2012; Thomson, 2005). If a person has severe xerostomia induced by disease (Sjögren's syndrome), therapy (radiation or chemotherapy), or by drugs (e.g., amitriptyline), which may increase the risk of ulcerations when wearing dentures and a loss of retention of the maxillary denture (Thomson, 2005). The risk of mucosal infection by *Candida albicans*, especially underneath a maxillary denture, is increased. Saliva substitutes such as Oral Balance® or MI Paste® can help with the lubrication and retention of a complete denture (Gil-Montoya *et al.*, 2008).

When caring for frail or functionally dependent older adults, an evaluation of their health history will help determine whether these problems will affect them. (See Chapter 14 for a more detailed discussion of xerostomia.)

Tips and techniques for treating frail or functionally dependent elders

Time of the appointment
Due to the circadian changes in platelet aggregation related to hemostasis, patients with cardiovascular disease should not be seen between 6 AM and 9 AM because of an increased risk of a cardiovascular event (Chursciel *et al.*, 2009). Patients with arthritis are preferably not seen before late morning or early afternoon due to stiffness of their joints in the morning (Walker, 2011). Patients with dementia should be seen in midmorning when they are fresh as tiredness can bring on unacceptable behaviors (Mancini *et al.*, 2010).

Length of the appointment
Many frail or functionally dependent older adults cannot sit for extended periods of time. Patients who are underweight may need pillows and support in the dental chair to cushion their spines. It is suggested that a dental visit should *not* be longer than 90 minutes from the time the patient leaves their residence to the time they return. They may require additional and shorter appointments for their prosthodontic procedures.

Patient positioning
Patients who have hiatus hernia, severe cardiopulmonary disease, or a variety of pulmonary diseases may not be comfortable when laid flat in a dental chair for the length of time of an appointment. Apart from asking directly, it may be useful to ask the patient how many pillows they sleep with or if their bed is propped up for sleeping.

Need for antibiotic prophylaxis
The 2007 American Heart Association guidelines revised the recommendations for antibiotic prophylaxis to reduce the risk of infective endocarditis (Wilson *et al.*, 2007). Persons with prosthetic valves, a previous history of infective endocarditis, a cardiac transplant, or who are significantly immunocompromized are best treated with prophylactic antibiotics for any invasive dental procedures such as extractions, deep scaling, crown lengthening, etc. The guidelines suggest that all others who are at risk should rinse with chlorhexidine gluconate 0.12% prior to any invasive procedures. Persons who have had a major joint replaced should have antibiotic coverage for the first 2 years after their replacement. If they have not had any complications, or dislocations, then further coverage is not recommended (ADA & AAOS, 2003). The antibiotic prophylaxis guidelines were revised because of a lack of evidence-based data that antibiotics were beneficial compared to the existing data of the danger of an allergic reaction to antibiotics or the potential for development of resistant organisms.

Use of local anesthetic with vasoconstrictor (epinephrine)
It has been suggested that the amount of epinephrine used in local anesthesia be limited to 0.036 mg of epinephrine. in patients with cardiovascular disease (Neves *et al.*, 2007). This translates to the approximate equivalent of two cartridges of 2% lidocaine (1.7 ccs) with 1 : 100 000 epinephrine (Brown & Rhodus, 2005).

Level of cognitive impairment
Since communication is an extremely important interaction between the patient and the dentist, the level of cognitive impairment influences treatment. Here are some areas to consider before beginning treatment. The clinician needs to determine if the patient can explain his or her chief complaint. Can the patient give an accurate medical history or do we need to procure it from their physician or significant other? Can the patient give us informed consent to proceed with treatment or will we need to obtain it from their legally appointed guardian for health affairs (healthcare proxy)? How will we be paid? Has the patient a legally appointed guardian for their financial affairs? Where is the patient living and is there anybody who can or will supervise their daily oral hygiene? Finally, will the patient be cooperative with you as the clinician?

Since prosthodontics usually requires multiple appointments, how do you assess the risk/benefit ratio of treatment, modified treatment, or no treatment? Will the patient benefit from the stress associated with these appointments? Will there be a need for physical or chemical restraint and who will give informed consent for that treatment?

These assessments are needed to determine whether the replacement of lost teeth is necessary and if it would be beneficial to the patient. The assessment will facilitate decision making with regard to replacement either with implants, a fixed partial denture (FPD), a removable prosthesis (RPD), or no replacement at all.

Case study 2

Frail older adult

Mr. Ray R. is 80 years old. He has been a widower for the past 5 years and lives in a communal home in a mid-sized town. He has little contact with his only son who lives on the West coast. He was referred for treatment to our clinic by his friend who drives and could bring him to his appointments. He has a limitation on what services he can afford, but his mouth is sore and he cannot eat comfortably. He has several major health problems. He is allergic to penicillin. He has hypertension and his blood pressure at the initial appointment was 195/98 mmHg. He has a history of hyperlipedemia. He had a mild stroke a year ago with full recovery of all functions. He has type 2 diabetes and monitors his blood sugar twice a day. This morning it was about 160 mg/dl. He had an inguinal hernia repaired 8 years ago. He had prostate cancer surgery 7 years ago. He has cataracts which need surgery. Mr. Ray R. is taking aspirin (enteric coated) 81 mg daily, to prevent any thrombus formation and reduce the risk of a cardiovascular event; Lasix® (furosemide) 40 mg daily, potassium chloride/potassium gluconate (KCL) 20 mEq twice daily, this is a loop diuretic that produces diuresis to lower his blood pressure; atenolol 50 mg daily, this is a selective beta-1 blocker which slows the heart rate and decreases myocardial oxygen demand; Zocor® (simvastatin) 20 mg daily, which is a HMG-CoA reductase inhibitor that lowers cholesterol; Glucophage® (metformin) 500 mg twice daily, this is an antihyperglycemic which improves glycemic control.

An oral examination revealed that he was not cleaning his teeth adequately, that the FPD on the maxilla was loose, and that tooth no. 8 had significant caries (Fig. 15.5). On the mandible, tooth no. 20 is fractured off at the gingival as are nos. 27 and 28 (Fig. 15.6), these teeth may be responsible for his discomfort. He also had caries and bone loss around teeth nos. 21 and 22. He said he had a mandibular RPD at one time but he had not worn it for some time. He also complained that his mouth was dry.

A radiographic examination revealed root canal therapy on his remaining maxillary teeth (Fig. 15.7). All the teeth were crowned with extensive caries underneath the crowns. There was an FPD, which extended from tooth no. 9 to tooth no. 13, and was unsupported on teeth nos. 9 and 11. Teeth nos. 12 and 13 were cantilevered. The FPD was removable. On the mandibular arch, teeth nos. 20, 27, and 28 were fractured off at the gingival and had periapical radiolucencies. Teeth nos. 21 and 22 were root treated and crowned and had some caries.

Case study questions

1 What is the indication for each of the medications prescribed for the patient? Do you have any concerns that the patient is taking his medications? Why or why not?
2 How will his medical problems impact dental treatment?
3 What additional information would you like to know about this patient and why?

What is the impact of his medical problems on his dental treatment?

Hypertension

Mr. Ray R. must see his physician prior to his next dental appointment. He will need his blood pressure monitored for all of his future dental appointments. He should not have more than 0.036 mg of epinephrine at one time when local anesthesia is used. This translates into approximately 2 carpules of 1.7 cc of lidocaine with 1 : 100 000 epinephrine. His appointments should be scheduled for mid-morning or early afternoon with attention to keeping stress to a minimum so as to avoid a cardiovascular event.

Diabetes

Mr. Ray R. will need to have breakfast and take his medication before he comes in for his dental appointments. We will need to assess how stable is his control of his blood sugar. We should expect some delayed healing after his extractions. We will prescribe a chlorhexidine rinse for him after his extractions.

Stroke

His stroke or cardiovascular accident (CVA) was due to a thrombus transiently blocking a vessel in his brain. He has many risk factors for another CVA, which include; his age, hypertension, high cholesterol, and having had a CVA previously. During treatment we need to monitor him for any signs of stroke such as headache and particularly confusion. We also need to limit the use of epinephrine and use a stress reduction protocol. One should try to limit his traveling time and his dental appointment to about 90 minutes, to reduce tiring him out and increasing stress.

Cataracts

His vision will be compromised because of the cataracts, so his oral hygiene may be poor until he gets the cataracts removed.

Dental treatment

Mr. Ray R. is in discomfort and he has several teeth which have their crowns broken off. An evaluation of his radiographic survey shows that he has caries on several other teeth. Due to a limitation of his finances and his health and mobility problems, the following rational treatment plans were offered.

Treatment plan no. 1 (emergency care – pain and infection)

- Extract all the remaining maxillary teeth
- Extract all the remaining mandibular teeth
- Wait 6 weeks for healing
- Evaluate the patient for the ability to benefit from new complete maxillary and mandibular complete dentures

Comment   This is the cheapest treatment plan which deals with his immediate problems.

Treatment plan no. 2 (limited care – restoration of function)

- Extract all of remaining maxillary teeth
- Extract teeth nos. 20, 27, and 28, and restore teeth nos. 21 and 22
- Prescribe the daily use of Prevident® 5000 gel
- Wait 6 weeks and construct complete maxillary denture and an interim mandibular denture

Comment   This treatment plan addresses his main complaint and improves his chewing ability.

Treatment plan no. 3 (comprehensive care)

- Extract all remaining maxillary teeth
- Extract nos. 20, 27, and 28 and restore teeth nos. 21 and 22, with new crowns
- Place an implant in place of tooth no. 27
- Prescribe the daily use of Prevident® 5000 gel
- Wait 6 weeks and construct complete maxillary denture and a cast removable partial mandibular denture
- After 3 months retrofit the denture with a locator attachment on the implant

Comment   This treatment plan addresses his immediate problems, stabilizes his mandibular arch and will improve his ability to chew.

Final treatment plan

After discussion with the patient and his friend, and a discussion with his physician, teeth nos. 27 and 28 were extracted immediately because it was determined that these teeth were the immediate cause of his discomfort. The patient returned the next week where the three treatment plans were presented. He had been to his physician who did not change his medications. The patient and his friend chose treatment plan no. 2 with modifications because he was interested in function and esthetics. The treatment modification was to construct an immediate complete maxillary denture and an interim all-resin RPD maintaining teeth nos. 21 and 22 (Fig. 15.8). He chose the immediate dentures because teeth nos. 21 and 22 were in occlusion with his FPD and this is what he chewed with so he did not want to lose that function. The treatment was successfully carried out with intravenous sedation for the surgery and the patient has returned on recall after 1 year (Fig. 15.9).

Evaluation of treatment

This treatment did improve the patient's quality of life. He is now pain-free and infection-free, and he has better function with more chewing pairs of teeth, which may help him choose more appropriate foods to control his diabetes. The use of Prevident® 5000 gel will help counter the effect of his medication-induced xerostomia as it is a high concentration fluoride that does not contain sodium lauryl sulfate, which would dry him out further.

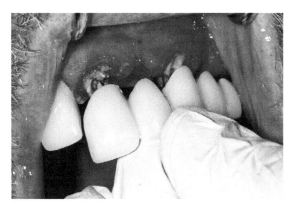

Figure 15.5 Maxillary arch, showing the patient's fixed partial denture, which is removable, and the extensive caries of the abutments (see Case study 2 for more details).

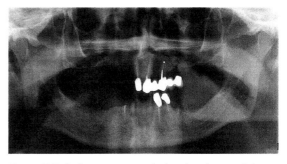

Figure 15.7 Orthopantomograph showing the remaining dentition (see Case study 2 for more details).

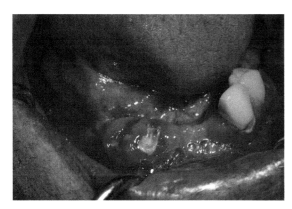

Figure 15.6 Mandibular arch, showing the loss of crowns on teeth nos. 27 and 28 (see Case study 2 for more details).

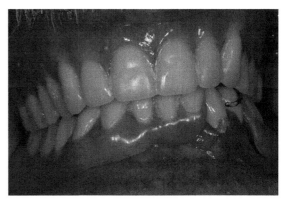

Figure 15.8 Shows the immediate maxillary complete denture and the immediate mandibular interim resin removable prosthesis (RPD) in occlusion which restored the patient's esthetics and function (see Case study 2 for more details).

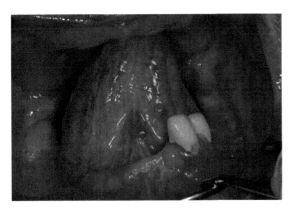

Figure 15.9 Shows the patient's healed arches after a year. He has not had any more caries on the abutments and states that he is using the PreviDent® 5000 gel (see Case study 2 for more details).

Evaluations for prosthodontic rehabilitation

After the clinician has gathered all of the required data from the patient and their caregiver, as well as from their physician, then the oral tissues should be evaluated. The face and neck should also be examined for any lesions, especially actinic damage. If lesions are identified and cause concern regarding the patient's health, or have potential to influence dental treatment, the patient should be referred to his/her physician for treatment. The temporomandibular joints should be palpated and auscultated for crepitus, clicks, or tenderness or pain over the joint.

An oral examination of the soft tissues of the mouth should follow, including looking under the tongue and in the tonsillar region. This should be followed by an examination and charting of the dentition supported by appropriate radiographs, periodontal probing, and determination of the existence of caries with pulp testing where appropriate. To establish an appropriate prosthodontic evaluation will usually require mounted study casts in centric relation.

A critical evaluation of the patient's ability to maintain daily oral hygiene independently or with the help of family or caretakers should be completed. The prognosis of treatment with a fixed or removable prosthesis will depend on this assessment. If the patient cannot maintain daily oral hygiene independently, then a fixed prosthesis is questionable. If there is no one to reliably help with the patient's daily oral hygiene, a

RPD may not be the treatment of choice and the long-term prognosis for the dentition will need to be evaluated. A flowchart for decision making when faced with caring for a patient who has a terminal dentition is shown in Fig. 15.10. The options are to extract the unsalvageable teeth and make an interim RPD and follow the patient or to make the decision that the patient cannot care for the teeth and so they all should be extracted. If esthetics is not an issue, or finances cannot support an immediate denture, then the patient will be without any dentures for 6 weeks to allow adequate healing until a set of dentures can be fabricated.

Systematic evaluation of the dentition

Using the mounted study casts, the clinician can evaluate how many tooth pairs remain in the dentition and how many are required to restore function. What are the expectations of the patient and his or her family regarding the restoration of esthetics? Does one need to do a diagnostic wax-up to determine the feasibility of restoring the dentition? What is the risk/cost/benefit of saving a particular tooth and can the patient afford the treatment and tolerate the procedure? For instance, if there are extensive caries which extend subgingivally, the tooth may need root canal therapy, crown lengthening, and a crown. If there is a heavily restored tooth on either side, an extraction and a FPD may be the treatment of choice. If there are healthy teeth on either side, an implant may be ideal. If there are other missing teeth on the opposite side, an RPD may be appropriate. In every situation, it must be determined how important the tooth/teeth are for the patient and whether they need to be replaced.

Designing removable partial dentures for frail and functionally dependent older adults

The following general principles are helpful when restoring the mouth. First, one should try to restore the dentition to optimal health within the constraints given by the patient's modifying factors (e.g., medical problems, medications, transportation, etc.). Second, one

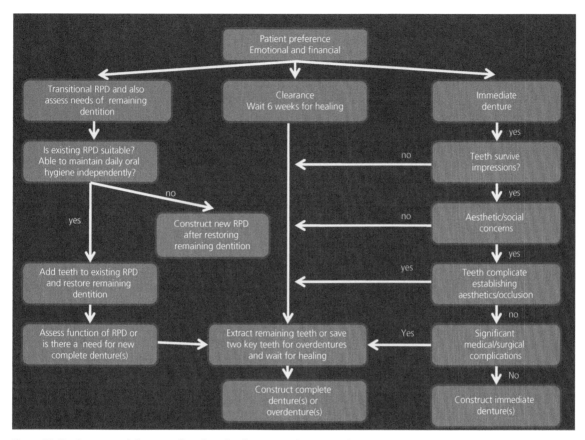

Figure 15.10 The terminal dentition flowchart for decision making. Modified from Dr. Lindsay Richards (University of Adelaide). RPD = removable prosthesis.

should identify the key teeth and build in a contingency plan for the failure of these teeth. A key tooth is one that can support itself or other teeth. If lost, a key tooth dramatically changes the treatment plan from:

- A FPD to a RPD.
- No RPD to a RPD.
- A tooth supported RPD to a distal extension RPD.

A key tooth is required to maintain an adequate chewing pair.

The following design principles for RPDs have been modified from concepts put forward by Budtz-Jorgensen for RPDs for frail older adults (Budtz-Jorgensen, 1966):

Do the least possible harm by preserving the existing dentition

It is wise to try and avoid distal extension RPDs, in which case one may try to save abutment teeth which have a poor prognosis by:

- Using a rest seat only on an at-risk distal abutment;
- Reducing the distal tooth and using it as overdenture support, may require root canal therapy and a restoration;
- And adding an implant as an overdenture support with or without an attachment.

When designing the major connector, it should be either at least 3 mm clear of the free gingival margin or if that is not possible, then the gingival margin should be covered.

If a distal extension RPD cannot be avoided, then it should be designed to incorporate stress distribution or stress breaking by the use of cast I bars or wrought wire circumferential clasps. In addition, the patient should have frequent recalls to assess the need for relines to prevent trauma to the abutment teeth.

RPDs should be easy to insert and remove

Many frail older adults are at risk to develop deficits in their neuromuscular coordination due to arthritis, stroke, Parkinson's disease, myasthenia gravis, dementia, etc. The clinician should design the RPD so that:

- The path of insertion and removal is simple and direct.
- The clasp design should not be complicated.
- The clasps should be sturdier so they are not easily distorted.
- The RPD may need to have grooves in the resin base for fingers, to assist removal from the mouth.
- In some situations, if the patient has significant changes to their hands as in rheumatoid arthritis, it may be necessary to design a removal tool so the patient will be able to independently remove the RPD.

Design of the RPD should be simple so that maintenance is easy

If anterior teeth are lost due to periodontal disease, there is usually a significant amount of bone loss. Without extensive grafting, it is not possible to restore this space with implants or a FPD. An RPD tends to rotate or torque the remaining anterior abutments; therefore tissue bars are often designed to support the RPD to prevent damage to the abutment teeth and the tissues. The use of attachments or bars should be used judiciously for frail older adults because their repair or replacement can be time-consuming, complex, and costly. Also, the patient's ability to keep their restored teeth clean can be problematic and the consequences may be caries at the margins of the crowns.

Design of the RPD should allow for potential failure of some of its units

Teeth with a guarded prognosis can be maintained if the RPD is designed so that if a tooth is lost, it can easily be added to the RPD. Therefore, if the anterior teeth are questionable and the patient wishes to try and maintain them, the major connector should be a plate rather than a bar. If the tooth with a guarded prognosis is a lone-standing molar, then the major connector to the tooth should not be cast metal but a mesh with acrylic resin, which will allow the addition

of a denture tooth without having to solder a retentive component to the RPD.

Flexible dentures – a new approach to RPDs

Many laboratories are advertising the benefits of a relatively new dental prosthesis; the flexible dentures. In our experience, they may be useful for frail older adults who need an interim RPD. They may also be useful for patients who have a limited ability to open their mouth (Samet *et al.*, 2007) because the patient has one of the following conditions:

- Scleroderma;
- Microstomia;
- Trauma or burns to the mouth.

The most common products currently available are:

- Opti-Flex® invisible clasp—acetyl resin;
- Valplast®—nylon;
- Cu-Sil®—silicone.

A description of each of these products follows:

- **Acetyl resin (Opti-Flex®).** This product is an acetyl resin, a polyoxmethylene. It is twice as stiff as nylon and is hot-pressed at a higher temperature, and so has less creep. It has fairly good dimensional stability and good color stability. Its water absorption is acceptable. It is possible to process acrylic resin onto it, but not easily.
- **Nylon (Valplast®).** The advantage of using Valplast® is that it can be completed in two appointments. It is easy to fit: simply put the denture in hot water and then into the patient's mouth. It is hot-pressed for processing. It is hypoallergenic and translucent. It is tough and resistant to brittle fracture. It is prone to creep so it loses retention over time and the clasps cannot be tightened. There is no long-term clinical data available on the life span of dentures made from Valplast®. The disadvantages are that it bonds poorly to acrylic resin and therefore it cannot be repaired or relined, it does stain over time, and it deteriorates.
- **Silicone (Cu-Sil®).** These are usually complete mandibular dentures which use a soft silicone gasket around the remaining natural teeth. These teeth are often periodontally involved and as there are no occlusal or incisal rests on the dentures, this is a slow way to - transition- the patient to a complete denture as additional remaining teeth are lost.

Complete dentures

Although the percentage of edentulous older adults is declining, those who are edentulous will remain so for the rest of their lives and the loss of teeth will continue for persons who are in the lower educational and socioeconomic groups. Douglass *et al.* (2002) stated that because of population growth, "More older adults will need complete dentures even though the percent of older adults who need dentures will decline."

Overdentures

When teeth are extracted, the bone resorbs. Ante Tallgren (1967, 1972) has shown that the restoration in the maxilla is 0.1 mm per year while in the mandible, it is 0.4 mm. One way to slow resorption is to use overdentures. Ettinger and Qian (2004) have shown that if the overdenture abutment teeth are cared for, the abutments can be maintained for many years. The natural roots support the denture, reduce its movement and in so doing, reduce the trauma caused by the dentures in function. Ideally an overdenture abutment tooth should have at least 6 mm of bone support, pockets no deeper than 3 mm, and at least 2–3 mm of attached gingiva (Lord & Teel, 1974). The abutments should be 2–3 mm in height with a dome-shaped contour (Graser & Caton, 1983). A clear advantage of using natural teeth for abutments is the simplicity of fabrication of the denture and the simplicity in maintaining the abutments and the denture. Use of daily high concentration (5000 ppm) topical fluoride gel or regular application of fluoride varnish is necessary to maintain the integrity of these natural tooth abutments.

Only if a patient is unhappy with the stability and retention of the dentures should attachments be used to stabilize the overdenture. The use of these attachments complicates the daily care and maintenance of the abutments with regard to repair or relines.

New or replacement complete dentures

To successfully wear new or replacement complete dentures, a person needs (Ettinger, 1978):
(a) Healthy tissue to support the dentures.
(b) Motivation, patience, and persistence in learning how to use the denture; especially the mandibular denture.

(c) Adequate neuromuscular skills to manipulate the dentures, especially the mandibular denture.

These three points are outlined in greater detail below.

Healthy tissues
A careful examination of the mouth is required to identify possible oral problems:

- **Sharp spiny crests of the ridge or sharp mylohyoid ridges causing pain.** These may require surgery to allow extension of the dentures or careful relief after the dentures are constructed. If comfort cannot be achieved, the use of a "permanent soft liner" such as a processed silicone may be the treatment of choice.
- **Exposed mental foramen causing pain.** There have been attempts to surgically move the nerve down from the surface, but often it has caused problems with hyperesthesia or numbness. Informing the patient and relieving the dentures can help to alleviate problems.
- **Neural trigger areas.** Marsland and Fox (1958) described a plexus of nerves in the deeper parts of the subepithelial connective tissue, which consisted of bundles of myelinated fibers parallel to the surface. If the epithelium thins out with age and denture wearing, the innervation will lie in a papilla close to the surface. These coiled nerve endings from extracted teeth have the appearance of "amputation neuromata" and can become trigger zones which are very sensitive to pressure from the denture. They tend to be more common in the mandible rather than in the maxilla. Alcohol injections or surgical intervention can alleviate the problem once it is diagnosed by palpation.
- **Calcified genial tubercles.** The origin of the genioglossus and the geniohyoid muscles on the mental spine of the mandible can become calcified and interfere with the lingual border of the mandibular complete denture. If there is discomfort, the denture can be adjusted. Occasionally, the patient will complain of swelling of the floor of the mouth and when questioned, will say while they were eating there was a "pop" and the floor of the mouth became painful and swollen. Usually this is due to a fracture of one of the calcified origins of the genioglossus, and the hematoma in the floor of the mouth will resolve itself (Glendenning & Hirschmann, 1977; Shohat *et al.*, 2003).

- **Root fragments of foreign bodies.** Continuous resorption of the residual ridge may result in the exposure of root fragments or foreign bodies (usually amalgam), which become uncomfortable. Once they have been identified with a radiograph they can be easily removed by a minor surgical procedure.
- **Infection by *C. albicans*.** If dentures are used continuously and are not removed at night while sleeping, the plaque on the tissue surface of a denture may become infected with *C. albicans* and cause either a generalized stomatitis (denture sore mouth) or a granular stomatitis (papillary hyperplasia) (Gendreau & Loewy, 2011; Webb *et al.*, 1998a). The inflammation of the mucosa is due to the toxins produced by *C. albicans* in the biofilm on the tissue surface of the denture, which causes a delayed hypersensitivity of the tissues (Ganguly & Mitchell, 2011). To treat the stomatitis, one must treat the biofilm on the denture as well as the infection of the tissues. The patient needs to remove the denture at night before going to bed. If they cannot do that for esthetic reasons (e.g., not wanting to be seen without dentures by their partner), then he/she needs to leave the dentures out of their mouth for at least 6 hours each day. Also the dentures need to be scrubbed gently with soap and water after each meal. The tissues can be treated with topical antifungals such as nystain ointment, clotrimazole lozenges or ketaconazole 2% cream (Webb *et al.*, 1998b). If compliance becomes a problem, then systemic treatment with fluconazole tablets can be effective (Arikan *et al.*, 1995). The denture needs to be cleaned in an ultrasonic bath and the patient needs to immerse the denture in chlorhexindine gluconate 0.12%, or in dilute sodium hypochlorite, or in a 1 : 750 dilution of benzalkonium chloride for at least 30 minutes each day. All three treatments work, but chlorhexidine is expensive and may stain the dentures. Sodium hypochlorite (household bleach) is cheap but if used over time, it can bleach the denture bases. The benzalkonium chloride is relatively cheap to dispense and a fresh solution should be used to soak the dentures each day, because if same solution is reused for several days, it has been known to grow gram-negative rods.

Once the supporting tissues for the denture are healthy, it is important to:
- Extend the denture bases to take advantage of all of the denture bearing areas, for maximum resistance and retention.
- Use special impression techniques such as **selective loading** or **two tray techniques** to capture the tissues in an undistorted position.
- If necessary, surgically improve the denture bearing area by removing hyperplastic tissue and freena, which interfere with the denture base in function.
- In selected patients who are healthy enough and can afford it, retrofit the mandibular denture with one (Schneider & Synan, 2011) or two implants (Allen *et al.*, 2011; Spitzl *et al.*, 2012) with attachments to stabilize the mandibular denture. The prognosis for osseointegration is guarded for elderly women with osteoporosis who have the greatest amount of resorption of residual bone, and if implants are placed, a longer period of osseointegration is required before they can be loaded (Gaetti-Jardim *et al.*, 2011).

Motivation to learn how to use dentures

If an older adult has never worn a complete mandibular denture, or if they have previously worn one for a long time, it takes a period of learning and accommodation before the patient can acquire the ability to wear the new mandibular denture. There is a group of older adults who have poor motivation to begin these skills (Allen & McMillan, 2003):
- Persons who are depressed;
- Persons who are grieving;
- Persons who are physically very frail;
- Persons who are confused or demented;
- Persons who have neuromuscular degeneration.

It is not wise to make new dentures for these patients. Relining their existing mandibular denture with a resilient silicone soft liner may help such a patient. Tissue conditioners can be used to make the patient comfortable and the soft-lined denture can be used as a functional impression for the reline (Haney *et al.*, 2010).

If patients have become so frail and their tissues so tender because their mandibular mucosa is unable to repair itself adequately, then the trauma induced by the denture in function means that the patient may not be able to wear the mandibular denture any longer. Ritchie and Fletcher in 1971 described a technique suggested by Everett for modifying the maxillary denture for these patients (Ritchie & Fletcher, 1971). The posterior teeth are removed and new teeth are reset at a position lower than the "normal" occlusal plane and in the curve of the mandibular edentulous ridge. The maxillary denture teeth should be able to touch the mandibular ridge when the patient closes their mouth.

A need for adequate neuromuscular skills

Wearing dentures is a learned art which depends on the patient's neuromuscular skills. Some patients will not be able to successfully wear a mandibular denture. These persons include patients (Ettinger, 1978):

- Whose tissues have degenerated due to poor health and extensive denture-wearing;
- Those with significant reduction in salivary flow rates due to disease, drugs, or therapies;
- Those whose pain threshold has been altered;
- Those whose neuromuscular skills have been deteriorated, e.g., post-CVA, Parkinson's disease, myasthenia gravis, etc.;
- Those whose cognitive skills have deteriorated, e.g., dementia, post-CVA, late stage Parkinson's disease, etc.

If these patients are wearing dentures, making even a technically perfect denture for them will not have a successful outcome because they cannot accommodate to the new dentures. Wyke (1974) has explained this process in the following manner:

> To wear a denture is a learned art which requires a will to learn and the acquisition of specific neuromuscular skills. When an initial denture or a remade denture is placed in the mouth, the person must consciously think about using his or her denture. The control is exercised mainly through the alpha motor neuron system directly from the cerebral cortex and the use of the denture requires continuous concentration. If control stays at this level, the wearing of dentures becomes intolerable. If a person does not have neuromuscular deficits, the control process becomes primarily reflex through the fusimotor-muscle spindle loop system, which controls mandibular posture. This ability allows the denture to be worn

unconsciously and successfully. Therefore, before new dentures are made, it is necessary to evaluate the motivation and neuromuscular skills of the older adult.

Treatment of patients with neuromuscular deficits

If a patient with neuromuscular deficits has been wearing dentures for a long period of time and they are worn and ill-fitting, simply remaking them may result in failure. If one can make incremental changes to the old denture prior to relining them, the patient may be able to accommodate to them. This technique has been called the copy denture method (Davis, 1994). Essentially, tissue conditioners can be used to stabilize the dentures on their tissues and, after a period of accommodation, centric records are made, the dentures are mounted, the teeth are replaced on the denture, and the denture is relined and delivered to the patient.

If the denture teeth are severely worn, the patient may complain that "my teeth are dull and need sharpening" or "I cannot chew any more" or "my face is falling in." When the vertical dimension of rest position is measured for these patients, it is usually greater than 5 mm. If a new denture is made at an increased vertical dimension of occlusion, these patients with neuromuscular deficits will not be able to accommodate to the dentures. However, if the dentures are stabilized with tissue conditioners and the occlusion rebuilt slowly over time with "occlusal pivots" (Watt & Lindsay, 1972) when the denture is relined and new teeth added, the patient can usually accommodate to the dentures.

Conclusion

The elderly population is changing and the younger dentate older adults tend to utilize dental care similar to those of the younger dentate age groups. Many, even when faced with extensive bone loss caused by periodontal disease and rampant caries, are no longer willing to accept the simple solution of the past, which was extraction of all the remaining teeth and the construction of complete dentures. Although the technical dental care for these older consumers is not different than that for younger adults, the decision-making process is much more complex and complicated by their chronic systemic diseases and the medications they take to treat them. Appropriate care for these persons requires a careful assessment of their needs and rational treatment planning, which ranges from no prosthesis to restoring lost teeth with fixed prosthodontics and implants.

References

ADA & AAOS (American Dental Association and American Academy of Orthopaedic Surgeons) (2003) Advisory statement: antibiotic prophylaxis for dental patients with total joint replacements. *Journal of the American Dental Association,* **134**, 895–9.

Allen, P.F., McKenna, G., Creugers, N. (2011) Prosthodontic care for elderly patients. *Dental Update,* **38**, 460–70.

Allen, P.F. & McMillan, A.S. (2003) A review of the functional and psychosocial outcomes of edentulousness treated with complete replacement dentures. *Journal of the Canadian Dental Association,* **69**, 662a–e.

Arikan, A., Kulak, Y. & Kadir, T. (1995) Comparison of different treatment methods for localized and generalized simple denture stomatitis. *Journal of Oral Rehabilitaion,* **22**, 365–9.

Bader, J.D, Rozier, R.G., McFall W.T., Jr., *et al.* (1991) Effect of crown margins on periodontal conditions in regularly attending patients. *Journal of Prosthetic Dentistry,* **65**, 75–9.

Berkey, D.B., Berg, R.G., Ettinger, R.L., *et al.* (1996) The old–old dental patient – the challenge of clinical decision-making. *Journal of the American Dental Association,* **127**, 321–32.

Brown, R.S. & Rhodus, N.L. (2005) Epinephrine and local anesthesia revisited. *Oral Surgery, Oral Medicine, Oral Pathology, Oral Radiology, and Endodontics,* **100**, 401–8.

Budtz-Jorgensen, E. (1966) Prosthetic considerations in geriatric dentistry. In: *Textbook of Geriatric Dentistry,* 2nd edn (eds. P. Holm-Pedersen & H. Loe), p. 453. Munksgaard, Copenhagen.

Budtz-Jorgensen, E. (ed.) (1999) *Prosthodontics for the Elderly: Diagnosis and Treatment.* Quintessence Publishing Co., Chicago.

Chalmers, J.M. & Ettinger, R.L. (2008) Public health issues in geriatric dentistry in the United States. *Dental Clinics of North America,* **52**, 423–46.

Chursciel, P., Goch, A., Banach, M., *et al.* (2009) Circadian changes in the hemostatic system in healthy men and patients with cardiovascular diseases. *Medical Science Monitor,* **15**, 203–8.

Davis, D.M. (1994) Copy denture technique. A critique. *Dental Update,* **21**, 15–20.

Douglass, C.W. & Watson, A.J. (2002) Future needs for fixed and removable partial dentures in the United States. *Journal of Prosthetic Dentistry,* **87**, 9–14.

Douglass, C.W., Shih, A. & Ostry, L. (2002) Will there be a need for complete dentures in the United States in 2020? *Journal of Prosthetic Dentistry,* **87**, 5–8.

Eklund, S.A. (1999) Changing treatment patterns. *Journal of the American Dental Association,* **130**, 1707–12.

Ettinger, R.L. (1978) Some observations on the diagnosis and treatment of complete denture problems. *Australian Dental Journal,* **23**, 457–64.

Ettinger, R.L. (1993) Cohort differences among aging populations: a challenge for the dental profession. *Special Care in Dentistry,* **13**, 19–26.

Ettinger, R.L. & Beck, J.D. (1984) Geriatric dental curriculum and the needs of the elderly. *Special Care in Dentistry,* **4**, 207–13.

Ettinger, R.L. & Qian, F. (2004) Abutment tooth loss in patients with overdentures. *Journal of the American Dental Association,* **135**, 739–46.

Gaetti-Jardim, E.C., Santiago, J.F., Jr., Goiato, M.C., *et al.* (2011) Dental implants in patients with osteoporosis: a clinical reality? *Journal of Craniofacial Surgery,* **22**, 1111–13.

Ganguly, S. & Mitchell, A.P. (2011) Mucosal biofilms of *Candida Albicans. Current Opinion in Microbiology,* **14**, 380–5.

Gendreau, L. & Loewy, Z.G. (2011) Epidemiology and etiology of denture stomatitis. *Journal of Prosthodontics,* **20**, 251–60.

Gil-Montoya, J.A., Guardia-Lopez, I. & Gonzales-Mioles, M.A. (2008) Evaluation of the clinical efficacy of a mouthwash and oral gel containing the antimicrobial proteins lactoperoxidase, lysozyme, and lactoferrin in elderly patients with dry mouth: a pilot study. *Gerodontology,* **25**, 3–9.

Glendenning, D.E. & Hirschmann, P.N. (1977) Fractures of the genial tubercles: two cases and a review of the literature. *British Journal of Oral Surgery,* **14**, 217–19.

Graser, G.N. & Caton, J.G. (1983) Influence of overdenture abutment tooth contour on the periodontium: a preliminary report. *Journal of Prosthetic Dentistry,* **49**, 173–7.

Guggenheimer, J. (2002) Oral manifestations of drug therapy. *Dental Clinics of North America,* **46**, 857–68.

Haney, S.J., Nicoll, R. & Mansueto, M. (2010) Functional impressions for complete denture fabrication. a modified jump technique. *Texas Dental Journal,* **127**, 377–84.

Jainkittivong, A., Aneksuk V. & Langlais, R.P. (2004) Medical health and medication use in elderly dental patients. *Journal of Contemporary Dental Practice,* **5**, 31–41.

Lord, J.L. & Teel, S. (1974) The overdenture: patient selection, use of copings and follow-up evaluation. *Journal of Prosthetic Dentistry,* **32**, 41–51.

Mancini, M., Grappasonni, I., Scuri, S., *et al.* (2010) Oral health in Alzheimer's disease: a review. *Current Alzheimer Research*, **7**, 368–73.

Marsland, E.A. & Fox, E.C. (1958) Some abnormalities in the nerve supply of the oral mucosa. *Proceedings of the Royal Society of Medicine*, **51**, 951–6.

Neves, R.S., Neves, I.L., Giorgi, D.M., *et al.* (2007) Effects of epinephrine in local dental anesthesia in patients with coronary artery disease. *Arquivos Brasileiros de Cardiologia*, **88**, 545–51.

Ritchie, G.M. & Fletcher, A.M. (1974) Complete denture replacement for geriatric patients. *Dental Update*, **1**, 287–93.

Samet, N., Tau, S., Findler, M., *et al.* (2007) Flexible, removable partial denture for a patient with systemic sclerosis (scleroderma) and microstomia: a clinical report and a three-year follow-up. *General Dentistry*, **55**, 548–51.

Schneider, G.B. & Synan, W.J. (2011) Use of a single implant to retain a mandibular complete overdenture on a compromised atrophic alevolar ridge: a case report. *Special Care in Dentistry*, **31**, 138–42.

Shelley, D., Russell, S., Parikh, N.S., *et al.* (2011) Ethnic disparities in self-reported oral health status and access to care among older adults in NYC. *Journal of Urban Health*, **88**, 651–62.

Shinozaki, S., Moriyama, M., Hayashida, J.N., *et al.* (2012) Close association between oral *Candida* species and oral mucosal disorders in patients with xerostomia. *Oral Diseases*, **18**(7), 667–72.

Shohat, I., Shoshani, Y. & Taicher, S. (2003) Fracture of the genial tubercles associated with a mandibular denture: a clinical report. *Journal of Prosthetic Dentistry*, **89**, 232–3.

Spitzl, C., Proschel, P., Wichmann, M., *et al.* (2012) Long-term neuromuscular status in overdenture and complete denture patients with severe mandibular atrophy. *International Journal of Oral & Maxillofacial Implants*, **27**, 155–61.

Tallgren, A. (1967) The effect of denture wearing on facial morphology. A 7-year longitudinal study. *Acta Odontologica Scandinavica*, **27**, 563–92.

Tallgren, A. (1972) The continuing reduction of the residual alveolar ridges in complete denture wearers: a mixed longitudinal study covering 25 years. *Journal of Prosthetic Dentistry*, **27**, 120–32.

Thomson, W.M. (2005) Issues in the epidemiological investigation of dry mouth. *Gerodontology*, **22**, 65–76.

Walker, J. (2011) Management of osteoarthritis. *Nursing Older People*, **23**, 14–19.

Watt, D.M. & Lindsay, K.N. (1972) Occlusal pivot appliances. *British Dental Journal*, **132**, 110–12.

Webb, B.C., Thomas, C.J., Wilcox, M.D.P., *et al.* (1998a) *Candida*-associated denture stomatitis. Aetiology and management: a review. Part I. Factors influencing distribution of *Candida* species in the oral cavity. *Australian Dental Journal*, **43**, 45–50.

Webb, B.C., Thomas, C.J., Wilcox, M.D.P., *et al.* (1998b) Candida-associated denture stomatitis. Aetiology and management: a review. Part 3. Treatment of oral candidosis. *Australian Dental Journal*, **43**, 244–9.

Wilson W., Taubert, K.A., Gewitz, M., *et al.* (2007) Prevention of infective endocarditis guidelines from the American Heart Association. *Journal of the American Dental Association*, **138**, 739–45, 747–60.

Wyke, B.D. (1974) Neuromuscular mechanisms influencing mandibular posture: a neurologist's review of current concerns. *Journal of Dentistry*, **2**, 111–20.

CHAPTER 16

Medical Complexities

Elisa M. Chávez

Department of Dental Practice, Pacific Dental Program at Laguna Honda Hospital, University of the Pacific, Arthur A. Dugoni School of Dentistry, San Francisco, CA, USA

Introduction

In this chapter we will review some of the most common systemic diseases and conditions that challenge older patients and discuss their management in dentistry. The method we will use for reviewing these classifications of diseases and conditions will be through a review of the medications prescribed for these conditions, viewing the medications as a proxy for the conditions themselves. Other chapters focus on coordinating care for patients with complex situations and the specifics of oral disease prevention for patients with complex needs. No one source can provide all the answers; multiple resources for patient management and professional development are required. A review of the references in this chapter's bibliography will provide additional information and resources for consideration in the management of patients with medical complexities. The websites listed may provide valuable updates to the information provided here.

Advanced age is not a contraindication to dental care. Some practitioners believe that seniors present with some inherent risk for dental care, but this is not the case. Many seniors who seek dental care in private practice are "well elders." Importantly, diseases that occur more commonly as people age are due to disease processes, not due to aging itself. They are age-prevalent, not age-related. This is true for systemic and oral diseases. Not all seniors will suffer from age-prevalent diseases, and many of those who do, have their disease(s) well under control. Some seniors are coping with multiple concomitant chronic diseases but fewer will fall into the frail patient category with conditions that have significantly impaired their physical and/or cognitive function. For some this a result of some acute event and for some a result of long-standing and poorly controlled disease. Identification of patients with multiple systemic diseases or even one known or unknown condition that may not be controlled is important in order to provide appropriate treatment planning and care. Rarely do the normal physiologic changes that occur with aging add to the medical complexity of dental treatment planning and care alone, but they can add to the overall complexity of providing care (see Chapters 6 and 7.) Rather than focusing solely on the age of a patient, the focus should be on the presence of disease(s) or disability that can impact oral health and the provision of oral health care.

Seniors are a more heterogeneous population with regard to health and function than are younger patients and there are several medical diseases and conditions that do occur with more frequency in senior populations. Even without preconceived notions about treating someone of advanced age, there may be uncertainty about how to manage patients with multiple diseases, conditions, and medications, or how to request appropriate consultations from other care providers. There may be concerns over appropriate treatment planning and dental management in the presence of these conditions.

Geriatric Dentistry: Caring for Our Aging Population, First Edition. Edited by Paula K. Friedman.

© 2014 John Wiley & Sons, Inc. Published 2014 by John Wiley & Sons, Inc.

Companion website: www.wiley.com/go/friedman/geriatricdentistry

Prescription and natural drug use as the window to systemic health

Patients take medications because they have underlying disease, or may self-medicate with over-the-counter products due to health concerns. Practitioners must be concerned about the drugs themselves as well as the diseases they are used to manage. Some medications are prescribed in the event of acute conditions such as angina. Some of the desired or undesired side effects of a drug may increase the risk for an adverse outcome in the dental clinic and require laboratory testing to assess risk – such with anticoagulants and immunno-suppressants or insulin and bisphosphonates respectively. Some will require consultation with the patient's physician or pharmacist regarding alteration of an existing drug regimen or use in concert with a needed dental treatment or prescription. Some medications and their side effects, or the disease they are used to treat, will require an alteration of a dental treatment plan or plan for prevention and maintenance. Some medications will have a direct impact on oral health. In all cases is it important to identify these potential risks and implications when we first evaluate a patient, on routine updating of medical histories, or upon review of any new diagnoses and medications with which a patient may present at any given appointment.

Polypharmacy

Polymedicine describes a patient taking many medications for many medical problems but the term poly-pharmacy often indicates the inappropriate use of multiple medications. A number of studies have demonstrated that seniors take more medications than any other age group – as much as a third of all prescriptions written. Several studies have demonstrated that as the number of prescription drugs a person takes is increased, the risk of adverse drug reactions (ADRs) also increases, to as much as 100% for those taking 8 or more. Some drugs commonly used in dentistry, corticosteroids, non-narcotic analgesics, and penicillin have some of the highest ADR rates. ADRs due to the use of nonsteroidal anti-inflammatory drugs (NSAIDs), also commonly used, is among one of the most preventable causes of untoward effects of medications. Among those aged over 65, the incorrect use of multiple medications and

ADRs can be a significant cause for acute hospitalizations. A 2005 American Association of Retired Persons (AARP) survey reported 67% of people aged 50–64, and 87% of those over 65 say they regularly take a prescription medication; among those the average number of prescriptions they report taking is four. US Centers for Disease Control and Prevention (CDC) data shows that, from 2007 to 2010, almost 40% of people aged 65 and older reportedly had taken five or more medication in the last 30 days. This is a significant increase compared with the 15.6% occurrence reported from 1988 to 1994.

There are seven kinds of ADRs: allergy, side-effect, drug toxicity, drug–drug interaction, drug–physiology interaction, drug–laboratory test interaction, and idiosyncratic. An ADR may occur with the administration of even a single drug (Jacobsen, 2001). These reactions may be relatively mild – such as a localized oral change like mucositis or xerostomia – or a life-threatening event such as anaphylaxis secondary to drug allergy or excessive bleeding due to a drug–drug interaction. Some drugs present an increased risk of an ADR in older individuals when administered alone, even when there are no drug interactions reported, such as with valium – a long-acting benzodiazepine. Because drug metabolism may be slower in older individuals, for reasons such as changes in body composition, they may remain sedated for a longer period of time than expected. The extended and unexpected length of sedation may present a risk on its own but it can also result in over-sedation if multiple doses are taken, even over an acceptable length of time. The risk increases for those with other systemic diseases such as diabetes, asthma, renal, or hepatic disease or those who are malnourished. Some of the more specific and preventable outcomes of the adverse drug events that occur in seniors are: falls, hip fractures, delirium, and urticaria. Approximately a fourth of these reactions are preventable and 95% are predictable because they are often exaggerations of expected side effects of these drugs. Those events may stem from some pharmacokinetic changes that occur with aging or that have occurred as a result of some disease. However, misuse and over- or under-use of medications is often the cause.

Improved patient–physician communication, including monitoring for and responding to symptoms, has been identified as an important strategy for the prevention of adverse drug events in outpatients and may reduce the frequency of these events. Seniors are one of the groups at risk for low health literacy, especially those aged over 85 and those who do not speak English or have English as their first language. Health literacy has been described as "The wide range of skills and competencies that people develop to seek out, comprehend, evaluate, and use health information and concepts to make informed choices, reduce health risks, reduce inequities in health, and increase quality of life" (Zarcadoolas *et al.*, 2005). There are many points in the healthcare system that may a present an opportunity for misunderstanding, miscommunications, and result in poor compliance and suboptimal outcomes related to health and oral health. And, apart from low health literacy some patients are unwilling to follow or incapable of following treatment recommendations and instructions to safely manage their medications. There are many social, psychologic, physical, and economic reasons for poor compliance and mistakes in drug usage that are not a result of aging but that may be more prevalent among older patients (see Chapter 6).

Tips for maximizing optimal medication compliance

Strategies for reducing medication errors include making certain the patient understands the reason a medication has been prescribed; the reason they should take it as directed; and that they can repeat how and how often to take the medication. Prescription bottles should not always be "child-proof" because arthritic or neuromuscular changes may make it difficult if not impossible for older adults to open child-proof bottle caps. Generics should be prescribed when possible in combination with a simple regimen in order to improve compliance (minimizing cost and complexity as barriers to compliance). Address physical and cognitive barriers to compliance by enlisting caregivers, friends, and relatives when appropriate. Provide clearly written and readable instructions, in large font, for the patients and caregivers to take home. Encourage the patient or caregivers to consult the pharmacist about their medication and to contact you if they have additional questions. Follow up with the patient to see if they are following the medication

regimen. If they are not, try to address the reason they are not or cannot. An example of why a patient might not be complying would be some unpleasant side effect the patient is unwilling to tolerate or cannot tolerate but which might be addressed by using a different drug or altering how and when the drug is administered. Document any issues of noncompliance in the patient record. If there is suspicion that lack of compliance is due to neglect or abuse, report to adult protective services or an ombudsman (see Chapter 19).

Systematic review of the medication list

Since patients may not have a firm understanding of the medications they are taking, or the diseases they are used to treat, it is important to be familiar with certain drugs or drug classes commonly used to manage some of the most commonly encountered systemic diseases and conditions in older patients. This will help identify potentials for problems in the dental management of these patients. These problems may arise from the use of the drug alone or because of the disease the drug is used to treat. For these reasons, a systematic method for reviewing a lengthy drug list will not only help highlight medication issues, but will also emphasize important considerations in caring for a medically complex population. See Table 16.1 for important points to review with patients taking multiple medications and points to address prior to writing a prescription.

The following sections will address classifications of drugs that may be needed in emergency situations and drugs on the medical history that may suggest potential risk during treatment.

Emergency drugs for emergency situations

Upon first review of a patient's medication list, determine if there are medications that may be required in the event of a medical emergency – such as nitroglycerin used for angina or bronchodilators inhaled during acute exacerbation of chronic obstructive pulmonary disease. These medications may be needed even before any care is provided to the patient and should

Table 16.1 Polymedicine checklist

Important drugs to identify from an existing drug list				Issues to identify prior to writing a new prescription		
*Drugs needed in the event of emergency**	*Drug classes, or the conditions they are used to treat, that presents an increased risk for an adverse event**	*Drug classes that may have specific oral lesions or conditions as side effect**	*Over-the-counter products with potential for adverse events**	*Potential for drug-drug interaction with the drug to be prescribed?*	*History of drug allergies and ADRs**	*Indications to reduce standard drug dosage or to use drugs with a different metabolic route**
nitroglycerin inhalers	**Anti-addictive** • Disulfiram • Methadone **Anticoagulants** • Warfarin • Clopidogrel • Aspirin **Chemotheraputics** • Vincristine • 5-fluorouracil [5FU] • Cisplatin **Corticosteroids** • Prednisone **Hypoglycemic and insulin** • Insulin • Sulfonylureas **Immunnosuppressants** • Methotrexate Cyclosporine Prednisone **Antidepressants** • MAO inhibitors • Tricyclic **Nonselective beta blockers** • Propanolol • Timolol **Recreational drugs** • Cocaine • Methamphetamines **Sedative hypnotics, narcotics, barbiturates** • Diazepam • Meperidine	**Xerostomia** • Antihistamines • Antidepressants • Calcium channel blockers • Diuretic **Fungal infection** • Antibiotics • Immunnosuppressant **Mucositis** • Anti-neoplastic **Gingival enlargement** • Anti-seizure • Calcium channel blockers • Immunosuppressant **Lichenoid reactions** • Diuretics **Delayed bone healing or necrosis** • Bisphosphonates (alendronate, zolendric acid)	**Increased bleeding** • Aspirin • Bilberry • Dong quai • Garlic • Ginger • Ginkgo biloba • Ibuprofen • St. John's Wort **Inhibit erythromycin and ketoconazole** • Echinacea • St. John's Wort **Increase HR/BP** • Ephedra • Bitter orange **Additive to anti-anxiety and sedation** • Valerian **Hepatotoxicity** • Kava-kava	Drugs to be prescribed should be cross-checked with the drugs on the existing drug list for risk of interactions to reduce such events	**Drug allergies** • Urticaria • Anaphylaxis • Edema **Signs of ADRs in seniors** • Delirium • Falls **Known side effects that are excessive or intolerable to patient** **Drugs with increased risk of toxicity and ADRs in aged** • Clindamycin • Cephalosporin • Diazepam • Tylenol® #3	**Impaired kidney function** Kidney function test: GFR: • <10ml/min 1 dose q 24h • 10–50ml/min 1 dose q 8–12 h • >50ml/min 1 dose q 8 h **Examples of drugs with renal elimination** • Amoxicillin • Tetracycline • Penicillin • Fluconazole **Impaired liver function** Liver function tests: ast/alt/liver transminases: • Normal=30–40 u/l • If >4 times normal, do not use drugs toxic to or metabolized by the liver Examples include: • Acetaminophen • Codeine • Lidocaine • Ibuprofen • Lorazepam • Erythromycin **85 years or older and/or weight below 100 pounds** • Reduce dosage by 50% or to the lowest therapeutic level

*These lists are not exhaustive. The drugs and conditions listed are examples.

ADR, adverse drug reation; GFR, glomerular filtration rate; q, every.

draw our attention to the underlying medical conditions, which may have an impact on our overall management of and treatment planning for this patient. These may not be patients who can tolerate lengthy appointments or may have guarded prognoses for their oral health due to other conditions related to their overall systemic health, such as xerostomia from medication use or dependence upon others due to limited functional ability. Patients should be reminded to bring medications that might be required in the event of a medical emergency with them to each appointment and to set them out when they come to the office, so that in the event they are needed, time is not lost in looking through their belongings for them. These drugs should also be available in an emergency kit.

Drugs that suggest potential risk

Hypoglycemic drugs and insulin

The second group of drugs to identify is drugs that may indicate to us that there is a higher chance for some adverse event in the dental office, either because of the drug itself, or because of the condition it is used to manage. Some drugs in this category have a narrow margin of safety and are highly titrated. One of the most common and recognizable in this group is insulin. Approximately 26% of all adults with diabetes take insulin to manage their disease. Diabetes was the seventh leading cause of death in 2010 for adults aged over 65 and is a major cause of heart disease and stroke, kidney failure, and blindness. The risk of death for patients with diabetes is twice that of age-matched individuals without the disease. Approximately 27% of US people over age 65 had diabetes in 2010 and 50% had pre-diabetes. Type 1 diabetes (DM1) accounts for about 5% of all adults with diagnosed diabetes. Risk factors include autoimmune, genetic and environmental and there is no known way to prevent its occurrence. Type 2 diabetes (DM2) is associated with older age, obesity, family history of diabetes, history of gestational diabetes, impaired glucose metabolism, physical inactivity, and race/ethnicity. DM2 accounts for approximately 90–95% of all diagnosed cases of diabetes in adults and usually begins as insulin resistance. In DM2 individuals, insulin is not used properly and as

the need for insulin rises, the pancreas gradually loses its ability to produce insulin. The remaining small percent of diagnosed cases of diabetes results from specific genetic conditions, surgery, ADRs, infections, pancreatic disease, or other illnesses.

Patients who have uncontrolled diabetes and/or require insulin to manage their disease are at risk of developing hyper- or hypoglycemia. A random blood sugar test done in the dental office can be useful to assess patient status just prior to treatment. A blood sugar level less than 140 mg/dl (7.8 mmol/l) is normal. The target for people with diabetes before meals is 70–130 mg/dl and the target 1–2 hours after meals is less than 180 mg/dl. Patients with values over 180 ml/dl may have symptoms of blurry vision, tiredness, thirst, or a sick to the stomach feeling. These patients should be referred to their physicians for a consultation and evaluation. A blood glucose level below 70 mg/dl indicates hypoglycemia and the patient should be given a sugar source. Hypoglycemia can strike rapidly and the patient may appear confused, shaky, sweating, anxious, and/or weak. Most cases of hypoglycemia can be managed by quickly giving the patient a source of glucose such as juice, full sugar soda, sugar, honey, candy, or glucose tablets. Check blood glucose again in 15 minutes. If it is still below 70 mg/dl another serving should be eaten and repeated until the blood glucose level is 70 mg/dl or above. If the patient will not eat for another hour or more they should have a snack after the blood glucose level is raised to 70 mg/dl or above. Note that patients taking acarbose (Precose®) or miglitol (Glyset®) must have the pure glucose tablets or gel because these drugs slow the rate of digestion of carbohydrates and, therefore, other sugar sources do not work quickly enough. If the patient loses consciousness they may require a glucagon injection and emergency services should be contacted. Severe hypoglycemia can lead to seizures, coma and even death.

Patients should be advised to follow their usual medication and diet regimen prior to dental treatments. If they may not be able to eat for some time after treatment – for instance following extensive oral or periodontal surgery or due to a long trip to and from home – a physician consultation should be completed to determine if this regimen can be altered on the side of mild hyperglycemia for a brief time to prevent hypoglycemia during the post-operative period. The use of insulin by a patient with DM1 or DM2 should also signal that this patient may be at risk of delayed healing or infection following surgery. As opposed to a random blood sugar test, which tells you only about that patient at the date and time of the test, a glycosylated hemoglobin test or HbA1c is used to assess long-term control for the patient with diabetes. The American Diabetes Association generally recommends an A1C level below 7%, or an average 150 ml/dL blood glucose range over a period of 3 months, if the patient is to have their disease controlled. If significant surgery is planned, a physician consultation should be requested in order to determine their long-term control and whether or not this patient would benefit from a peri-operative course of antibiotics. For patients who do not have well-controlled diabetes, inquire whether or not their kidney function is impaired as a result of their disease, especially if they have been diagnosed with diabetes for many years. In these cases it is important to consider whether prescription dosages need to be changed as a result of impaired renal function. Renal function is an important factor in drug metabolism and the drug's effect on the patient. Serum creatinine levels are generally regarded as an indicator of renal function. However, serum creatinine level is not a reliable measure in older adults because serum creatinine levels are a function of muscle mass. Muscle mass is reduced with advancing age and there may not be the mass that is assumed by this test. Another test for renal function is the glomerular filtration rate (GFR). GFR is a test used to check how well the kidneys are working. A glomerular filtration rate (GFR) of less than 50 ml/min per 1.73 mm^2 is a predictor for drug-related problems. See Table 16.2 for prescribing guidelines for medications metabolized in the kidney.

Patients with diabetes who have developed impaired renal function due to nephropathy may also suffer from retinopathies and neuropathies which may present additional challenges for these patients related to oral health and dental care, such as challenges to mobility or difficulty reading or following post-operative or hygiene instructions. And, many studies have demonstrated that patients with poorly controlled diabetes are at risk for poor oral health in general and periodontal disease in specific. Patients with long-standing or poorly controlled diabetes also have a higher prevalence of other systemic conditions that can also have implications for oral health care

and patient management. See Table 16.2, for a review of diabetes and its associated conditions, and some implications for oral health and oral health care. Clearly the recognition of an important group of medications, like insulin and hypoglycemic drugs, in a medication list can be an important point from which to consider the medical complexities with which this patient may present, as well as about the dental complexities we may encounter in their care.

Anticoagulants

Anticoagulants are drugs commonly used in the prevention of cardiac and cerebrovascular events such as myocardial infarct, atrial fibrillation, and stroke, and they should draw attention in review of a medication list. Stopping or altering the medication to complete dental/oral surgical treatment may present a risk to the patient and a physician should be consulted if altering the medication is thought to be necessary. Whether or not the drug regimen is altered, the appropriate lab work should be done to prevent the chance of excessive bleeding during or following a procedure. A PFA-100 can be requested for patients taking aspirin therapy, and a prothrombin time (PT) [normal range is 10–12 s, although this can vary] and international normalized ratio (INR) [normal range is 1–2, and takes into account the variation in PT results from laboratory to laboratory] should be requested no more than 48 hours prior to surgery for those patients taking warfarin (Coumadin®). While there are no recommended treatment modifications for patients taking clopidogrel (Plavix®), there is still the potential for complications that arise as a result of this type of anticoagulant therapy such as excessive bleeding and ecchymosis following procedures, and the rare occurrence of neutropenia and thrombocytopenia. The general health condition of the patient as well as the specific procedure that is being recommended should be taken into consideration when evaluating the risk of providing treatment to a patient on anticoagulants. If the patient is having extensive oral surgery, has multiple medical conditions, or other conditions or medications that may impair coagulation, it may be best to treat at an INR of 3.0 or less, or refer the patient to an oral surgeon and/or complete the treatment in a hospital setting if significant bleeding is anticipated following surgery. Practitioners should use their knowledge of the patient as well as knowledge about their own skills in making these

Table 16.2 Diabetes and associated diseases: impact on oral health care

Potential complications of diabetes with dental implications and considerations	Quick facts as they relate to aging and diabetes
Heart disease *Angina* • **Unstable:** urgent care only, possibly in hospital setting, palliative care where possible • **Stable:** caution with use of vasoconstrictors, stress reduction management and sedation may be appropriate, if patient is on anticoagulants, excessive bleeding may be a risk, nitroglycerin should be readily available. If the patient still has chest pain after the third dose of nitroglycerin – call 911 • If patient is taking nonselective beta blockers: limit epinephrine use to two cartridges of 1/100 000 epinephrine, avoid retraction cord with epinephrine and avoid anticholinergic medications *Congestive heart failure* • If condition is uncontrolled or symptomatic, urgent care only but with careful cardiac monitoring and possibly in a hospital setting • If condition is controlled and asymptomatic, proceed with routine dental care • Stress reduction management and sedation may be appropriate • If patient is taking nonselective beta blockers: limit epinephrine use to two cartridges of 1/100 000 epinephrine, avoid retraction cord with epinephrine, and avoid anticholinergic medications • Administration of epinephrine can result in arrhythmia for patients taking digoxin • Patient may not be able to lay back in the dental chair *History of myocardial infarction* • If MI less than 1 month ago, urgent care only in consultation with a physician • If MI more than 1 month ago, keep stress low, limit epinephrine use • If patient is taking nonselective beta blockers: limit epinephrine use to two cartridges of 1/100 000 epinephrine, avoid retraction cord with epinephrine, and avoid anticholinergic medications *Orthostatic hypotension* • **Symptoms and signs:** dizziness, confusion, blurred vision, feeling faint and falls or syncope • Raise patients slowly to the upright position after reclining in the dental chair • Support patients as they stand • If patient reports feeling faint, elevate their feet above their heart (Trendelenburg position)	• The rate of heart disease is 2–4 times higher in patients with diabetes than in those without • Heart disease was documented as the cause of 68% of diabetes related deaths in 2004 • Heart disease was the leading cause of death in all adults over 65 years of age from 1997 to 2007 and 2010 • Individuals with diabetes have 2 times the risk of heart failure as those without diabetes • Orthostatic hypotension risk increases with age and can occur even in the absence of cardiovascular disease

Hypertension

- Defer elective dental treatment if BP is uncontrolled (>180 systolic, >110 diastolic) and refer immediately to a physician for evaluation
- **Symptoms and signs**
  - BP >140/90
  - Patients may be asymptomatic, others may have dizziness, facial flushing, fatigue, headaches, nervousness, or nose bleeds
  - Oral side effects:
    - (a) altered taste due to drug metabolism
    - (b) gingival enlargement (calcium channel blockers)
    - (c) lichenoid reactions (ACE inhibitors)
    - (d) salivary dysfunction and xerostomia (potentially from a wide list of medications)
- There are no contraindications to care or use of local anesthetic if BP is well controlled
- Monitor BP before and after administration of local anesthetic
- Excessive use of epinephrine can increase BP
- Stress reduction management and sedation may be appropriate

- An estimated 67% of patients with diabetes are on medication for hypertension or have BP >140/90
- Almost half of all people over 65 have chronic hypertension
- Almost one third of people with hypertension are unaware they are hypertensive

Stroke (CVA)

- If patients have been prescribed anticoagulants to prevent future CVAs, use laboratory tests appropriate to the medication given to evaluate risk of bleeding
- Provide emergency treatment as needed but minimize stress of appointment
- Keep appointments short and monitor blood pressure, limit use of epinephrine and avoid epinephrine-impregnated retraction cords
- If there is a known or suspected cognitive impairment, consult the physician with regard to patient ability to make treatment decisions
- Delay elective dental care and definitive treatment planning to 6 months post stroke to allow time for maximum rehabilitation to be reached and considered in the overall treatment plan; consider physician consultation to determine if patient has reached peak of rehabilitation potential in all areas, physical and cognitive (see Chapters 7 & 19)
- Identify if patient requires assistance with ambulation or transfers in the dental office to reduce the risk of falls

- The rate of CVA is 2–4 times higher than in patients with diabetes than without
- Strokes were responsible for 16% of diabetes related deaths 2004
- Stroke (CVA) was the third leading cause of death in all adults aged over 65 from 1997 to 2007 and fourth in 2010

Blindness

- Identify if patient requires assistance with ambulation or transfers in the dental office to reduce the risk of falls
- Provide appropriate oral post-operative instructions and, if possible, utilize family and friends to assist with written instructions that will go home with the patient

- Diabetes is a leading cause of blindness in people aged 20–74
- People with diabetes are 40% more likely to develop glaucoma
- People with diabetes are 60% more likely to develop cataracts

Kidney disease

- See Table 16.1 for dosage guidelines
- Avoid nephrotoxic drugs: e.g., high dose acetaminophen, acyclovir, aspirin, NSAIDs
- Patients undergoing dialysis should not be scheduled for dental care the same day as dialysis

- Diabetes is the leading cause of kidney failure
- The prevalence of CKD is growing most rapidly in people aged 60 and older
- The 1988–1994 NHANES study reported a prevalence of 18.8% in people over age 60 with CKD, and this increased to 24.5% in their 2003–2006 study

(Continued)

Table 16.2 (*Continued*)

Potential complications of diabetes with dental implications and considerations	Quick facts as they relate to aging and diabetes

Avoid taking BP on an arm with a shunt in place, but do monitor blood pressure
• Approximately 2–9% of people receiving hemodialysis develop endocarditis; however, antibiotic prophylaxis is recommended for patients with nonvalvular cardiac devices (i.e., hemodialysis shunts) only if they must undergo incision and drainage of an abscess, but not for routine procedures. Antibiotic prophylaxis to prevent endocarditis is recommended for all invasive procedures in these cases:
  ◦ cardiac transplant with valvulopathy
  ◦ congenital heart diseases
  ◦ previous history of endocarditis
  ◦ presence of prosthetic heart valves (may also have risk of increased bleeding if taking anti-coagulants)
  ◦ **Standard oral prophylaxis:** 2 g amoxicillin po 1 h prior to the procedure; **or**
  ◦ **If patient is allergic to penicillin:** 600 mg clindamycin po 1 h prior to the procedure (alternatives: 2 g cephalexin* or 2 g cefadroxil* 1 h prior to procedure, or 500 mg azithromycin or 500 mg clarithromycin 1 h prior to the procedure)
  ◦ **If intolerant of oral medications:** 2 g ampicillin IM or IV 30 min prior to procedure; **or**
  ◦ **If patient is allergic to penicillin:** 600 mg clindamycin IV 30 min prior to procedure (alternative: 1.0 g cefazolin* IM or IV 30 min prior to the procedure)
See AHA guidelines for complete details and recommendations regarding premedication:
• Patients on hemodialysis and those with or preparing for transplants, may require corticosteroid supplementation – consult physician
• Patients who are preparing for or have had a transplant may require antibiotic prophylaxis – consult with physician. If possible address oral health prior to the start of immunosuppressive therapy and transplant. If the patient's dentition is good and will be maintained, an aggressive program to prevent new and recurrent dental disease is required. Only emergency dental procedures and oral hygiene should be performed in the 6 months post transplant
	• Greater than 45% of all new ESRD patients have diabetes
	• More than 50% of new ESRD patients are aged 65 or older
	• In 2007, diabetic nephropathy was the cause of ESRD in an estimated 22% of kidney transplant recipients in the USA
	• The 5-year survival rate for those with transplants is almost twice that of those on dialysis
	
	http://kidney.niddk.nih.gov/kudiseases/pubs/kustats/#4

Nervous system disease • Neuropathy may include altered intraoral sensations such as burning, tingling, paresthesias, and others • Identify patients requiring assistance with ambulation or transfers in the dental office to reduce the risk of falls **Dental disease** • Periodontal disease • Oral pathology – *Candida*, trauma, lichen planus, burning mouth syndrome, hyposalivation	• Occurs in 60–70% of patients with diabetes • Severe disease is a major contributor to lower-extremity amputations • Greater than 60% of nontraumatic leg/foot amputations occur in people with diabetes • Periodontal disease occurs 2–3 times more in people with diabetes than those without and it may factor into poor glycemic control

*Note: cephalosporins should not be used in patients who have had anaphylaxis, angioedema, or urticaria in response to penicillin.
ACE, angiotensin-converting enzyme; BP, blood pressure; CKD, chronic kidney disease; CVA, cerebrovascular accident; ESRD, end stage renal disease; IM, intramuscular; IV, intravenous; MI, myocardial infarction; NHANES, National Health and Nutrition Examination Survey; NSAIDs, nonsteroidal anti-inflammatory drugs; po, by mouth.

treatment decisions. Surgical technique to minimize trauma and tearing of adjacent tissues can minimize risk of excessive bleeding. When possible, suturing to primary closure is appropriate. This is especially true for a patient who may also be cognitively or physically impaired and cannot follow post-operative instructions to minimize bleeding. The use of topical hemostatic agents such as gel foam, Surgicel®, or Thrombostat® should also be considered. Carefully review post-operative instructions with the patient, and their caregiver, to be sure that the caregiver does not inadvertently disrupt the clotting process after the patient has left the office.

Bisphosphonates

Bisphosphonates are another class of drugs that are important to identify in a medication list. Oral bisphosphonates (e.g., alendronic acid [Fosamax®] and ibandronate [Boniva®]) are commonly used to manage patients with osteoporosis; sometimes intravenous bisphosphonates (e.g., Boniva and zoledronic acid [Reclast®]) may be used quarterly or yearly . Osteoporosis occurs more commonly in women but carries a significant risk of fracture for all people with the disease. Hip fractures in particular have a high mortality and morbidity rate. These are documented by Hung *et al.* (2012):

> Older adults who experience hip fractures often have poor outcomes, including functional decline, institutionalization, and death. Among older adults who sustain hip fractures, approximately 13.5% die within 6 months and 24% within 1 year. The increase in mortality risk persists beyond 10 years after hip fracture, with higher excess mortality risk among men than women. Among those who survive 6months, only 50% recover their pre-fracture ability to perform activities of daily living (ADLs) and only 25% recover their ability to perform instrumental ADLs. Following a hip fracture, older adults are 5 times more likely than age-matched controls without hip fracture to be institutionalized at 1 year.

Oral bisphosphonates reduce fractures by an estimated 35–50% annually. According to the 2004 Surgeon General's report, half of all Americans over 50 could have osteoporosis and low bone mass by 2020. Bisphosphonates have other important indications:

Breast cancer, multiple myeloma, prostate, renal, lymphatic, lung, and others cancers may also receive treatment with intravenous bisphosphonates (e.g., zoledronic acid [Zometa®] and pamidronic acid [Aredia®]). According to the US Centers for Disease Control and Prevention (CDC), cancer was the second leading cause of death for people aged over 65 from 1997 to 2007 and in 2010. Bisphosphonates may be a critical element in managing these diseases. In the dental management application, they also pose a risk of bisphosphonate-related osteonecrosis (BON) following bony oral surgical procedures, recurrent trauma, such as from an ill-fitting prosthesis, and even spontaneously due to untreated dental disease. Osteonecrosis itself is necrosis of the bone due to an inadequate blood supply. BON of the jaw defined as "exposed, necrotic bone in the maxillofacial region persisting for more than eight weeks in a patient who is taking, or has taken, a bisphosphonate and has not had radiation therapy to the head and neck" (Edwards *et al.*, 2008). Sometimes the patients are asymptomatic and the condition is only observed in radiographs. Sometimes there is pain, infection, and exposed bone, or even fracture and severe pain or paresthesia. The exact mechanisms and risk factors behind BON are not clear. However, identification of this class of drugs from a medication list is important in diagnoses and treatment planning as well as gaining consent for treatment. Risk factors for developing BON may include age over 65, DM, corticosteroid use, and smoking. Risk for oral bisphosphonate users generally does not occur earlier than 5 years into treatment; however, some cases of BON have been reported in just under 2 years from the start of treatment. There appears to be more risk for patients taking the intravenous form of the drugs for cancer therapy resulting in increased incidence, greater severity, and less response to treatment compared with those cases that have resulted from the oral form. Patients for whom bisphosphonates are administered via the intravenous route receive much higher doses of the medication, and much more of the drug is absorbed when administered intravenously.

There is little research to support definitive recommendations for assessing risk of developing BON, or recommendations to prevent it if bony surgery is needed, or to treat it if it occurs. The American Dental Association Council on Scientific Affairs has made some recommendations for BON associated with oral bisphosphonate use (ADA, 2008). Patients who have received oral bisphosphonates should be informed of the potential risk for BON although it appears to be small. Treatment alternatives to surgery should be discussed. Prophylactic antibiotics are not indicated unless there is some other risk of infection. Chlorhexidine rinses may be used pre- and post-surgery. Limiting surgery to a small area or the extraction of a few teeth initially to assess patient response should be considered, unless there is an emergency situation. Patients should be advised that untreated disease can also result in BON, so prevention of oral disease is critical as is seeking treatment as soon as a problem is suspected. Ill-fitting prostheses can also result in necrosis so they should be examined regularly. If BON occurs, debridement may be necessary. Recommendations for the management of cancer patients on intravenous bisphosphonate therapy and patients with BON have been published by The American Academy of Oral and Maxillofacial Pathology, the American Association of Oral and Maxillofacial Surgeons, and the American Society for Bone and Mineral Research and The American Academy of Oral Medicine (see Bibliography).

Immunosuppressants, chemotherapeutics, and radiation

Patients who are taking intravenous bisphosphonate medication to treat cancer may also be taking other chemotherapeutics, which can place them at risk for additional complications related to oral health and dentistry. These are another class of drugs which should be of special interest in assessing risk for dental care. A physician consultation and review of relevant laboratory values should be completed prior to treating patients taking immunnosuppressants, such as cyclosporines (Sandimmune®), azathioprines (Imuran®), or high dosage corticosteroids (prednisolone), as they are at risk for poor healing and possibly excessive bleeding following treatment, as well as opportunistic and refractory diseases. Peri-operative antibiotics may be considered prior to invasive procedures. Some patients may require additional local or systemic measures to prevent excessive bleeding. Some may require supplemental steroid support to tolerate extensive procedures. These patients may be suffering other adverse side effects of their treatment such as nausea or fatigue and may not be motivated to pursue, or be able to tolerate, general dental treatment at this time. Acute infections should be managed aggressively and palliative treatment provided until laboratory tests reach at least minimum values, as described below, for reduced risk of bleeding and infection post-operatively. Minimums will vary depending upon the procedure. The provider's surgical ability and ability to manage outcomes should also be considered. Some general laboratory values to consider as adequate to provide routine dental care are: platelet count greater than 60 000 per mcl; WBC greater than 2000 cells per mcl; and absolute neutrophils greater than 1000 per mcl. These should be considered on a case-by-case basis and taken into account along with any additional known risks for bleeding or infection. The oncologist should be involved in the dental treatment decision-making as dental and cancer treatment proceed.

Individualized oral hygiene/prevention regimens should be created for patients preparing to undergo chemotherapy or radiation treatments whenever possible before the treatments begin. If that is not possible, preventive interventions should be accomplished while the patient is undergoing chemotherapy or radiation therapy to minimize the adverse effects of the cancer treatment on their oral health, such as the destruction caused by xerostomia. What can be accomplished will vary as a function of the patient's ability to tolerate the oral hygiene/prevention regimens. Patients may also develop mucositis as a result of their treatment. Management could include antifungals and topical anesthetics such as viscous lidocaine, or coating products such as Kaopectate® or sucralfate to provide some pain relief. Cryotherapy or sucking on ice chips before or during chemotherapy has also shown been shown to reduce mucositis in some studies of patients taking chemotherapeutic drugs suchs as 5-fluorouracil and vinblastin, among others (Karagözoğlu & Filiz Ulusoy, 2005; Rocke et al., 1993).

However, mucositis can become so severe that narcotics and /or hospitalization is required because the individual is unable to maintain his/her nutrition and subsequently has a high risk of infection. The goal is to not only maintain oral health during this time, but to maximize the patient's potential to complete his/her cancer treatment by maintaining oral comfort so that oral health and nutritional intake can be maintained. Importantly, not only patients with cancer are on immunosuppressants. They are also used to manage conditions such as rheumatoid arthritis, systemic lupus erythematosus, multiple sclerosis and organ transplant as examples. The same considerations apply for any patient on immunosuppressive therapy, regardless of the diseases being treated.

When possible, provide needed dental treatment and plan a preventive program prior to beginning any immunosuppressive therapy so that known and typically routine problems such as caries or denture sores are not made to wait for treatment and risk becoming acute issues for these compromised individuals. This will require consultation with the oncologist. This is especially important for patients who will undergo treatment for head and neck cancer where radiation will be a treatment modality. These patients have the added risk for osteoradionecrosis following any bony trauma or surgery (at ~5500 CGy), as well as severe xerostomia during and post treatment than can lead to severe radiation caries. Irreversible salivary gland damage can occur with less than 25 Gy. Those patients are also at risk for mucositis, secondary infections, altered or loss of taste, tooth sensitivity, and trismus. Thoughtful oral care, analgesics and nutritional support measures aim to limit the severity and impact of these side effects. Fluoride trays can serve two purposes. They can be used to apply a fluoride gel (1.1% neutral sodium fluoride) daily to prevent radiation caries. They can also be worn empty during radiation to reduce risk and severity of mucositis adjacent to metal dental restorations, but this should be approved by the oncology team. If oral surgery is needed post radiation therapy, the ports of radiation must be assessed to determine risk of osteonecrosis. If the patient received more than 5500 cGy to the area in question, teeth should be maintained endodontically rather than extracted. If extractions cannot be avoided, or if they received more than 6000 cGy, hyperbaric oxygen therapy may be an option to reduce the risk of post-surgical osteoradionecrosis. Prior to radiation therapy, prostheses must also be made and followed carefully. Sores from ill-fitting prostheses can result in necrosis post radiation. Any dental disease or infection in patients who will have, or have had, head and neck radiation should be managed aggressively and prevention of new disease is critical. Educate and advocate toward excellent oral hygiene practices and make the routine as easy as possible. These patients face significant physical and psychologic challenges during treatment. These challenges can compromise an individual's motivation and ability to succeed in this area. Maintaining nutrition is also a priority and there must be recognition that while their dietary regimens (e.g., high caloric, frequent meals or liquids) may place them at risk for caries, the priority must be on their overall health and care should be taken not to contradict medical orders with preventive recommendations. Even basic hygiene practices such as flossing and brushing may need to be modified in the face of severely reduced platelet counts that place the patient at risk for severe bleeding with minimal abrasion, even from a toothbrush.

Antidepressants

Recent CDC data reports 17% of women and 10% of men over 65 years old take antidepressant medications. The onset of depression in seniors may be in conjunction with the onset of diseases or may be a sequella of events which impair their physical or cognitive function or alters lifestyle such as cancer or stoke. Sometimes seniors are coping with the passing of friends and loved ones. Sometimes family members are geographically dispersed and the older adult feels isolated. The presence of depression can also negatively impact the motivation to follow through with dental treatment and even oral hygiene. Elders may be taking antidepressants that can result in xerostomia, placing them at additional risk for caries and other infections or oral pathology. Tricyclic antidepressants (e.g., amitriptyline [Elavil®], nortriptyline [Pamelor®]) can interact with epinephrine to create a hypertensive crisis. It is recommended to limit epinephrine use to two cartridges and avoid epinephrine that is more concentrated than 1/100 000.

Some patients with depression may rely on alcohol or recreational drugs, or abuse of prescription drugs, to manage their depression. An estimated 20% of Americans with a mood disorder such as depression also suffer with substance abuse. Patients should be asked to list all the drugs they use, including recreational, as these substances can interact with medications that are administered or prescribed in dentistry. Used in excess these substances can lead to additional oral and systemic problems. Kidney or liver damage may occur as result of substance abuse. Patients may have issues with pain control, drug metabolism, risk for increased bleeding or susceptibility to opportunistic infections. Importantly patients who are taking anti-addictive drugs or who are in sobriety should not be given medications that may trigger an adverse reaction or relapse to their addiction. Examples of such medications include: narcotics, sedatives, or medications containing alcohol. These patients should be warned that even many mouthwashes contain alcohol and should not be used. Some people who cannot swallow tablets may require a liquid form of the drug and some medications such as pain relievers, fever reducers, or antihistamines contain alcohol. This can occur in both over-the-counter and prescription medications. A pharmacist can confirm if the prescription you want to order contains alcohol. For patients with a history of substance abuse issues, consultation with their physician may be indicated to help ensure adequate pain control is achieved without risk of an adverse event.

Depression can be mistaken for, and often occurs in conjunction with, dementia. Both can be characterized by an inability to concentrate, emotional disturbances, and personality changes such that they interfere with daily life. In contrast to dementia, delirium is a *temporary* state of mental confusion resulting from reversible causes such as high fevers, intoxication, or other systemic causes. Any patient who presents with sudden changes in cognition, orientation, and behavior should be referred to a physician for immediate evaluation. When there is evidence of a cognitive impairment, a variety of tests are typically done to rule out other diseases, including depression, which may account for the changes in cognition and personality. There are an estimated 5 million people with Alzheimer's disease (AD) in the USA, or 1 in 8 older adults. AD is the most common cause of dementia and the sixth leading cause of death. Deaths from AD rose 66% from 2000 to 2008. The disease slowly destroys cognitive skills. There are three findings in brain tissue that characterize AD: amyloid plaques, neurofibrillary tangles, and the loss of neurons. The trigger to the process is unknown. There may be a combination of genetic, environmental, and lifestyle factors that lead to the disease.

Understanding the type of dementia and the expected progression of the disease is important in management as well as treatment planning. For example, vascular dementia can occur as a sudden onset. Previously called multi-infarct dementia, and the second most common cause of dementia, it results from bleeding into brain tissue or blockage of blood flow to the brain resulting in damage. The damage may be limited to one or two areas of cognition. If these future events can be prevented – with anticoagulant therapy for example – then the scope and severity of the patient's dementia may remain stable. Advancement is possible, but it is not a given as it is for progressive diseases such as AD or Parkinson's-related dementia. Individuals will eventually rely on others for their basic activities of daily living. There are no treatments at present that cure or reverse the course of AD. Drugs used in the management of AD are donepezil hydrochloride (Aricept®), rivastigmine tartrate (Exelon®), and galantamine (Razadyne®) for mild to moderate severity and memantine (Namenda®) or Aricept for advanced severity. If these are present on the medication list but there is no mention of AD, inquire if the patients have been told they have some cognitive impairment, i.e., memory loss or difficulty with tasks or chores they used to do routinely. The therapies available only slow the onset of symptoms or target behavioral symptoms but cognitive function will decline; all areas of cognition will be impacted. And as the disease advances, patients may be prescribed antidepressants, antipsychotics, and anxiolytics, all of which can impact oral health and the provision of dental care. Ideally patients would have a dental evaluation when they are diagnosed with AD in the early stages of the disease when the patient is better able to cooperate, follow instructions, and make decisions. Any restorative or prosthodontics treatment should be completed as early in the disease as possible. A thorough preventive plan, including 3-month recall and prophylaxis with fluoride applications can be put in place. The plan must change as the disease progresses. For instance, introducing an electric toothbrush in an early stage is more likely to be successful than at a later stage. A caregiver can slowly be introduced into the oral hygiene routine. Perhaps they can provide reminders and cues to start, and then move to more direct assistance or total assistance with oral hygiene as the disease advances. As the disease progresses, these patients will be at greater risk for caries, oral pathology and periodontal disease. This is due to lack of motivation and understanding, reliance on others for oral care, dietary restrictions, and requirements due to dysphagia as well as behavior that may prevent oral care. Patients who return to the dentist in more advanced stages of AD after a period of neglect of their oral health have a guarded prognosis for the outcome of treatment and acceptance of care. Patients in advanced stages may also suffer orofacial trauma from falls and other accidental injury. These patients cannot follow post-operative instructions because of their advanced condition, so care needs to be taken to prevent injury after anesthesia and to minimize post-operative bleeding if treatment is required. Treatment goals in later stages may be to maintain existing teeth as long as possible, with or without the use of prostheses as the patient can tolerate, and to preserve comfort and dignity.

There are many causes of dementia and some are progressive, so to say only that a patient has dementia does not say anything about the patient's ability to tolerate, cooperate with, adapt to, and maintain dental treatment we may provide. A diagnosis of dementia should not be a deterrent to treatment and is not a contraindication to dental care. Understanding the disease presentation and likely course, as well as evaluating each patient as an individual, is critical. Patients may be completely cooperative and appropriate or combative and unapproachable. These may be transient or permanent situations. Behavior may depend upon the procedures in question. An individual may be cooperative for routine cleanings but not be cooperative enough for procedures that are more complex and may require more time in the dental chair. Patients with dementia may have different responses to different caregivers and dental providers; they may cooperate with some people but not with others. Gathering input from other providers, caregivers and family members prior to finalizing treatment plans for patients with dementia can be valuable. This is also an opportunity to discuss the limitations of treatment due the kind and severity of dementia as well as the behavioral or sedation interventions that may be required to complete desired or needed treatment.

Over-the-counter and natural medications

Finally, inquiry about over-the-counter medication or natural product use is important. Many of these have the potential for adverse effects such as increased bleeding or sedation but patients view them as harmless because they are "natural" and/or do not require a prescription. Used correctly and alone they may not pose a risk for routine dental care, but in combination with other drugs or diseases that pose these same risks, or with medications they counteract, their effect can result in adverse situations. For example Ginkgo, which may be taken to address cognitive disorders or vertigo, may increase the risk of bleeding for those on anticoagulant or antiplatelet therapy. Echinacea, which may be used to stimulate the immune system, can inhibit the actions of erythromycin and ketoconazole. Kava-kava, which may be used for anxiety or insomnia, may have an additive effect on alcohol or other central nervous system depressants. These are just a few examples of natural products older adults may be using that can create potential risks in the dental office. Depending upon the health literacy of the patient, they may not recognize these risks and may not mention their use of these products unless they are asked directly.

Conclusion: an interdisciplinary approach

As some of our older patients will present with complex medical as well as socioeconomic situations, working as a part of an interprofessional team is critical to success. Just as no single resource has all the answers, no single practitioner should feel compelled to address every medical or dental issue on their own. The general dentist can coordinate a team of dental and medical specialists working together to keep or return the patient to good oral health even in the face of compromised systemic health. Healthcare providers can share knowledge and resources to devise effective strategies aimed at maintaining oral health and total well-being over the patient's lifetime. The approach to geriatric oral health must be dynamic and inclusive of the entire health team to meet the diverse and changing needs of these individuals and this population over time. (See Chapter 20 for further discussion of the dentist as part of the interdisciplinary team.)

Case study 1

Mr. Hernandez

Mr. Hernandez is a 64-year-old man who comes to your office for an initial exam. He had a cerebrovascular accident (CVA) 6 weeks ago. He has hypertension, diabetes type 2, and chronic obstructive pulmonary disease (COPD). His wife reports he has difficulty chewing and swallowing and his doctor has recommended a pureed diet with thickened liquids. She thinks he may have a dental problem and would like him to be able to eat food other than puree. The patient has significant dysarthria and cannot relay a chief concern himself. Although there a few restorable caries and evidence of moderate to advanced periodontal disease, there are no acute dental or oral conditions evident.

Case study questions

1 Do you think this patient's diet is a result of his oral condition?
2 Do you think his dietary restrictions may have some implications for the provision of dental care and/or his oral health?
3 Do you think this patient can make decisions for himself?
4 How might you determine this?
5 Would you recommend a definitive treatment plan at this time?
6 Would you wait? How long would you wait? Why?
7 What other questions would you ask about his condition or what treatment he is receiving at this time?
8 How might the answers impact your treatment plan?

Case study 2

Mrs. Andrews

Mrs. Andrews is a 70-year-old woman who presents for a routine dental cleaning. She comes in every 3 months and is always pleasant and talkative. She has no history of cognitive impairments. She has well controlled hypertension and type 2 diabetes (DM2) and has had multiple sclerosis (MS) for 25 years. She has been in a wheelchair ever since you have known her. She is usually accompanied by her niece. When she comes to the office today her niece reports that her aunt is "not herself." Mrs. Andrews repeatedly asks you your name and asks "What am I doing here?" Her blood pressure is unusually low. She appears confused and agitated this morning.

Case study questions

1 What might be the causes of this sudden change?
2 What questions might you ask?
3 What actions would you take in this case?

Case study 3

Mr. Sullivan

Mr. Sullivan is a 75-year-old man with Alzheimer's disease – a progressive dementia. There is no other significant history. He has poor oral hygiene and lives in a skilled nursing facility. He comes to your office with an escort from the facility for an initial dental examination. He has recently moved to the facility from his own home within the last 3 months. He is able to answer basic questions and respond to simple commands but he becomes visibly agitated after about 20 minutes. He cannot provide any dental history. His daughter reported to the facility that he lost his lower partial denture and he has a broken lower left molar. Your findings include intraoral *Candida*, an upper denture with poor retention and stability, and excessive adhesive in place, root-carries teeth nos. 20B, 21B, and 22F, and no. 30 tooth broken below the gingival crest. You determine he will need to have no. 30 extracted, three fillings, and scaling and root planning of his remaining mandibular teeth nos. 20–27 and new prostheses.

Case study questions

1 What additional questions do you need to ask and of whom?
2 Do you think he can cooperate for your treatment plan?
3 What if he cannot?
4 What might the options be for helping him receive the treatment he needs?
5 Do you think he can maintain his oral health after you have restored it?
6 What measures might you suggest?

Case study 4

Mrs. Tsang

Mrs. Tsang is a 68-year-old woman who comes to your office for an initial dental examination. She has brought all her medications with her and they include: nifedipine, glucophage, glyburide, Zoloft®, Vioxx®, and baby aspirin daily, Ativan® before bed, nitroglycerin prn, and Tylenol prn. She is not able to tell you exactly why she takes these medications but this is not due to cognitive impairments.

Case study questions

1 What diseases or conditions do her medications suggest?
2 Are there any medications on this list that might be needed in an emergency?
3 Are there any medications that might have a potential for some adverse outcome during or following her dental care?
4 Do any of the diseases or conditions they are used to treat have some potential for some adverse outcome during or following her dental care?
5 Do any of these medications have a direct impact on oral health?
6 Do any have an indirect effect on oral health?
7 Do any have direct or indirect effects on the dental plan or treatment?
8 Are there any that might interact with prescriptions you may need to write such as antibiotics or pain medications?

Clinical examples

Clinical example 1

78-year-old man

The 78-year-old patient has Parkinson's disease with some cognitive impairment. He also has a h/o seizures and hypertension. It is not clear from review of the records if he is able to make his own decisions. He does not seem to speak but appears to nod yes or no appropriately indicating he has understood the conversation. We will consult his physician to see if there is some surrogate decision maker who should be informed of our findings and recommendations. We will also inquire about his seizure control since removable partial dentures (RPDs) are planned. His blood pressure was within normal limits (WNL) at this appointment, but we will also inquire if his blood pressure is well controlled.

- **Chief complaint:** None apparent, the patient was referred by his physician in his skilled nursing facility for a "routine exam." The patient nodded no when asked about tooth or gum pain or discomfort. He nodded yes when asked if he was able to eat well. The date and location of his last dental visit is unknown. He nods yes when asked if he ever had partial dentures, but shrugged when asked if he knew where they were or when he had them last.

- **Initial exam:** panoramic image (pano), 5 periapical (PA).
- **Extraoral exam:** The temporomandibular join (TMJ) is within normal limits (WNL), no popping, clicking or crepitus. There is no apparent tenderness to palpation, no apparent lymphadenopathy, swellings or masses.
- **Intraoral exam:** His salivary flow is good; there is some pooling of saliva. There are no lesions, swellings, or masses. He has a coated tongue, heavy calculus, and plaque. There is good ridge support for prostheses and no caries. There is advanced horizontal alveolar bone loss but no mobility of teeth nos. 2, 15, 22 and 27. There is class I mobility no. 26 and class II mobility nos. 23, 24, 25.
- His oral motor function appears somewhat impaired and his facial tone appears diminished as well. These are likely to decline further as his Parkinson's disease advances. This may impact his ability to use dentures, so maintaining abutments for partial dentures will be important in this case. He may also have a diminished ability to tolerate extensive dental procedures in the future as his disease progresses. He will likely need increasing levels of assistance with oral hygiene as well.
- This patient is missing teeth nos. 1, 3–14, 16–21, 28–32
- The patient has no caries
- The patient has generalized advanced chronic periodontal disease
- The patient has no apparent prostheses

Treatment plans to consider

1 No treatment
2 Scaling and root planing, no prostheses: goal is to maintain all existing teeth
3 Scaling and root planing, extract nos. 2, 15, 23, 24, 25, 26, upper denture, lower partial
4 Scaling and root planing, extract nos. 23, 24, 25, 26, upper and lower partials
In all cases, unless the patient refuses, a daily plan for oral care should be implemented and should be expected to change over time. A 3-month recall with regular fluoride varnish should be implemented. Should he develop caries, additional preventive prescriptions and regimens may need to be considered.

Clinical example 2

A 67-year-old man

A review of health history reveals many significant findings including cerebrovascular accident (CVA) 2 months ago, deep vein thrombosis, hypertension, and depression. The patient is on anticoagulant therapy, a calcium channel blocker, and a tricyclic antidepressant. He has hemiplegia and hemiparesis of his dominant side. He also has dysphagia and some dysarthria. His diet was recently upgraded from tube-fed to puree and thickened liquids. He is currently in a rehabilitation center. It is unknown at this time if he will be able to return to independent living.

- **Chief complaint:** He reports that he has a hole in his upper left (UL) tooth, which he stuffs with cotton so food does not get in it but, otherwise, there is no pain or discomfort. However he is most concerned with missing teeth nos. 8 and 10. He lost the partial he had in the hospital. He says his last dental visit was 5–6 years ago.
- **Initial exam:** Four bitewings (BWs), 3 periapicals (PAs), panoramic image (pano).
- **Extraoral exam:** Click left temporomandibular join (TMJ), no tenderness to palpation, no apparent tenderness to palpation, no apparent lymphadenopathy, swellings or masses.
- **Intraoral exam:** Slight decreased salivary flow. Oral hygiene (OH) fair, moderate plaque but heavy calculus (likely due to length of time since last dental visit). Patient has a few missing teeth, two in the upper anterior, and there is a large cavity in no. 15 as well mesial no. 16. These appear to be nonrestorable. There is generalized moderate and localized advanced horizontal alveolar bone loss nos. 23–26.
- The patient is missing teeth nos. 1, 3, 4, 8, 10, and 14
- The patient has two teeth, nos. 15 and 16, nonrestorable caries.

- The patient has generalized moderate, localized advanced chronic periodontal disease (lower anterior teeth).
- The patient has no prostheses.

Since his main concern is missing anterior teeth, consider making an upper acrylic partial denture for him. This should not interfere with his diet or require stressful procedures and will address his esthetic concern. Otherwise, consider urgent dental care only, until 6 months post-CVA and then proceed with routine dental care if he has been medically stable. At 6 months post-CVA, reassess treatment plan with regard to oral motor function and any other rehabilitative progress he may have made since his CVA. However, should teeth nos. 15, 16 become symptomatic, consider urgent extractions.

Suggested treatment

The following suggested treatment is assuming that the patient is interested in pursuing treatment.

Phase 1: immediate needs

1 Upper acrylic partial denture to replace teeth nos. 8 and 10.
2 If teeth nos. 15 and 16 become urgent issues extract; otherwise consider temporization, if possible and if it is not likely to exacerbate the situation. Whether extractions are done now or later, inform his primary care physician of the need and the plan, and limit use of epinephrine due to his prescribed tricyclic antidepressant. Order laboratory work as indicated to avoid excessive bleeding from the extractions. Suture to primary closure if possible. Consider referral to an oral surgeon if you determine this patient would be best managed by a specialist in this case.

Phase 2: post 6 months CVA

3 Prophy, probe, fluoride, and oral hygiene instructions (OHI); re-examine for caries
4 Scaling and root planing
5 One-month periodontal and prosthodontic re-evaluation
6 Three-month recall

Review findings with the patient and explain the recommendation to wait on some procedures until he has some time to recover. He should let you know right away if he experiences any pain or discomfort or other problems in the interim.

The patient should also be made aware that the calcium channel blocker, combined with impaired oral hygiene, places him at risk for gingival enlargement, and that limited hygiene combined with his diet places him at risk for caries. If he will agree, he should continue to try to brush his own teeth as he is able with help from occupational therapy, and he should have an order for someone to brush his teeth for him once daily. In addition he should have a prescription for 1.1% neutral sodium fluoride toothpaste twice daily in place of regular toothpaste. He should not rinse out but spit out the excess when he is finished brushing.

Bibliography

Bibliography is intended as a reference list for content.

Adult Meducation. (2006) *Dimension 1. Social and Economic Factors.* From http://www.adultmeducation.com/Social andEconomicFactors.html. Accessed April 18, 2014.

Alzheimer's Association (2014) *Alzheimer's Facts and Figures.* From https://www.alz.org/alzheimers_disease_facts_and_figures.asp. Accessed April 18, 2014.

Alzheimer's Association (2014) *Types of Dementia.* From http://www.alz.org/dementia/types-of-dementia.asp. Accessed April 18, 2014.

American Dental Association: http://ada.org. Accessed April 18, 2014.

American Optometric Association: http://www.aoa.org/x6814.xml. Accessed April 18, 2014.

Barrett, L.L. (2005) *Prescription Drug Use Among Midlife and Older Americans.* AARP, Washington, DC. From http://assets.aarp.org/rgcenter/health/rx_midlife_plus.pdf. Accessed April 18, 2014.

Centers for Disease Control and Prevention (2007) *Working Together to Manage Diabetes: A Guide for Pharmacists, Podiatrists, Optometrists, and Dental Professionals.* US Department of Health and Human Services, Atlanta.

Chavez, E.M. Systematic review of the medication list: a resource for risk assessment and dental management. *CDA Journal of the California Dental Association,* **36**(10), 739–45.

Edwards, B.J., Hellstein, J.W., Jacobsen, P.L., *et al.* (2008) Updated recommendations for managing the care of patients receiving oral bisphosphonate therapy: an advisory statement from the American Dental Association

Council on Scientific Affairs. *Journal of the American Dental Association*, **139**(12), 1674–7.

Friedlander, A.H., Norman, D.C., Mahler, M.E., *et al.* (2006) Alzheimer's disease psychopathology, medical management and dental implications. *Journal of the American Dental Association*, **137**(9), 1240–51.

Halter, J.B., Ouslander, J.G., Tinetti, M.E., *et al.* (eds.) (2009) *Hazzard's Geriatric Medicine and Gerontology*, 6th edn. McGraw-Hill Co., New York.

Hancock, P.J., Eptein, J.B. & Sadler, G.R. (2003) Oral and dental management related to radiation therapy for head and neck cancer. *Journal of the Canadian Dental Association*, **69**(9), 585–90.

Harrison, L.B., Sessions, R.B. & Hong, W.K. (eds.) (2009) *Head and Neck Cancer: A Multidisciplinary Approach*, 3rd edn. Lippencott Williams & Wilkins, Philadelphia.

Heft, M.W. & Mariotti, A.J. (2002) Geriatric pharmacology. *Dental Clinics of North America*, **46**(4), 869–85.

Henry, R.G. & Smith, B.J. (2009) Managing older patients who have neurologic disease: Alzheimer's disease and cerebrovascular accident. *Dental Clinics of North America*, **53**, 269–94.

Hersh, E.V. & Moore, P.A. (2008) Adverse drug interactions in dentistry. *Periodontology*, **46**, 109–42.

Hung, W.W., Egol, K.A., Zuckerman, J.D. & Siu, A.L. (2012) Hip fracture management: tailoring care for the older patient. *JAMA: The Journal of the American Medicial Association*, **307**(20), 2185–94.

Jacobsen, P.L. (2001) Adverse drug reactions. In: *Essentials of Oral Medicine* (ed. S. Silverman), pp. 107–10. BC Decker, London.

Jacobsen, P.L. & Chavez, E.M. (2005) Clinical management of the dental patient taking multiple drugs. *The Journal of Contemporary Dental Practice*, **6**(4), 144–51.

Johns Hopkins Health Alerts: http://www.johnshopkinshealthalerts.com/reports/prescription_drugs/3363-1.html. Accessed April 18, 2014.

Karagözoğlu, S. & Filiz Ulusoy, M. (2005) Chemotherapy: the effect of oral cryotherapy on the development of mucositis. *Journal of Clinical Nursing*, **14**(6), 754–65.

Kocaelli, H., Yaltirik, M., Yargic, I. & Ozbas, H. (2002) Alzheimer's disease and dental management. *Oral Surgery, Oral Medicine, Oral Pathology, Oral Radiology, and Endodontics*, **93**, 521–4.

Krueger, K.P., Berger, B.A. & Felkey, B. (2005) Medication adherence and persistence. In: *National Quality Forum. Improving Use Of Prescription Medications: A National Action Plan*, pp. D1–D41. National Quality Forum, Washington, D.C 2005:D1–D41.

Lamaster, I.B. & Northridge, M.E. (eds.) (2008) *Improving Oral Health for the Elderly: An Interdisciplinary Approach*. Springer, New York.

Lamaster, I.B., Lalla, E., Borgnakke, W.S. & Taylor, G.W. (2008) The relationship between oral health and diabetes mellitus. *Journal of the American Dental Association*, **139** (Suppl 5), S19–S24.

Laudenbach, J.M., Jacobsen, P.L., Abdel, M.R., *et al.* (2011) *Clinician's Guide to Oral Health in Geriatric Patient*, 3rd edn. The American Academy of Oral Medicine, Baltimore.

Lexicomp Online: http://www.lexi.com/institutions/products/online/. Accessed April 18, 2014.

Little, J.W., Falace, D.A., Miller, C.S. & Rhodus, N.L. (eds.) (2013) *Dental Management of the Medically Compromised Patient*. Elsevier, St. Louis.

Lockhart, P.B., Bolger, A.F., Papapanou, P.N., *et. al.* (2012) Periodontal disease and atherosclerotic vascular disease: does the evidence support an independent association? A scientific statement from the American Heart Association. *Circulation*, **125**, 2520–44.

MedlinePlus (2013) *Multi-infarct Dementia*. From http://www.nlm.nih.gov/medlineplus/ency/article/000746.htm. Accessed April 18, 2014.

Merck & Co. (2005) *The Merck Manual of Health and Aging: The Comprehensive Guide To the Changes and Challenges Of Aging – For Older Adults and Those Who Care For and About Them*. Random House, New York.

Miller, N.S., Belkin, B.M., Gold, M.S. (1991) Alcohol and drug dependence among the elderly: epidemiology, diagnosis, and treatment. *Comprehensive Psychiatry*, **32**, 153–65.

Murphy, S.L., Xu, J. & Kochanek, K.D. (2013) *National Vital Statistics Reports. Deaths: Final Data for 2010*, **61**(4). From http://www.cdc.gov/nchs/data/nvsr/nvsr61/nvsr61_04.pdf. Accessed April 18, 2014.

National Center for Health Statistics (2013) *Health, United States, 2012 with Special Feature on Emergency Care*. From http://www.cdc.gov/nchs/data/hus/hus12.pdf#091. Accessed 4/18/2014.

National Diabetes Education Program (2012) *Working Together to Manage Diabetes: A Guide for Pharmacy, Podiatry, Optometry and Dental Professionals*. Centers for Disease Control and Prevention, McLean, VA.

National Diabetes Information Clearinghouse (NDIC) (2011) *National Diabetes Statistics, 2011*. From http://diabetes.niddk.nih.gov/dm/pubs/statistics/. Accessed April 18, 2014.

National Diabetes Information Clearinghouse (NDIC) (2012) *Kidney Disease Statistics for the United States*. NIH Publication No. 12-3895. From http://kidney.niddk.nih.gov/kudiseases/pubs/kustats/. Accessed April 18, 2014.

National Institute of Dental and Craniofacial Research (NIH) (2014) *Oral Complications of Cancer Treatment: What the Dental Team Can Do*. NIH Publication No. 09-4372. From http://www.nidcr.nih.gov/OralHealth/Topics/CancerTreatment/OralComplicationsCancerOral.htm. Accessed April 18, 2014.

National Institute on Aging (NIH) (2014) *Alzheimer's Disease Medications Fact Sheet*. From http://www.nia.nih.gov/alzheimers/publication/alzheimers-disease-medications-fact-sheet. Accessed April 18, 2014.

Natural Medicines Comprehensive Database: http://naturaldatabase.com. Accessed April 18, 2014.

Patterson, T.L. & Jeste, D.V. (1999) The potential impact of the baby-boom generation on substance abuse among elderly persons. Special section on mental health and aging. *Psychiatric Services*, **50**(9), 1184–8.

PDRHealth *Physicians' Desk Reference*: http://pdrhealth.com. Accessed April 18, 2014.

Pham, C.B. & Dickman, R.L. (2007) Minimizing adverse drug events in older patients. *American Family Physician*, **76**(12), 1837–44.

Plassman, B.L., Langa, K.M., Fisher, G.G., *et al.* (2007) Prevalence of dementia in the United States: the aging, demographics, and memory study. *Neuroepidemiology*, **29**(1–2), 125–32.

PubMed Health: http://www.ncbi.nlm.nih.gov/pubmed-health/. Accessed April 18, 2014.

Rocke, L.K., Loprinzi, C.L., Lee, J.K., *et al.* (1993) A randomized clinical trial of two different durations of oral cryotherapy for prevention of 5-fluorouracil-related stomatitis. *Cancer*, **72**(7), 2234–8.

Rockwood, K., Stolee, P. & Robertson, D. (1994) Frailty in elderly people: an evolving concept. *Canadian Medical Association Journal*, **150**(4), 489–95.

Ruggiero, S.L., Dodson, T.B., Assael, L.A., *et al.* (2009) American Association of Oral and Maxillofacial Surgeons position paper on bisphosphonate-related osteonecrosis of the jaw – 2009 update. *Journal of Oral and Maxillofacial Surgery*, **35**, 119–30.

Scully, C. & Ettinger, R. (2007) The influence of systemic diseases on oral health care in older adults. *Journal of the American Dental Association*, **138** (Suppl 1), S7–S14.

Ship, J.A. (2003) Diabetes and oral health an overview. *Journal of the American Dental Association*, **134** (Suppl 1), S4–S10.

Southerlans, J.H. & Taylor, G.W. & Offenbacher, S. (2005) Diabetes and periodontal infection: making the connection. *Clinical Diabetes*, **23**(4), 171–7.

Taylor, G.W. & Bornakke, W.S. (2008) Special review in periodontal medicine, periodontal disease: associations with diabetes, glycemic control and complications. *Oral Diseases*, **14**, 191–203.

Turner, M.D. & Ship, J.A. (2007) Dry mouth and its effects on the oral health of elderly people. *Journal of the American Dental Association*, **138** (Suppl), S15–20.

US Centers for Disease Control and Prevention (CDC): www.cdc.gov. Accessed April 18, 2014.

US National Libriary of Medicine: http://nlm.nih.gov. Accessed April 18, 2014.

Wilson, W., Kathryn, A., Tauber, M.G., *et al.* (2007) Prevention of infective endocarditis: Guidelines From the American Heart Association: *Circulation*, **116**, 1736–54.

Wynn, R.L., Meiller, T.F., Crossley, H.L. (2012) *Drug Information Handbook for Dentistry*, 18th edn. Lexicomp, Hudson, OH.

Zarcadoolas, C., Pleasant, A., & Greer, D.S. (2005) *Health Promotion International*, **20**(2), 195–203.

PART 5

Care Delivery

CHAPTER 17

Delivery Systems

Diane Ede-Nichols

Department of Community Dentistry, Nova Southeastern University College of Dental Medicine, Fort Lauderdale, FL, USA

NURSING HOMES

One of the most dentally underserved populations in the USA is the nursing home (NH) population. Some have suggested that NH residents are invisible to the dental profession. Often among the most physically and cognitively impaired individuals in the health-care system, dental needs are not met or are over-looked for a number of reasons. This area is addressed in greater detail in Chapter 19. Our chapter will describe the different types of long-term care facil-ities and how to work with many aspects of providing oral health services in long-term care facilities, including contracts and affiliation agreements, med-ical records, dental records, billing systems, advanced directives, and treatment delivery options, among other important topics.

Although the number of Americans over the age of 65 has increased dramatically over the past decade by 5.4 million or 15.3% (US Department of Health and Human Services, 2014), a relatively small percentage of those persons (4.1%) reside in an institutional setting such as a NH at any given time. However, recent projections indicate that the number of Americans needing long-term care will double between 2000 and 2050 (CDC, 2009). As a result, consumers along with their families, legislators, healthcare providers, and other interested parties will require current and accurate information in order to plan a continuum of health care that gives consideration to the best possible oral healthcare delivery system for each person.

Definitions

The healthcare needs of the aging population vary considerably, as does the location that these needs are provided. Described below are the different types of facilities that are available to provide care to the elderly or debilitated.

Assisted living facility

A residence that provides services but emphasizes the residents' privacy and choice. Housing may consist of an apartment or a room with locking doors and bath-rooms. Resident units often contain a full kitchen. Most assisted living facilities (ALFs) provide breakfast and dinner to all residents; some provide all three meals. Personal care services are available on a 24-hours-a-day basis. Care services include some assistance with activities of daily living (ADLs) and instrumental activities of daily living (IADLs) such as shopping, house cleaning, or laundry. However, it does not include nursing services such as the administration of medication. ALFs emphasize inde-pendence and generally provide less intensive care than that delivered in a NH. Some residents may elect to hire aides to assist them. The cost structure for ALFs varies widely; some require a large buy-in fee (several hundred thousand dollars and above) as well as ongoing monthly fees (several thousand dollars). Typically, this option is a choice for older adults who sell their homes and have financial resources available. Other ALF models require a substantial monthly fee but no buy-in. ALFs may be independent or part of a continuing care community (CCC or "triple-C"),

Geriatric Dentistry: Caring for Our Aging Population, First Edition. Edited by Paula K. Friedman.

© 2014 John Wiley & Sons, Inc. Published 2014 by John Wiley & Sons, Inc.

Companion website: www.wiley.com/go/friedman/geriatricdentistry

where residents may "age in place" – staying at the same community, but transitioning from independent living to assisted living to skilled nursing care facilities as their health needs change.

Intermediate care facility

An intermediate care facility (ICF) is a NH that provides health-related care and services to individuals who do not require acute or skilled nursing care and is recognized under the Medicaid program for reimbursement. Specific requirements vary by state and are subject to different regulations and coverage requirements than for institutions that do not provide health-related care and services.

Long-term care

Long-term care (LTC) is defined as a range of medical and/or social services designed to help people who have disabilities or chronic care needs. Services may be short- or long-term and may be provided in a person's home, in the community, or in residential facilities (e.g., NHs or ALFs).

Nursing home

A nursing home (NH) is a facility licensed by the state to offer residents personal care as well as skilled nursing care on a 24-hours-a-day basis. In addition to nursing care and personal care, the NH provides room and board, supervision, medication, therapies, and rehabilitation. Rooms are often shared, and communal dining is common.

Skilled nursing facility

A skilled nursing facility (SNF) is a NH that is certified by Medicare to provide 24-hour nursing care and rehabilitation services in addition to other medical services.

Contracts and affiliation agreements

In 1987. President Ronald Reagan signed into law the first major revision of the federal standards for NH care since the creation of both Medicare and Medicaid in 1965 (known as OBRA '87). This revision is known as Federal Regulation 42 CFR 483. This legislation changed the public's expectations of NHs and the care provided. Since 1987, any NH or SNF that establishes

eligibility for Medicare or Medicaid funding must provide services so that each resident can "attain and maintain her highest practical physical, mental, and psychosocial well-being" (Turnham, 1987). The dental service specifications of 42 CFR 483 are outlined as follows:

- Both skilled nursing facilities (SNF) and nursing facilities (NF) must provide the following dental services (US National Archives and Records Administration, 2012):
  1 Provide or obtain from an outside resource routine and emergency dental services to meet the needs of each resident.
  2 The Medicare resident may be charged an additional fee for routine and emergency dental services.
  3 The facility must if necessary, assist the resident:
     (i) in making appointments; and
     (ii) arranging for transportation to and from the dentist's office; and
  4 Promptly refer residents with lost or damaged dentures to a dentist.

Nursing homes that receive Medicare or Medicaid reimbursement are required by law to perform and record an oral examination as part of a comprehensive physical exam done for each new resident admission. This examination is part of a Minimum Data Set that must be completed within 14 days of a resident being admitted to a facility, and then must be done on an annual basis (Schwartz, 2002).

To comply with the above regulations, LTC facilities will seek to have an affiliation agreement, or contract, with a dental group or single providers to provide the dental services for their residents. According to the CDC's *The National Nursing Home Survey: 2004,* many services provided to NH residents are delivered through formal contracts with outside providers (CDC, 2009). Of all facilities who provide oral and dental services for their residents, 62.5% are provided by outside groups (CDC, 2009). When creating such an agreement or contract, the dental group or provider should meet with the facility's chief executive officer (CEO), director of nursing (DON), director of social work (DSW), chief financial officer (CFO), and legal counsel. In most instances the provider will need to apply for and receive medical staff privileges by completing a packet of required documentation.

All of the important issues should be addressed prior to signing the affiliation agreement such as expectations of both parties, compensation, billing, space, equipment, supplies, schedule, and access to charting systems.

Record keeping

Medical charts

All NH facilities must maintain a comprehensive medical chart on every patient that is admitted into the facility. The medical chart may be an electronic health record (EHR) or a paper chart. The paper chart is usually maintained in a binder and kept in the nurses' station of each floor or ward. If the chart is electronic, computer terminals are usually accessible in the nurses' stations or in an area specifically for providers. The purpose of the chart is to provide the nursing staff with a medical and daily care plan for each resident and to record every event that occurs over the course of the day for each resident. Although different facilities may utilize different versions of the chart, the basic information is the same. In each chart you will find the following information.

Patient information or 'face" sheet (Fig. 17.1)

Occasionally a photograph of the resident may be included on the inside front cover of the hard chart or in front of the "face" sheet.

The "face" sheet is usually the first page of the chart and multiple copies of it may also be present. This "face" sheet is very important as it provides all of the billing information needed including home address, social security number, Medicare or Medicaid number, and type of insurance coverage for the patient, if any. It may also include a snapshot of the patient's medical diagnoses and whether or not they have advanced directives. It is duplicated so that the consultant may take a copy for their records.

Advanced directives section

Advanced directives are legal documents that provide a way for people to communicate to family, friends, and healthcare providers their wishes should they not be able to make healthcare choices for themselves. Advanced directives typically involve the election of a healthcare proxy via a document called a durable power of attorney for health care.

This proxy (the person elected to hold this responsibility) will make healthcare decisions for the patient. It is expected that the healthcare proxy will have had conversations with the person for whom they have been appointed to determine that person's wishes in the event critical health issues occur and the person is not able to direct care decisions themselves.

Also included in advanced directives is a living will. A living will expresses the person's view about efforts to sustain their life. The person can accept or refuse medical care and specify certain conditions including:

- The use of dialysis and breathing machines.
- A desire to not be resuscitated if breathing or heartbeat stops. This is known as a DNR (**D**o **N**ot **R**esuscitate) order. (The person can also direct that they do want to be resuscitated.)
- Whether the person wants tube-feeding to sustain life.
- Whether the person wants to be an organ or tissue donor.

Before a healthcare practitioner may provide any form of treatment, it is necessary to determine whether the patient is their own guardian and is capable of making their own healthcare decisions (i.e., whether they have been determined to be competent). If they have selected a healthcare proxy, then that individual must give their consent in order for the patient to be seen. On occasion, a NH resident may be capable of making their own healthcare choices but may have a family member or friend handling their finances. It is important to discuss the fees for dental care with that individual as well in order to prevent future misunderstandings.

History and physical section

As stated earlier, upon each and every admission to a NH the admitting physician is required to perform and document a comprehensive medical history and physical. In this section, the providing oral healthcare practitioner can review the patient's medical history, review of systems, medications, and treatment plan for care. This information is critical to know before any oral health care is provided.

Progress notes

In this section of the chart every practitioner who has an encounter with the patient or resident must enter what has been done in that visit. It is important

Facility		Date/Time Admitted

Patient Name	Medical Record Number	Sex Marital Status

Address Phone Number	Date of Birth Age SSN	Religion Race

Room Number	Previous Admission/Discharge	Admitted From Hospital	Hospital From/To Dates

Payor Source	Policy Number	Medicare Part A/B Effective Dates

Insurance Information	Policy Number Phone Number Authorization Number Level

Pharmacy   Phone Number   Medicare Part D Plan Name   Policy Number

Attending Physician

Alternate Physician   Referring Physician

Podiatrist   Dentist

Next of Kin: Relation: Home: Work: Cell:

Responsible Party for Healthcare Decisions: Relation: Home: Work: Cell:

Guarantor: Relation: Home: Work: Cell:

Additional Contact: Relation: Home: Work: Cell:

Advance Directives:

Diagnoses

Discharge Date/Time	Discharge To	Discharge Code

Date of Last Payer Change: Date Printed:

Figure 17.1 Patient information sheet.

to include the date, time, and treating service at the top of the note. The note should follow the SOAP (Subjective, Objective, Assessment and Plan) format. Clearly defining and recording the next step in the dental treatment plan is very helpful to the facility in assisting the provider with the next visit. It may be useful to include a statement of general disposition of the patient at the end of treatment such as "the patient left the dental area in stable condition."

Doctors' orders section

Upon admission to a NH, the facility assumes responsibility for the total care of the NH resident. Similar to a hospital admission medication lists, nursing requirements, diet, vital signs, activities, and bathing must be planned and ordered by the appropriate healthcare provider for the resident. The doctor's order section is where all of the orders for each patient are recorded. This is also where the oral healthcare provider will write orders for medication needed in the treatment of dental disease.

In most charts, a medication list compiled and printed by the pharmacy will follow the doctors' order section. Typically each month a new medication list will be generated.

Consult section (Fig. 17.2)

The dental team will often be asked to consult on a resident for a specific reason such as pain, swelling, or malodor. When this occurs, the oral health practitioner should complete a consultation form. These forms are either in the chart or available at the nurses' station and may be in duplicate or triplicate form. The top section of the form should provide the reason for consult and the medical history. The portion for the consultant to complete should include the findings upon examination of the resident expressed in the SOAP format. The original usually remains in the chart and the consultant takes one copy for their records.

Laboratory result section

In this section all recent laboratory results may be found. This section should be considered when reviewing the patient's medical history. It may be necessary to evaluate therapeutic levels of specific medications such as warfarin and phenytoin (Dilantin®), blood glucose levels, or the presence of an anemia or low platelet count prior to rendering treatment.

Dental chart

Each NH facility will have a different approach to maintaining the dental records. Some facilities will include a specific section for dentistry within the medical chart. It is often necessary to maintain conventional dental radiographs in a separate filing system. Other facilities will ask the dental team to maintain their own charts and also make notes about procedures done in the medical chart. Of course electronic health records may eliminate the need for separate charts and storage of conventional radiographs if digital radiographs are employed.

Treatment delivery options

During the contract negotiation between the dental provider and the facility, it is important to determine what types of procedures may be realistically accomplished as well as what physical space, equipment, and supplies will be made available for oral care. Various treatment delivery system options exist. These include the following options.

On-site operatory

An on-site dental treatment room is ideal. However, it is not the typical situation as many NH CEOs view the costs of equipping the dental treatment room too great given the utilization rate, space limitations, and fiscal constraints. The oral health practitioners are usually on-site no more than 1 day per week. As a result, the dental operatory is likely to remain empty most of the time.

Minimally, the dental treatment room should be lockable and contain the following:
* Sink and running water.
* Cabinetry for storage and possibly dental charts.
* High and low speed hand pieces, air/water, and suction.
* A dental chair may or may not be needed depending on the number of wheelchair-bound patients are in the facility.
* A good intraoral light source.
* Radiographic and developing capacity, either conventional or digital.
* Sterilization capacity.

Sticker here

Consulation form

Name: _____   Date: _____

Consultant/Provider: _____

Reason for Referral: _____

_____

_____

Patient Information: _____

_____

_____

_____

_____

Signature/Title: _____   *Date:* _____

Consultant's report

_____

_____

_____

_____

_____

_____

_____

_____

_____

_____

_____

_____

_____

Signature/Title: _____   *Date:* _____

Return Appointment: _____

White: Patient chart   **Yellow**: Consultant   **Pink**: Referring physician

Figure 17.2 Consultation form.

- Appropriate dental supplies for anticipated procedures.
- Telephone.
- Emergency medical equipment if emergency support is not readily available.
- Computer if the chart is electronic.

Bedside

Both consultation and minimal treatment procedures can be provided at the bedside. A bedside consultation prior to treatment may provide useful information about the cognitive state and cooperation level of the resident.

The following will be needed to perform a bedside consultation:

- Light source such as: head lamp, penlight, or flashlight
- Gloves, mask, and protective eyewear
- Gauze
- Tongue blade or disposable mirror.

Always knock on the door before entering a NH resident's room even if the door is open. It is important to remember their room is now their home and they deserve to have their privacy respected to the greatest degree possible in an institutional setting. Identify yourself to the patient and ask about their chief complaint. Always ask permission to examine the patient. If they say no, after a few requests respect their autonomy, make a note in their chart, and try again at another time.

If a resident appears to be nonresponsive or showing signs of dementia or organic brain disease, assessing their level of alertness may be useful when considering future treatment and the best modality for that treatment. By asking the questions noted in Table 17.1, the level of alertness and orientation of the resident may be assessed.

As the level of alertness and orientation decrease, the ability to perform dental services may decrease as well. It is important to document your findings to support any recommendations for alternative treatment modalities such as oral sedation, intravenous sedation, or general anesthesia. It is also generally best to do as much as possible as soon as possible. As cognitive and/or medical status declines, treatment only becomes more difficult.

A thorough soft and hard tissue intraoral and extraoral head and neck examination should be completed. Be certain to remove any prosthesis that may be present to adequately visualize the tissues. Additional

Table 17.1 Alert and oriented (A&O)

Question	A&O × 3	A&O × 2	A&O × 1	A&O × 0
Do you know what day it is?	YES	NO	NO	NO
Do you know where you are?	YES	YES	NO	NO
Do you know your name?	YES	YES	YES	NO

Key: A&O × 3 = 3 answers correct. A&O × 2 = 2 answers correct. A&O × 1 = 1 answer correct. A&O × 0 = 0 answers correct.

treatment procedures may be done bedside by bringing in the supplies and equipment necessary for the procedure. Impressions, wax try-ins, and bite registrations are relatively uncomplicated done bedside. Oral prophylaxis with hand-scalers and extractions, as well as other dental procedures, can also be done bedside, but are much better-suited to the controlled environment of the dental treatment room. Although a dental treatment room is preferable, with appropriate planning, it is remarkable how much can be accomplished with relatively minimal equipment bedside.

Multi-purpose room/beauty salon

Many NHs will not have a dedicated space available for the provision of oral health care. The NH staff may suggest the use of a multi-purpose room, such as a resident lounge or conference room or, more commonly, the beauty salon.

Treatment may be provided in these venues utilizing portable dental equipment. The practitioner may want to consider a storage area in the vicinity to store some of the needed equipment or supplies dedicated to that facility. It will be important to establish areas for clean equipment and supplies and an area for dirty instrumentation or contaminated disposable supplies and sharps. Careful planning is a prerequisite for successful provision of care whenever service is provided in an alternative venue where familiar and complete equipment and supplies are not available.

Note Regardless of the location that dental treatment is provided, all dentures fabricated for NH residents must be labeled with their name. In NH environments, dentures are often left on food trays, may get wrapped up in bed linens or within towels, or may be mistakenly taken by another resident from a bedside table while the owner of the dentures is sleeping. Denture labeling is quick, easy, inexpensive, and can avoid costly and time-consuming denture remakes.

Patient referrals to outside resources

Each NH resident is a unique and special individual being the sum total of their life experiences, education, economic status, medical, and mental status, etc. Understandably not all NH residents will be able to be treated in the NH setting and may require outside referral for appropriate treatment.

Nursing home residents who are minimally disabled and have dental needs beyond the scope of practice of the NH provider may be referred to an outside practitioner's office for care. This will involve arrangement for transportation and possible accompaniment by a staff member on the part of the NH.

Severely complex, compromised, and/or noncompliant NH patients may require some type of sedation or general anesthesia to be able to safely and appropriately receive dental treatment. This occurs most often in emergency or life-threatening situations such as severe infection, aspiration risk, or noncompliance. Prior to making a referral, a risk-benefit analysis must be done in conjunction with the primary-care provider to determine the best setting for the dental service.

It is useful to keep a referral list of needed oral healthcare specialists that might include an oral pathologist, oral and maxillofacial surgeon, dental specialists, general practitioner with hospital privileges, and a university- or hospital-based dental program.

Billing

During the contractual phase to become a NH oral healthcare provider, billing issues must be discussed and resolved before any agreement is signed. Questions such as, primary-payer source; who will bill – the facility or the provider; and do residents have personal spending accounts, should be clarified.

Most NH residents enter into a facility using multiple sources of payment such as private resources, Medicare and Medicaid. However, after a period of time approximately 60% rely totally on Medicaid dollars to pay for their care (DHHS, 2009).

Medicaid provisions for adult dentistry vary from state to state within the USA. It may be important to understand the Medicaid guidelines for the state where the treatment is being provided in order to make an informed decision on whether to become a Medicaid provider.

Meticulous and accurate record-keeping is the key to successful billing no matter where the oral healthcare services are provided.

Summary

Providing oral health care in the NH environment can be one of the most rewarding and satisfying career options available to practitioners. There is no question that the need is great and that access to dental care is very limited in many locations for this population.

It is not always an easy task as one must consider the special nuances of the population being treated in addition to providing quality oral health care. The overall experience for the provider and the patient may be greatly enhanced by following the few basic principles found in Box 17.1.

Box 17.1 Basic principles that can enhance the overall experience for provider and patient

- Always be courteous to the patients, their family members, and the NH staff. You may need to enlist their support for patient cooperation; getting the patient dressed, into a wheelchair, transported to the dental treatment area, following of postoperative instructions; etc.
- Due to changes in memory and recall it may be helpful to engage the NH resident in conversations that involve their past personal history. Most residents are eager to share their life experiences and are grateful for a willing listener.
- Remember that hearing impairment is common among the elderly and has been reported to be almost 70% in NH residents (Berg & Morgenstern, 1997). When addressing a NH resident be certain to speak clearly and slowly while facing them directly without a mask if possible.
- Allow the NH resident time to respond to questions asked or commands given. Keep in mind changes in the neurologic system may slow down processing. Often it isn't that they did not hear but rather that they are taking longer to respond.
- Always grant the NH resident autonomy. If they do not wish to visit with the oral healthcare provider accept their refusal, document, and try again at a later time. If their need is urgent or emergent, discuss with the nursing staff and patient care provider alternative ways to engage the patient and resolve the problem.

Case study

Mrs. Elsie Farbman is an 82-year-old widowed female who has been coming to Sunnyside Dental Office for the last 25 years. Her medical history is presented below. During this time she has had multiple dental procedures completed including endodontic therapy, post and core placement, crown and bridge placement, and two implants placed and restored. Over the last 10 years she has been returning faithfully every 6 months for oral prophylaxis, radiographs and examination when indicated. At her last dental visit there were no significant dental findings and the patient was without complaints. Her periodontal status and home care were noted as being excellent. Mrs. Farbman surprisingly failed to schedule her last 6-month recall appointment and a reminder card was sent to her home address on record.

Today the office manager at Sunnyside Dental Office received a telephone call from Mr. David Farbman, Elsie's son, who informed the office that 8 months ago his mother fell at home and fractured her left hip. Since that time she has undergone hip replacement surgery, rehabilitative therapy and is now residing in Sunnyside Skilled Nursing Facility (SNF) just down the street. He lives over 1500 miles away and, while speaking to his mother, she complained of a "terrible toothache." Mr. Farbman would like to know if it is possible for an oral healthcare practitioner to visit his mother at the SNF to address her problem.

Over the past several decades Sunnyside Dental Office has established a working relationship with Sunnyside SNF due to the proximity of the two facilities. You have just joined Sunnyside Dental Office. While you are aware of this relationship, this is the first time you have been asked to see a patient at the Sunnyside SNF. All of the Sunnyside Dental senior personnel are at a dental meeting being held on a cruise ship in the Caribbean and are not available for consultation.

Past medical history

Past medical history as recorded in the dental chart (updated 18 months ago):
- 82-year-old pleasant white female
- Alert and orientated (A&O) × 3
- Ambulates independently
- Comes unaccompanied to the dental office every 6 months for oral prophylaxis

Illnesses:	(+) Hypertension; hyperlipidemia; mild angina; osteoporosis; osteoarthritis
Medications:	(+) Hydrochlorothiazide 50 mg od
	(+) Lovastatin 40 mg po q pm
	(+) Boniva 150 mg PO once a month
	(+) Baby aspirin 81 mg od
	(+) Naprosyn 500 mg PO bid prn joint pain
	(+) Nitrostat 0.4 mg sublingually prn chest pain
Hospitalization:	(+) childbirth × 2 in 1951and 1954; (+) hysterectomy 1987
Allergies:	(+) Penicillin, shellfish
Social history:	Worked at the telephone company before marriage; homemaker since
	Denies alcohol (ETOH) but admits to drinking a 6 oz. glass of sherry once a week.
	Denies tobacco and recreational drugs
Family history:	Widow for past 12 years
	Two children (one deceased)
	Mother deceased – (+) hypertension (HTN)
	Father deceased – (+) myocardial infarction (MI), HTN
	Siblings × 1 deceased
Vital signs:	Blood pressure 140/90 mmHg
	Heart rate: 82 beats per minute
	Resting rate: 17 beats per minute

Case study question

1 What approach will you take to help Mrs. Farbman? (See also Figure 17.3.)

od, once a day; pm, at night; po, by mouth; q, every.

There is great satisfaction in providing a much needed service that others are not trained or willing to do. Additionally, the NH residents and their families are eternally grateful for the care given. This population can be well-spring of knowledge and information as well as a personal tour guide through past history. Each NH resident is an individual with a unique and interesting past. Listen, enjoy, and have fun!

There are many factors to take into consideration when treating NH patients. Each patient is a unique individual and should be treated as such. Please consider all aspects of care as an oral healthcare professional before seeing the patient. Consider if you will need additional information or not. The more information you have available to you the more successful you will be and the more pleasant the overall experience will be for everyone.

HOME VISITS

As the population of the USA ages, the number of homebound elders also increases. Advances in medicine and dentistry have resulted in a significant increase in overall longevity and in the number of dental visits and procedures done, especially for the "Baby Boomer" generation. As the physiologic changes related to aging and disability occur resulting in decreased ambulation, many of these previously reliable dental patients may not seek dental care for significant periods of time. Failure to receive routine dental care puts them at risk for increased dental disease including pain, bleeding and infection. One possible solution may be to go to the patient if the patient cannot come to the oral healthcare practitioner.

Treating a person in the home allows the oral healthcare practitioner to assess much more than the oral condition of the patient. A home visit will provide a greater understanding of the following:
- Level of family support.
- Patient's living conditions; signs of neglect.
- Patient's support network; availability of community based services.
- Functional capacity of the patient; watching the elder perform ADLs.
- Nutritional status of the patient; check pantry and refrigerator if possible.

- Elder abuse; look for signs of abuse and how the caregiver treats the elder.
- Possible linkages with home care agencies.

Home visits can be done either by a private practitioner or as part of a group that specializes in providing care to the home bound. In either case special consideration must be given to the equipment and supplies that will be needed. Organization will be the key to a successful home visit.

Procedures that can be provided in the home include:
- Exams, X-rays, and diagnoses
- Treatment planning
- Hygiene (professional cleanings), fluoride trays, and cancer screenings
- Denture fabrication and adjustment, night guards
- Emergency dental treatment

Preparation for the home visit

If the oral healthcare practitioner is part of an organized dental team that routinely does home visits, protocols and procedures should be clearly defined and understood prior to any visit.

A solo or private practitioner may be asked to visit one of their long-term patients of record in their home for a dental emergency or for routine examination and care if needed.

There are several key points to keep in mind prior to doing a home visit. Safety must be a primary concern not only for the patient but for the dental team as well:
- Prior to the visit determine the "chief complaint" or purpose of the visit.
- Make certain the address and telephone numbers are correct and obtain directions if needed.
- Ascertain who else will be present at the home in addition to the patient. Request a family member or friend to be there and be certain to have their contact information.
- Never go alone. Always take a member of your dental team with you.
- Plan the visit during the daytime if possible.
- Bring the patient's chart and any anticipated equipment and supplies needed.
- Proper consent forms will be required to be signed by the patient or their healthcare proxy.

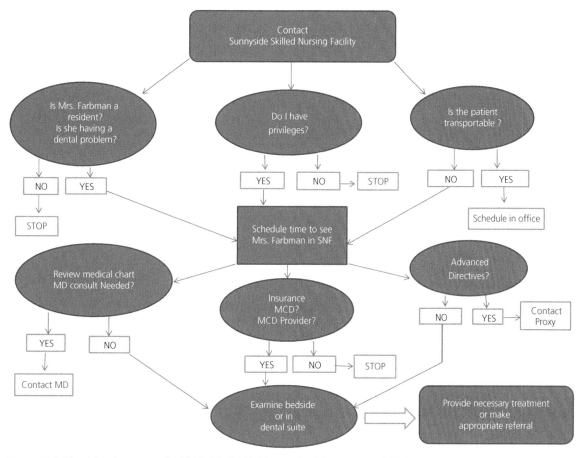

Figure 17.3 Algorithm for case study. MCD, Medicaid; MD, medical doctor; SNF, skilled nursing facility.

The visit

Upon arriving at the patient's home it is important to be aware of your surroundings. It may be helpful to the patient and their family or caregiver if attention is paid to the surroundings and necessary recommendations made:
- Park your car in a well-lit and easily accessible spot.
- Be certain to wear proper attire and with proper identification. Remember you are a visitor and should demonstrate professionalism and courtesy.
- When entering the property note cluttered walkways, stairs, and overgrown trees and shrubs. Make certain to note if any steps are faulty and could result in a fall.

- Is there good lighting at the entry way?
- Are hallways clearly lit and uncluttered?
- Are throw rugs tacked down and carpet in good condition?
- Are telephones easily accessible and clearly marked with emergency numbers?
- Are smoke detectors present and working?
- Does the patient have a system in place for accurate dosing of medications?
- Do you notice any frayed electrical wires on appliances or extension cords?

Although these do not directly relate to dental care working in a safe environment is necessary for all members of the dental team as well as the patient. You may decide not to return to the home unless safety issues are addressed.

Other important treatment issues to consider include:

- Where will the patient be treated: in bed, a chair, at the kitchen table?
- Will there be sufficient space to maintain a clean and dirty area while performing the procedure?
- Is there an adequate intraoral light source present?
- Will hand pieces and suction be available?
- How will sterilization be completed?
- What mechanisms are in place for proper disposal of bio-hazardous waste?
- Be certain to clean up after the procedure and leave the area as it was when you began.

Record keeping

No matter where oral care services are provided it is important to properly document all of the procedures done. Consideration must be given to storage of the personal health records of the patients. All health records are protected under The Health Insurance Portability and Accountability Act of 1996 (HIPAA) Privacy and Security Rules (US Department of Health and Human Services, 1996). When transporting patient records all efforts must be made to keep the records in a safe and protected environment where healthcare information cannot be breached.

Billing/house/extended care facility call

As a private practitioner when providing treatment out of the office there is a CDT code for the professional or hospital visit.

Code D9410 includes visits to nursing homes, long-term care facilities, hospice sites, institutions, etc. Report in addition to reporting appropriate code numbers for actual services performed (ADA, 2011).

For patients who are eligible for Medicaid coverage the Medicaid guidelines for the state in which the service is provided must be followed.

1 A facility licensed by the state to offer residents personal care as well as skilled nursing care on a 24-hour-a-day basis including room and board, supervision, medication, therapies, and rehabilitation is known as which of the following?
   A Assisted living facility
   B Nursing home
   C Intermediate care facility
   D None of the above

2 Many nursing homes that receive Medicare or Medicaid reimbursement will seek an oral healthcare practitioner to perform an oral examination as part of a comprehensive physical exam with each new resident admission. Which of the following is true:
   A This examination is part of a Minimum Data Set that must be completed within 14 days of a resident being admitted to a facility.
   B If an oral healthcare practitioner is not available the nursing home may elect not to provide the oral examination.
   C This examination is mandated by federal law.
   D A & C
   E B & C

3 A set of legal documents that provide important information to family, friends, and healthcare providers concerning the nursing home resident's wishes should they not be able to make healthcare choices for themselves are known as which of the following?
   A Advanced directives
   B Patient's orders
   C Patient information form
   D Patient progress notes

4 You are asked to consult on a nursing home resident because a staff member noticed a swelling on the right side of the jaw that was not previously there. Following the guidelines for a bedside visit you find the patient to be nonresponsive to any of your questions. The patient only mumbles yes when you call her name. You would consider this patient to be which of the following?
   A Alert and oriented × 3
   B Alert and oriented × 2
   C Alert and oriented × 1
   D Alert and oriented × 0

5 Although not the traditional methodology for oral health care, a visit to patient's home to provide care may be needed. In addition to the provision of

a dental service what other assessments may also be made?

A Nutritional status of the patient

B Family support of the patient

C Elder abuse

D Environmental safety

E All of the above

6 Which of the following is recommended when traveling to a patient's home to provide oral health care?

A Always wear identification

B Go alone

C Request a family member to be present

D Leave the patients dental records on the front seat of your automobile

E A & C

7 Traveling to a patient's home to provide oral health care is a very commendable thing to do. However, you are not permitted to bill for your time taken from the office to treat the patient.

A True

B False

References

American Dental Association (ADA) (2011) *Code on Dental Procedures and Nomenclature (CDT)*, 2011-2012. From http://www.ada.org/8832.aspx. Accessed April 7, 2014.

Berg, R. & Morgenstern, N.E. (1997) Physiologic changes in the elderly. *The Dental Clinics of North America Clinical Decision Making in Geriatrics*, **41**(4), 651–68.

CDC (US Centers for Disease Control and Prevention) (2009) *The National Nursing Home Survey: 2004*. Vital and Health Statistics, Series 13, No. 167, June 2009. From http://www.cdc.gov/nchs/data/series/sr_13/sr13_167.pdf. Accessed April 7, 2014.

Hawes, C., Mor, V., Phillips, C.D., *et al.* (1997) The OBRA-87 nursing home regulations and implementation of the Resident Assessment Instrument: effects on process quality. *Journal of the American Geriatric Society*, **45**(8), 977–85.

Schwartz, M. (2002) Dentistry for the long term care patient. *Dentistry Today*. From http://www.dentistrytoday.com/practice-management-articles/long-term-care/1378. Accessed April 7, 2014.

Turnham, H. (1987) *Federal Nursing Home Reform Act from the Omnibus Budget Reconciliation Act of 1987 or simply OBRA '87 Summary*. From http://www.allhealth.org/briefingmaterials/obra87summary-984.pdf. Accessed June 24, 2012.

US Department of Health and Human Services (1996) *Health Information Privacy*. From http://www.hhs.gov/ocr/privacy. Accessed April 7, 2014.

US Department of Health and Human Services (2014) *Administration on Aging: Aging Statistics*. From http://www.aoa.gov/AoARoot/Aging_Statistics/index.aspx. Accessed April 7, 2014.

US National Archives and Records Administration (2012). *e-CFR 2010*. From http://www.gpo.gov/fdsys/pkg/CFR-2013-title42-vol5/pdf/CFR-2013-title42-vol5-sec483-55.pdf. Accessed April 7, 2014.

CHAPTER 18

Portable Dentistry

Harvey Levy

Frederick Memorial Hospital, Frederick, MD, USA

Introduction

The purpose of this chapter is to offer practical tools, tips, and techniques for establishing and conducting a successful and much needed portable dentistry practice to serve the growing unmet needs of our aging population, especially the frail, medically complex, homebound individuals. In this chapter, we share the "best practices" that have evolved from many years of developing and refining systems that work, both for the patient and the dental team.

We first need to differentiate portable dentistry from mobile dentistry. Portable dentistry is what occurs when the dentist treats patients at locations not outfitted with the needed medical and dental equipment, such as nursing homes, private homes, and institutions. The dentist transports dental supplies and equipment from the office to the location. Mobile dentistry, on the other hand, mostly involves equipment with wheels. At the hospital or surgical center most of the needed equipment is already in the building, and is merely wheeled into the patient's room, the emergency room, or the operating room. Mobile dentistry and working in an operating room are beyond the scope of this chapter. This chapter will discuss the essential elements of portable dentistry.

Radiographs

For an initial evaluation, the most important diagnostic tools are the Aribex NOMAD-Pro® handheld X-ray unit, coupled with the DEXIS® instant digital imaging software and sensor installed on a laptop (Figs 18.1 & 18.2).

The NOMAD-Pro® handheld X-ray unit is cordless and weighs just over 5 lbs. It looks like a police officer's radar gun, and is practical for taking X-rays in any location. Its battery is capable of exposing 1000 films, and a second battery is provided with the equipment. The NOMAD®, an older unit, weighs just over 8 lbs. The estimate price of under $7000 is cost-effective if used for more than one operatory, eliminating installation construction, ease of relocating, being serviced, or used away from a fixed operatory wall.

DEXIS® digital images are instantly obtained and provide excellent resolution, which enables performing root canals and quickly identifying fractured root tips in a portable setting. Digital images have the further advantage of being readily archived and easily e-mailed.

When a laptop is not available, the backup for portable imaging is the inexpensive Ergonom-X® self-developing Dental Film, which requires between 60 and 90 seconds of processing (Fig. 18.3). It comes with its own in-packet chemicals, and requires no extraneous developing equipment or electricity. Because it contains no tin or aluminum foil, backwards or herringbone pattern errors are precluded.

Suction

Operating rooms have better evacuating units than most dental offices. Out in the field, treatment requires suction units with enough capacity to complete all the necessary work on one patient. Such units must be lightweight, portable, and easily cleansable. A single canister unit (Fig. 18.4) fills up

Geriatric Dentistry: Caring for Our Aging Population, First Edition. Edited by Paula K. Friedman.

© 2014 John Wiley & Sons, Inc. Published 2014 by John Wiley & Sons, Inc.

Companion website: www.wiley.com/go/friedman/geriatricdentistry

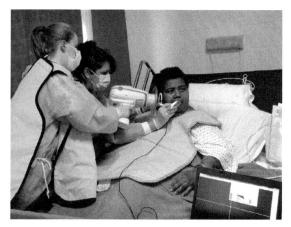

Figure 18.1 An over 500 lb patient in an assisted living facility. (Aribex NOMAD-Pro® and DEXIS® images.)

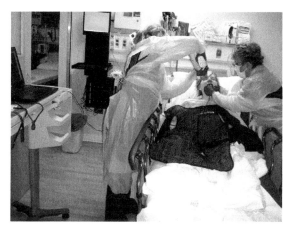

Figure 18.2 A contagious patient in an isolation room setting. (Aribex NOMAD-Pro® and DEXIS® images.)

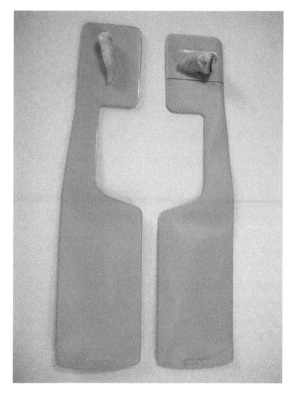

Figure 18.3 Ergonom-X® self-developing Dental Film.

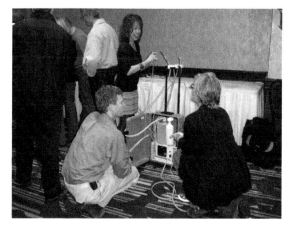

Figure 18.4 Aseptico portable cart with suction, single canister, and single water bottle.

quickly and requires halting dental treatment to empty it out, whereas a multiple canister unit allows for a simple toggle switch. This same capacity limitation holds true for the water source. A single one-liter water bottle requires halting the handpiece or scaler while the water is replenished. Dual bottles have double the capacity and generally do not require interrupting use of the handpiece or scaler.

Portable and mobile carts

There are a variety of portable and mobile dental carts that can be quickly assembled/disassembled and transported.

Portable carts

ASI Medical makes the Triton®, which looks like a small suitcase, is plumbing-free, and easy to transport in a car or van. Just as portable and with

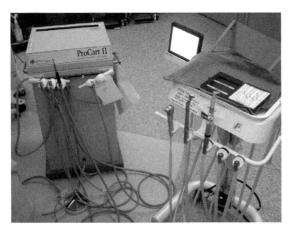

Figure 18.5 Mobile carts: DNTL Works Port-Op II (left); Forest Dental Cart model 5910 (right).

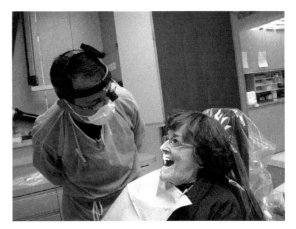

Figure 18.6 Head lights.

convenient carrying cases is Mobile Dental Systems' Port-Op III®. Aseptico also provides popular plumbing-free lightweight models that are easily transported, set up and maintained, such as the one in Fig. 18.4. These compact and compartmentalized "set-up and go" units readily pack up to travel in a car across town, or in an aeroplane across the world on mission trips.

For simple prophylaxis cleanings, the small rechargeable portable prophy handpieces are excellent. In states where hygienists can perform off-site exams and cleanings without a dentist present (see Chapter 19), the units are light enough to be carried by the hygienist without an assistant.

It is essential to have a backup prophy unit on hand in the event of a nonfunctioning unit or one where the battery has run down. In its absence, a failed or discharged prophy head is likely to require a second visit to the patient, causing increased expenditure of resources (time and expense for the patient and/or dental professional).

Mobile carts (Fig. 18.5)
Aseptico's rolling AMC-20® has two water canisters, instead of one, making it ideal when being moved and used within a facility. Another excellent two-canister, four-wheeled mobile cart is DNTL's ProCart III®. These units are designed to be wheeled, rather than disassembled, and hand-carried to a site.

Lighting

Carts may come with a wide variety of light sources. Based on experience with all kinds of lighting – attached vs. free-standing, battery-powered vs. electric – dental professionals generally prefer to selection to those that fit around the user's head without umbilically connecting him or her to the wall (Fig. 18.6).

The under-$30 Panther Vision PowerCap® by Lowes has up to three lights shining straight ahead. It allows head movements to follow the patient's moving head, keeping the teeth always well lit. These inexpensive and practical "light hats" are also useful in cars and homes for emergencies. Our favorite of all head lights is the Ultralight Optics lights due to the low cost, light weight, and high multi-use versatility.

Patient chairs (Fig. 18.7a,b)

Chairs run the gamut from $5 discount store folding stools to our favorites – the sophisticated and readily movable DentalEZ Airglide® J-chairs or DentalEZ Nu-Simplicity® chairs. In a dental office, these Airglide® J-chairs or Nu-Simplicity® chairs with hovercraft technology move around on a cushion of air, allowing patients to remain in the comfort of their own wheelchair or gurney if they wish. The cost range of $5000–8000 is reasonable when you factor in the unique versatility of movement and transport. Options within nursing homes include the beauticians' chairs.

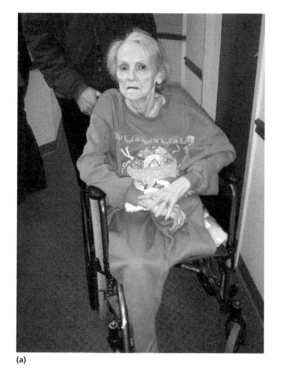

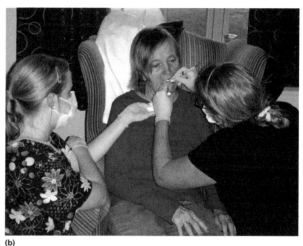

(a)   **(b)**

Figure 18.7 Patients can sit in their own wheelchair (a) or chair (b).

In private homes, the patient or caregiver will make the selection from what is available and comfortable for the patient within the home. It is helpful to always have a portable folding chair in the provider's car, and to bring it in when needed.

Lathe

Denture adjustments are easy with the proper lathe to supplement the handpieces. These are included with some of the portable and mobile carts, and can also be purchased at a hardware store. It is important to carry a second lathe or a backup dremel (such as a Sears portable cordless drill) to be able to adjust removable appliances if the first one fails.

Computer equipment

A paperless workflow is becoming increasingly important, and eventually will become mandatory. Whether you are logged on to your office system via the internet, or make do with a pen/flash/USB drive to upload upon your return to the office, a reliable laptop is essential. You need fast access to your patient database to read their chart, and the ability to upload X-rays and clinical notes to the patient's file. The Dentrix® system integrates seamlessly with all other software and hardware in the practice, including the DEXIS® instant digital imaging software. Of course, individual preferences may vary.

Wraps and props

Wraps and props are often necessary for completing dental care on patients who are unable to cooperative. Velcro® hand restraints are vital in preventing a thrashing hand from causing an accident while the dental practitioner is holding a drill, needle, or other sharp instrument. Whether the hand movements are behaviorally intentional or medically involuntary, they can cause disaster. Specialized Care Company (www. SpecializedCare.com) makes the Rainbow Wrap®

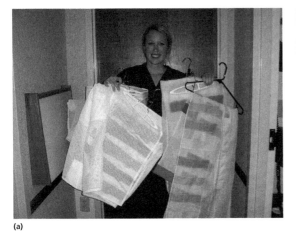

(a)

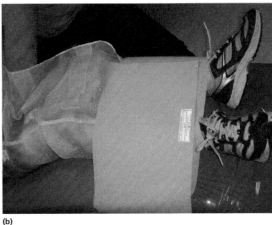

(b)

Figure 18.8 Rainbow Wrap® (a) and Rainbow® Knee Belts (b).

stabilizing system, soft hand restraints in conjunction with wraps made of colorful breathable mesh, all of which are adjustable with Velcro® (Fig. 18.8a). They are available in seven sizes and are able to effectively and gently immobilize most patients. Velcro® Rainbow® Knee Belts (Fig. 18.8b) are knee/leg stabilizers, and there are also head/forehead stabilizers, very effective in reducing sudden jerky movements. All these wraps are easy to apply, inexpensive, and readily washable.

Specialized Care Company's Open Wide® mouth rest (see Fig. 8.13 later in this chapter) is an inexpensive, disposable, and well-designed pair of tongue depressors in foam, used as a first tool for initially opening and maintaining the mouth open. Other mouth props commonly used include the unilateral Molt mouth gag by Hu-Friedy (Fig. 8.9), and the bilateral Jennings mouth prop by 3i (Fig. 8.10), often used by ENT physicians for their exams and intraoral procedures. There are dozens of other props in the market including McKesson, Logibloc®, lip retractors, and many more.

A special mouth prop serves a five-in-one function. The Isolite® safely props the mouth, retracts the cheek, retracts the tongue, removes the saliva, and serves as an excellent five-level light source (Fig. 18.11). When using the Isolite® in the office or in the field, the assistant can be on standby. It hooks up to the suction unit and light source on the cart, and provides a propped, clear, illuminated, dry, and isolated field that improves the patient's and practitioner's comfort and chance of success.

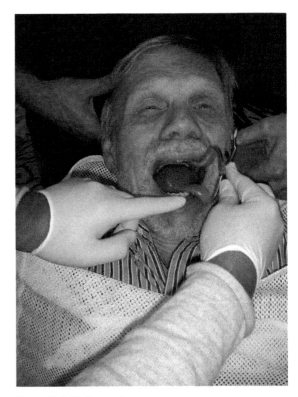

Figure 18.9 Molt mouth gag.

Headrests

Headrests range from the assistant's chest or lap to wheelchair tilting devices with double articulating headrests. Removable headrests that can be clamped

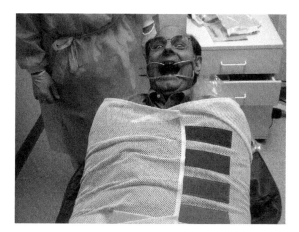

Figure 18.10 Rainbow® wrap and Jennings prop.

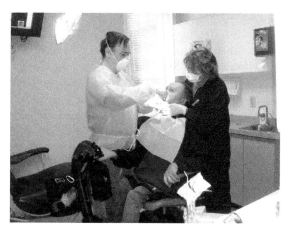

Figure 18.12 Assistant serving as patient's headrest.

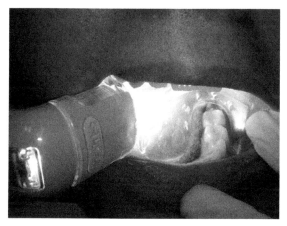

Figure 18.11 Isolite® 5-in-1.

on to many surfaces, including the backs of most chairs or wheelchairs, work very well. An equally good, if not preferable, choice, however, is a live human being – a caregiver's or an assistant's hands and chest can immobilize and stabilize the patient's head better than any product available for purchase (Fig. 18.12).

Maintenance and repairs

A good maintenance person or company is worth their weight in gold. Ideally at least one designated person should be responsible for routine cleaning, lubricating, and maintenance of any reusable equipment, especially the suction, water source,

handpieces, and hoses. A good working relationship with your dental supplier, including periodic preventive maintenance visits, will reduce malfunctions and breakdowns. It is worthwhile to schedule semi-annual preventive maintenance visits with your supplier's representative. The adage for equipment maintenance is a lot like car maintenance, where you can pay a little now, or a lot later.

Vans

Vans are wonderful for a serious practitioner of mobile dentistry or organization that can fund, monitor, and support the effort. Details are beyond the scope of this chapter, but vans must be mentioned as a viable, low-overhead option for delivering treatment in addition to, or instead of, a conventional dental office.

Sedation

Not every patient is able to cooperate in a way that enables treatment to be accomplished. A typical means of gaining cooperation in elderly patients is via a sedative pill or elixir. Common pills include the benzodiazepines diazepam (Valium®), triazolam (Halcion®), or lorazepam (Ativan®). These work extremely well as sedatives, but the dentist must be mindful of any synergistic or antagonistic reaction with other medicines the patient may be taking. Often the sedative dose must be reduced due to the patient's existing medical condition, concomitant drugs, body frailty, and the increased half-life of many of these pharmacologic agents in the elderly.

To prevent overdose, the American Society of Dentist Anesthesiologists (ASDA), DOCS, and other organizations advise to "dose low and dose slow," titrating up as needed. (Another version of this recommendation is "Start low, go slow".) The best reversal agent for respiratory depression from excessive or over-dosage is 2 ml Romazicon® (flumazenil). This benzodiazepine reversal agent is part of an emergency kit, and is designed to be given intravenously. However, in case of an emergency, sublingual injections have been highly successful, be it from an intraoral or extraoral insertion. It is important to check the expiration dates on all medications in the emergency kit on a regular basis and to ensure the availability of unexpired reversal agents at all times.

Many anxious patients benefit from the anxiolytic effects of nitrous oxide (laughing gas) analgesia (Fig. 18.13), whether portable or fixed at the location.

When used in addition to local anesthetic, wraps, props, and a sedative, the success rate for completion of the procedure with nitrous oxide is extremely high. At the end of the procedure, we often reverse the anesthetic effect of a mandibular block by injecting Septodont's OraVerse®, to prevent lip, tongue or cheek biting.

In our experience with 35 000 anxious or uncooperative patients, we were able to complete the needed dental care 96% of the time using gas, drugs, wraps, and props. The other 4% of patients were successfully treated via general anesthesia in the operating room.

Level of care

Once the diagnostic data is obtained, we develop a treatment plan that ranges from minimal care to comprehensive care. Minimal care is limited to ensuring that the patient is both pain-free and infection-free. That includes treating what is urgent or affecting their quality of life (Fig. 18.14).

Comprehensive care has no limitations other than the dentist's skills and comfort level, plus the capability of the portable dental equipment and facility. For selected cases, the majority of the dental work is handled at the off-site facility using portable dentistry, while one or two visits may be made to a dental office or operating room via medical transportation. That combination offers the best of both worlds for nonambulatory patients requiring and agreeing to more extensive dental care. For nonambulatory patients or patients for whom transportation is

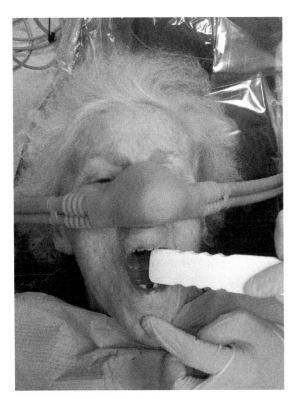

Figure 18.13 Nitrous oxide mask and Open Wide® mouth rest.

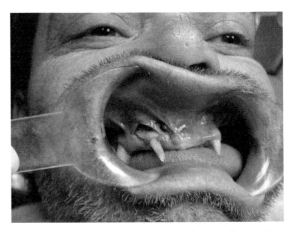

Figure 18.14 At the very least, we aim for pain-free and infection-free treatment.

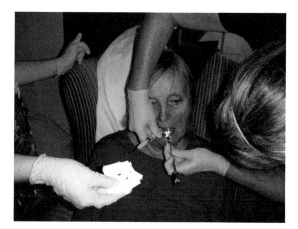

Figure 18.15 Portable hygiene kit with hygienists treating an Alzheimer's patient in a nursing home.

difficult, the goal is to achieve as much as possible at their residential site (long-term care facility, home, acute care setting). A consultation, examination, and cleaning/prophylaxis are usually achievable in these settings with minimal armamentarium.

To perform a thorough oral exam with full intraoral radiographs and a good prophylaxis cleaning, a minimal portable dental set-up suffices (Fig. 18.15). This treatment may be performed by a hygienist alone (under "General Supervision"), if state practice acts allow.

Periodontal scaling may require additional equipment if more than simple hand instruments with portable prophy cups are used, since electricity, suction, and availability of compressed air may be necessary. Fabrication of full or partial dentures is readily performed, with the dentist's comfort level and the patient's cooperation being determining factors. Similarly, denture repairs, adding teeth to existing complete or partial dentures, and denture relines are procedures that do not require extensive equipment and can be accomplished in the patient's residence.

Restorative and surgical care are best performed with the aid of a good assistant. Some facilities may provide nurses or other personnel, but when the dentists brings his or her own staff, the established teamwork, communication flow, and familiarity with procedures generally ensures faster and smoother running of the dental service. The dental staff is familiar with the equipment, with the necessary clerical chores (paper and/or computer), and with the clinician. There is a high premium on familiarity that includes efficiency, comfort, and rate of success. There

is also the equally important element of personal and professional satisfaction achieved in completing dental treatment for someone who otherwise would not have access to care and be left at risk for emergency services only, usually accompanied by pain and/or infection.

Inventory control

In the field, having what you need, when you need it, is the secret to success in portable dentistry. Redundancy is essential. If a perishable item is depleted or a piece of equipment fails, you need to have a backup. The best way to ensure the backup is in place is to assign someone to be responsible for maintenance and inventory control. That person should have an assigned backup as well.

In a successful portable practice, everything has a backup. This includes perishable and disposable goods, autoclavable and reusable supplies, all equipment including cart, computer, and X-ray units, auxiliary staff, and even the dentist. The patient care provided should not be compromised or curtailed because the portable dental setup was incomplete or faulty. Murphy's Law ("Anything that can go wrong will go wrong") has no place in portable dentistry.

Fees

Fees vary depending on frequency of visits, distance traveled, whether staff accompanies you, whether you see other patients that same session, overhead, and other fixed and variable factors. In our practice, we charge our usual fees for services rendered plus $260 travel allowance. It is important to know in advance who will be responsible for the fee, and who will be making the decisions regarding further fees and treatment plan approval for any additional work to be done. The responsible party or Power of Attorney must be identified and consulted to ensure consent and payment.

Opportunity

We are increasingly hearing about dentists not being fully scheduled, having idle time and empty chairs, or having their practices encroached by specialists or mid-level providers. The best way to re-expand a practice is to broaden the portfolio of offerings. Portable dentistry reaches an enormous number of patients that cannot readily come to a conventional dental office, and these numbers will increase as Baby Boomers reach geriatric age.

Patients in nursing homes, private homes, institutions, assisted living arrangements, and other locations are in dire need of dental services, and can arrange to pay for such needed dental care. There is a limitless amount of dental work to be done for these patients (Fig. 18.16). They are waiting for you to make your availability known. There is very little competition, and your schedule will soon be filled beyond capacity. It's up to you to recognize the many golden opportunities to treat patients in their golden years.

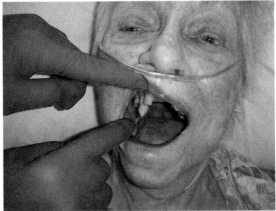

(a)

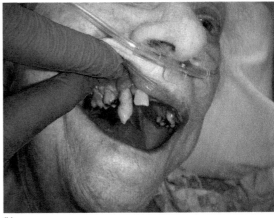

(b)

Figure 18.17 Ella Mae's tooth no. 6 is extruded and acutely painful. She joked that she was very "long in the tooth." (See Case study 1 for more details)

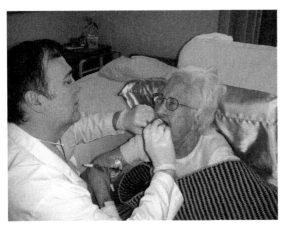

Figure 18.16 Bed-bound patient having a denture fabricated and delivered at a facility.

Case study 1

Ella Mae

Ella Mae is a 90-year-old female, bed-bound from a hip fracture. Her upper right cuspid has extruded and is preventing her from closing her mouth, causing pain upon chewing (Fig. 18.17a,b). We examined and X-rayed her bedside, using DEXIS® instant imaging with a NOMAD® handheld unit (Fig. 18.18). We then anesthetized and extracted tooth no. 6, allowing the patient to eat and talk without further pain (Fig. 18.19).

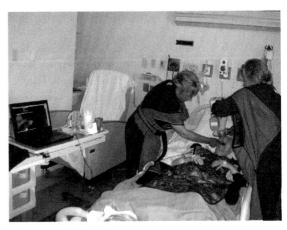

Figure 18.18 DEXIS® instant digital imaging with NOMAD® handheld portable X-ray unit and a laptop computer. (See Case study 1 for more details)

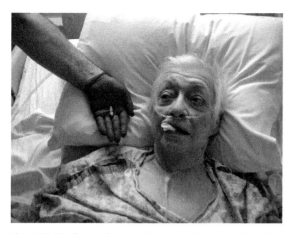

Figure 18.19 The tooth is anesthetized and extracted bedside, providing relief of pain, and restoring normal function to Ella Mae's quality of life. (See Case study 1 for more details)

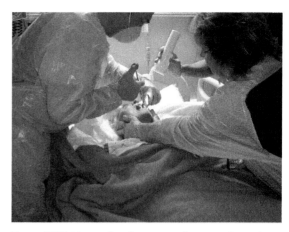

Figure 18.21 The teeth to be extracted are anesthetized. (See Case study 2 for more details)

Case study 2

Marguerite

Marguerite is a 102-year-old female in hospice care with chronic obstructive pulmonary disease (COPD), nosocomial pneumonia, pleural effusion, renal insufficiency, and ambulatory dysfunction with osteoporosis and leg wounds. A tooth supporting her upper left cantilever fixed bridge fractured, leaving the bridge dangling in her mouth (Fig. 18.20). She was unable to close her mouth or function, and was in pain from the fractured, infected root plus the mobile bridge. We examined the patient bedside, then exposed and processed Ergonom-X® self-developing Dental Film with a NOMAD-Pro® handheld X-ray unit. We anesthetized the fracture roots, and removed them along with the bridge (Figs 18.21, 18.22, 18.23).

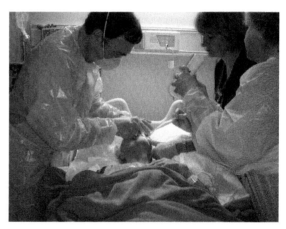

Figure 18.22 The fractured teeth are extracted bedside. (See Case study 2 for more details)

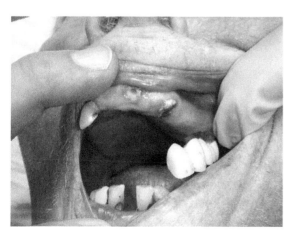

Figure 18.20 Two teeth supporting a bridge fracture, causing pain upon closure. (See Case study 2 for more details)

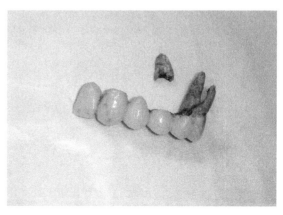

Figure 18.23 The bridge and fracture teeth are removed. (See Case study 2 for more details)

DISCUSSION QUESTIONS

Answers are found at the end of the book.

1 What drugs are commonly used to relax agitated or anxious patients?
2 What are some alternatives to conventional X-ray systems that are used in portable dentistry?
3 What is used to prevent patients' thrashing movements from harming someone or preventing completion of a needed procedure?
4 What kinds of props are used to maintain the patient's mouth open during a procedure?
5 What are some the primary differences between mobile dentistry in a hospital compared to portable dentistry in homes, nursing homes, and other off-site facilities?
6 Why is redundancy so important in portable dentistry?

Bibliography

Arevalo, O., Chattopadhyay, A., Lester, H. & Skelton, J. (2010) Mobile dental operations: capital budgeting and long-term viability. *Journal of Public Health Dentistry*, **70**(1), 28–34.

Arevalo, O., Saman, D.M., Bonaime, A. & Skelton, J. (2010) Mobile dental units: leasing or buying? A dollar-cost analysis. *Journal of Public Health Dentistry*, **70**(3), 253–7.

Bee, J.F. (2004) Portable dentistry: a part of general dentistry's service mix. *General Dentistry*, **52**(6), 520–6.

Carr, B.R., Isong, U. & Weintraub, J.A. (2008) Identification and description of mobile dental programs. *Journal of Public Health Dentistry*, **68**(4), 234–7.

Douglass, J.M. (2005) Mobile dental vans: planning considerations and productivity. *Journal of Public Health Dentistry*, **65**(2), 110–13.

Fiske, J. (2000) The delivery of oral care services to elderly people living in a non-institutionalized setting. *Journal of Public Health Dentistry*, **60**(4), 321–5.

Hamilton, J. (2007) Mobile dentistry: entrepreneurial boom sparks debate. *AGD Impact*, **35**(12), 38–46.

Henry, R.G. & Ceridan, B. (1994) Delivering dental care to nursing home and homebound patients. *Dental Clinics of North America*, **38**(3), 537–51.

Issrani, R., Ammanaqi, R. & Keluskar, V. (2012) Geriatric dentistry – meet the need. *The Gerodontology Society*, **29**(2), e1–e5.

Lee, E.E., Thomas, C.A. & Vu T. (2001) Mobile and portable dentistry: alternative treatment services for the elderly. *Special Care in Dentistry*, **21**(4), 153–5.

Levy, H. (2008) Can't do this? Think again. *Maryland State Dental Association Newsletter*, **43**, 8.

Levy, H. (2008) Impossible dentistry made simple. *DOCS Digest*, **(4)** 12–14.

Levy, H. (2010) The myths about special-needs patient care. *Dentaltown Magazine*, **11**(8), 62.

Levy, H. (2011) Management of special-needs patients: There's always a way, Part 1. *The New Jersey Academy of General Dentistry Wisdom*, **10**(4), 5–7.

Levy, H. (2011) Management of special-needs patients: There's always a way, Part 2. *The New Jersey Academy of General Dentistry Wisdom*, **11** (1), 6–8.

Levy, H., Ceridan, B. & Moore, P. (1995) Dentistry in alternative settings. *Academy of General Dentistry, Dental Audiodental Series*, Medical Information Systems Inc., Port Washington, *New York*, **2**, 8.

MacEntee, M., Kazanjian A., Kozak, J.F., *et al.* (2012) A scoping review and research synthesis on financing and regulating oral care in long-term care facilities. *The Gerodontology Society*, **29**(2), e41–e52.

Morreale, J.P., Dimitry, S., Morreale, M., *et al.* (2005) Setting up a mobile dental practice within your present office structure. *Journal of the Canadian Dental Association*, **71**(2), 91.

Appendix: Resources

ADSA
877-255-3742
www.adsahome.org

Aribex NOMAD Handheld X-ray
801-226-5522
www.aribex.com

Aseptico
866-244-2954
www.aseptico.com

Colgate-Palmolive
800-2Colgate
www.ColgateProfessional.com

Dental Elite
888-228-7706
www.dentalelite.com

DentalEZ Group
866 DTEINFO
www.dentalez.com

DEXIS X-Ray Systems
888-883-3947
www.dexis.com

DOCS Education
877-325-3627
www.DOCSeducation.org

DUX Dental
800-833-8267
DUXDental.com

Ergonom-X Dental Film
Lenty Dental Sales
800-635-3689
lentysales.com

Hu-Friedy
800 HUFRIEDY
www.hu-friedy.com

Isolite Systems
800-560-6066
www.isolitesystems.com

Lexi-Comp
800-837-5394
lexi.com
wolterskluwerhealth.com

Porter Instrument – Nitrous Oxide
888-723-4001
www.porterinstrument.com

Septodont
800-872-8305
oraverse.com

Special Care Dentistry Association
312-527-6764
www.scdaonline.org

Specialized Care Co.
800-722-7375
www.specializedcare.com

Ultralight Optics
323-316-4514
ultralightoptics.com

Walter Lorentz Surgical/Biomet 3-i
574-267-6639
www.biomet.com

Dr. Levy's on-line courses: www.DentalEdu.TV, or direct link from
http://www.drhlevyassoc.com/clinicians/clinicians.htm

CHAPTER 19

Promoting Oral Health Care in Long-Term Care Facilities

Mickey Emmons Wener[1], Carol-Ann Yakiwchuk[2], and Mary Bertone[3]

[1] *School of Dental Hygiene, Faculty of Dentistry, University of Manitoba, Winnipeg, MB, Canada*
[2] *Faculty of Dentistry, University of British Columbia, Vancouver, BC, Canada*
[3] *Centre for Community Oral Health, Faculty of Dentistry, University of Manitoba, Winnipeg, MB, Canada*

Introduction

Along with longer life spans comes the increased likelihood that many of us will experience challenges managing routine activities of daily living (ADLs, which include independently moving between locations, transferring, eating, using the toilet, and performing personal hygiene tasks). Dependent older adults reside in a variety of settings, such as at home, in an assisted living residence, in hospital for rehabilitation or an extended stay, or in a long-term care (LTC) facility. The majority of elders prefer to receive care at home and enter a facility only when their health concerns become unmanageable (Canadian Healthcare Association, 2009). A renewed focus on improving quality of life and deinstitutionalizing care has led to new models of elder-centered continuous care communities (see Appendix 19.1, Resources for Promoting Oral Health in Long-Term Care). As demands grow for assistance at all levels of LTC, a variety of informal and formal caregivers are needed, including family and friends, a myriad of healthcare providers, and advocates such as social workers.

Mouth care is the foundation of maintaining the oral health of older adults in LTC (Stein & Henry, 2009). Brushing teeth, cleaning dentures – all seemingly simple tasks – become quite complex when individuals are no longer able to care for themselves. Daily mouth care needs vary greatly – from a reminder that it's time to brush, to keeping the mouth comfortable during palliative care (see also Chapter 2,

Palliative Care Dentistry). Advocating for oral health in LTC is of increasing importance as mouth care is at risk for widespread neglect, perhaps as a function of the fact that oral health professionals (OHPs) are typically not part of the healthcare team (MacEntee, 2011). How can we work together to ensure that vulnerable elders have dignity and comfort, are able to eat a nutritious diet, and are not putting their overall health at risk?

The content of this chapter is based on the collective experience of a team of dental hygienists promoting oral health in LTC. Oral health promotion is an "upstream" approach, heavily weighted toward prevention and addressing existing problems early, before more complex treatment is required "downstream." Our practical approach to oral health promotion for dependent older adults is illustrated in Fig. 19.1, a model using colored rings (oral health promotion strategies) of increasing size stacked on a center cylindrical post (oral health of the older adult). In sequence, from bottom to top in Fig. 19.1, they include: **(i) standards, (ii) commitment, (iii) education and training; (iv) assessment and professional care; and (v) daily mouth care**. The size of the ring gives stability with the larger ones forming the base from which to build a solid structure. The model recognizes that the base is not necessarily the first ring to be set. For example, education and training may occur first to inform others about oral systemic health and outcomes of poor daily oral hygiene, which then leads to action

Geriatric Dentistry: Caring for Our Aging Population, First Edition. Edited by Paula K. Friedman.
© 2014 John Wiley & Sons, Inc. Published 2014 by John Wiley & Sons, Inc.
Companion website: www.wiley.com/go/friedman/geriatricdentistry

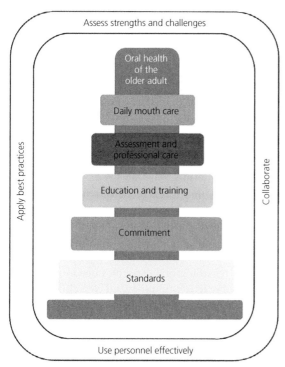

Figure 19.1 An oral health promotion model with application to a variety of long-term care (LTC) settings. Created by Wener, Bertone, and Yakiwchuk, 2012

in the form of being committed to change or developing standards. Until all the rings are in their designated position, the structure is less stable, and correspondingly, the individual's oral health is less protected. Surrounding the rings are the principle actions in which oral health promotion occurs; these include **(a) assess strengths and challenges; (b) collaborate; (c) use personnel effectively; and (d) apply best practices**. These four critical environmental elements are described in the following section.

Assess strengths and challenges

The first step in assessing the oral health promotion environment is to assess the LTC environment. Be aware of the caregiving milieu as settings vary greatly based on size, management, and funding; and, similarly, individual needs vary based on general health, functional and cognitive abilities, and social and financial supports. Barriers to achieving oral health for dependent older adults are pervasive and well-documented (Canadian Dental Association, 2009; Jablonski *et al.,* 2005; MacEntee *et al.,* 2008; McNally & Lyons, 2004; Matthews *et al.,* 2012; Pronych *et al.,* 2010; Stein & Henry, 2009). This growing population has complex medical issues, many of which require medications that cause dry mouth (xerostomia) (see Chapter 2, Palliative Care Dentistry, and Chapter 14, Xerostomia, for additional information). Although oral disease is rampant due to competing concerns and financial challenges, families often relegate dental care to the lowest priority. Loss of function and autonomy is a major "tipping point" in an individual's oral health status. Being dependent on others for daily mouth care, acquiring oral hygiene products, and arranging for access to dental care contributes to poor oral health. Families and friends, who are the sole caregivers for 70% of the elderly in the USA (US Dept. of Health and Human Services, 2009), are often stressed with multiple responsibilities and limited resources. Caregivers have heavy workloads, view mouth care as an unpleasant, often strictly cosmetic task (Dharamsi *et al.,* 2009; Forsell *et al.,* 2011), and can significantly overestimate residents' ability to independently care for their own mouths (Forsell *et al.,* 2009; Stewart, 2013). LTC facilities may have mouth care protocols, but often they are not enforced by the facility or by regulatory agencies (Seniors' Oral Health Secretariat, 2011; Weintraub, 2011). Educational preparation for promoting oral health, from administrators to front-line staff, is woefully inadequate. OHPs themselves often have little preparation and expertise in providing this specialized care, are unfamiliar with and unwilling to explore the LTC milieu (Nunez *et al.,* 2011), and have limited experience being part of a healthcare team (Institute for Oral Health, 2008; MacEntee, 2011). Add to these barriers the lack of integration between dental and medical care, discriminatory ageism (stereotypical prejudicial attitudes and practices regarding older people), and the frequently present physical and cognitive challenges that impact upon the abilities of elders, and we are in the midst of the perfect storm for oral and overall health problems. A chilling example of the result of oral neglect is seen in the following newspaper article excerpt:

Nursing home fined $100,000 for death. The resident, a 76-year-old woman who required total assistance with daily living activities, died from a dental abscess that led to cardiopulmonary arrest, according to the California Department of Public Health. The CDPH investigation revealed that the woman was not given a dental exam because "the facility thought the resident had dentures" (Jackson, 2007).

Collaborate

Interprofessional practice is becoming the cornerstone of improved patient outcomes (Institute of Medicine, 2011a; World Health Organizaiton, 2010). Fostering environments that support collaboration and team communication to discuss perspectives, goals, and roles brings stakeholders together, increasing readiness to move forward with promoting oral health (Yoon & Steel, 2012). Reconnecting the frequently ignored health of the mouth with overall health and wellness to establish common ground and support quality of life is the all-important first step. It takes a person-centered, proactive care team of elders, their families, decision-makers, caregivers, and advocacy bodies such as the Alzheimer's Society to help create an environment supportive of oral healthcare. On a day-to-day basis, team communication is crucial to ensure feedback and best care. For example, did the home care worker let the family know that the denture is broken and needs repair? Did the dental hygienist providing clinical care connect back with the unit nurse to follow-up on strategies to promote better daily care? Did the dietitian's recommendation of sugar-laden liquid meal substitutes to assist in weight gain result in appropriate changes to the mouth care protocol?

Collaboration

Collaboration is an interprofessional process of communication and decision making that enables the separate and shared knowledge and skills of healthcare providers to synergistically influence the client/patient care provided. (See Way & Jones in Canadian Interprofessional Health Collaborative, 2007, and Way *et al.*, 2001.)

Use personnel effectively

Promoting oral health requires a motivated, caring champion to act as an advocate (MacEntee *et al.*, 1999, 2008). OHPs need to support or be champions, and likewise, care providers need to recognize the important roles that OHPs can play (Table 19.1). Including OHPs on the healthcare team can increase the likelihood of improving oral health through increased visibility, active participation, and regular evaluation of results (Chalmers *et al.*, 2009; Thorne *et al.*, 2001). Other caregivers are well-positioned to champion oral health, such as the nurse trying to prevent ventilator-acquired pneumonia (VAP) or the concerned administrator who has just experienced a critical incident stemming from poor oral health. Decisions regarding oral care roles need to be based on scope of practice, training, and cost-effectiveness. Remuneration can significantly impact how personnel are utilized. For example, if OHPs are compensated strictly on a fee-for-service basis for specific clinical services provided, this can limit their ability to participate in health promotion activities. Whereas, a salaried OHP position can provide the flexibility needed to provide caregiver education, respond to an on-unit request for mouth care coaching, or to participate in an interprofessional healthcare meeting. There is no

---

Table 19.1 Roles in long-term care (LTC) can extend far beyond clinical care

---

Oral health professional roles in LTC

Oral assessment
- Assess oral problems initially, quarterly and as needed
- Consult with and refer to other professionals
- Develop individualized treatment and daily mouth care plans

Clinical oral care
- Liaise with caregiving staff and families
- Provide preventive and therapeutic care
- Provide restorative and surgical care

Mouth care training
- Build (i) oral health knowledge and connect to overall health; (ii) assessment and care skills; and (iii) positive attitudes
- Network and collaborate to establish partners and commitment

Policy and protocol development
- Support quality assurance and care with best practices

proven personnel formula; however, with expertise in oral health promotion, dental hygienists have been identified as being well suited for the LTC environment as they have the requisite skills, are prevention-focused, and are increasingly able and willing to practice as primary healthcare professionals in alternative settings (Coleman *et al.*, 2006; Glasrud *et al.*, 2005; Monajem, 2006).

Apply best practices

While bringing available evidence to bear on decision making, keep in mind the efficacy and the effectiveness of any intervention – "Does it work?"; "Will it work?" Feasibility can only be addressed by direct involvement of the care provider and recipient. For example, a therapeutic mouth rinse may be proven effective, but is the individual actually capable of swishing and spitting and avoiding swallowing or aspirating the rinse? Do LTC personnel know the rationale for its use and assume responsibility for including it in daily mouth care? Guidelines do exist for best oral care practices for dependent older adults; however, there is no widely recognized and standardized evidence-based protocol (MacEntee *et al.*, 2012). Much of what is done in practice combines research and protocols from a variety of sources with personal experience and preference. It is an area ripe for research and regulation, and brings us to the first ring of the model: **Standards**.

Standards (health promotion ring 1)

My mother has just entered long-term care and I am appalled at the lack of oral care provided. What exactly am I allowed to do? What standards exist regarding oral health?

Registered Dental Hygienist

I am pretty sure that we have mouth care policies, but I don't recall ever seeing them.

Healthcare Aide

Reports of over two-thirds of residents without their own toothbrush, or caregivers wearing gloves with visible feces from a previous task to brush a resident's teeth (Coleman & Watson, 2006), are telling signs of the oral healthcare crisis in LTC. What governance

Table 19.2 Terminology

- *Acts and Regulations:* Care required by law
- *Standards*: Expected level of care
- *Guidelines:* Means to meet standard of care
- *Policy:* Rules governing care
- *Protocol:* How care is to be provided

Table 19.3 Regulatory requirements direct and shape practice

Explore legislation in your jurisdiction that:
- Establishes oral health standards for long-term care (LTC)
- Governs the scope of practice of oral health professionals
- Provides financial coverage of dental care for elders
- Protects vulnerable persons, the mentally competent, and the disabled
- Clarifies abuse, restraint and neglect
- Establishes rights for those in LTC
- Defines informed consent for decision making by individuals or guardians
- Describes how to physically transfer individuals safely
- Governs home care provisions and respite for caregivers

measures are in place at the national, state/provincial, regional or facility levels in your jurisdiction to protect and promote an elder's oral health in LTC? And more importantly, are these measures monitored and enforced for quality control?

The foundation of our LTC oral health promotion model upon which all of the other rings rest, represents a range of recognized measures and requirements for providing and evaluating the quality of mouth care including legislated acts and regulations, standards, guidelines, policies, and protocols (Table 19.2). Care providers need to be knowledgeable about relevant legislation that establishes standards, governs the scope of practice of OHPs, and protects vulnerable cognitively impaired older adults as these requirements impact upon how care is provided (Table 19.3).

Oral health in LTC legislation
US Federal Law, the Omnibus Budget Reconciliation Act (OBRA) of 1987, requires facilities that accept Medicare or Medicaid residents to do the following (Guay, 2005; Haumschild & Haumschild, 2009):
- assess oral health using the Minimum Data Set (MDS) tool;

- complete an oral examination within 45 days of admission and annually thereafter;
- provide for dental care;
- provide daily oral hygiene care; and
- offer annual staff in-service training sessions.

More than half of the US states have requirements beyond OBRA requirements. For example, Minnesota regulations include that a facility must arrange on-site dental services for residents who cannot travel, establish a resident's daily oral care plan during the initial assessment, and provide the necessary supplies and assistance for daily oral care (Minnesota Administrative Rules, 1995). In Canada, the government provides medical care for all permanent residents (*Canada Health Act*), but does not cover home and institutional care for the frail. There is no Canadian national or provincial infrastructure for oral healthcare for elders, and little national consistency in the actual delivery of health care, including LTC, which is provincially regulated (McNally & Lyons, 2004). All of the Canadian provinces but none of the territories have legislation that can be interpreted to incorporate or mandate oral healthcare services in LTC facilities (Abi-Nahed, 2007). Only 2 of the 10 provinces were found to have established government LTC standards that included oral care: Ontario (*Long-Term Care Homes Act*) and British Columbia (*Community Care and Assisted Living Act*), while others are anticipating regulatory change.

To become a licensed LTC facility, governments require yearly on-site inspections to determine if established standards, such as those required by OBRA, are being met (Castle, 2012). Even where oral care requirements are legislated, there are still significant gaps in care observed including many with poor oral health, long periods of time without being seen by a dentist or lack of help with daily mouth care (Frenkel *et al.*, 2000; Henry, 2005; Seniors' Oral Health Secretariat, 2011). Problems enforcing oral care standards have been reported and include lack of awareness of the regulation, lack of collaboration, not expecting inspectors to assess mouth care, and very limited investigation of daily mouth care during scheduled site inspections (Jiang & MacEntee, 2013). Experts call for a more explicit framework to systematically assess oral healthcare programs in LTC (MacEntee, 2011). The ONiIE (Oral Neglect in Institutionalized Elderly), yet to be operationalized, is an assessment tool that defines neglect for 29 oral conditions, which could help provide enforceable guidelines for quality assurance monitoring of LTC facilities (Katz *et al.*, 2010). Legislated government funding of oral health in LTC could improve oral care (Helgeson & Smith, 1996), improve integration with other publicly funded health services (MacEntee *et al.*, 2012), ease consent for treatment from guardians, and increase the number of OHPs willing to provide care (Seniors' Oral Health Secretariat, 2011).

Oral care guidelines

When health departments, facilities, or home care agencies have standardized policies and procedures, such as valid assessment and daily care plan tools, caregivers' involvement in maintaining residents' oral health can improve (Berry *et al.*, 2011; Chalmers *et al.*, 2009). OHPs can play an important leadership role in their development, including educating key decision-makers regarding why particular directives are important. The challenge in developing policies is that there is no consensus on an ideal oral care protocol due to a lack of scientific evidence based in the real world of LTC, multiple factors influencing individual needs, and the wide variety of available oral hygiene products, tools and techniques (Berry *et al.*, 2011). For example, in the development of the *Oral Health Care Guideline for Older People in Long-Term Care Institutions*, 12 of the 16 recommendations were based on expert opinion, with only 4 based on research evidence (De Visschere *et al.*, 2011). For guideline documents, see Appendix 19.1 (Resources for Promoting Oral Health in Long-Term Care). For policy example see Appendix 19.2 (Example of Oral Health Promotion Guidelines for a Long-Term Care Facility).

Elders access to care legislation

Access to care is maximized by allowing professionals to practice to the full extent of their education in a variety of settings (Institute of Medicine, 2011b). The ability of US dental hygienists to practice independently in LTC varies greatly between states, and is an increasingly topical issue (Jablonski *et al.*, 2005). To help address access to care, Minnesota's 2001 legislation allows dental hygienists who are in a collaborative agreement with a dentist to practice without the presence, diagnosis, and treatment planning of a dentist in settings other than dental offices. In Canada, significant regulatory reform in the vast majority of the 10 provinces allows dental hygienists to initiate care as primary healthcare professionals. This has led to a growing number of mobile dental hygiene practices able to visit private homes and LTC facilities.

A lack of existing and enforced public policies and guidelines for the provision of accessible oral health care is putting dependent older adults in LTC at risk. OHPs and concerned others must advocate at all levels for legislated, measureable, and enforced standards that support vulnerable elders' oral health (Canadian Dental Association, 2008; MacEntee *et al.,* 2008; McNally *et al.,* 2012; Petersen & Yamamoto, 2005; Weintraub, 2011). The bottom line is that many believe that achieving oral health is important in LTC, but few follow through. This gap forms the impetus for champions committed to promoting oral health.

Commitment (health promotion ring 2)

Everyone is concerned about the health of older adults. No one is quite sure who is responsible for their ORAL health.

All too often, administrators and caregivers are unclear of the role they should play and why it is necessary to improve their oral healthcare program (Dharamsi *et al.,* 2009; McKelvey *et al.,* 2003). **Commitment**, the second health promotion ring, provides a crucial foundation toward supporting oral health change for dependent older adults. By serving as strong advocates and meeting with all stakeholders, OHPs can help everyone involved understand the significance of their roles and potential impact of their improved efforts. As commitment builds, the OHP champion's role can transition toward empowering and inspiring leadership in others through education, collaboration, and mentorship (Table 19.4). Through transformational leadership, OHPs can positively impact caregivers' attitudes, behavior, and performance toward sustainable change, while creating the synergy and connectivity necessary within the organization to build momentum (Daft, 2008).

What appears contingent on sustaining oral healthcare improvements is a strong consideration for the organizational context within the caring environment (MacEntee *et al.,* 2008; Thorne *et al.,* 2001). What

Table 19.4 Assessing your readiness to be an oral health champion

- Do you have a passion for working with older adults?
- What skills do you bring to the situation?
- What resources and training do you require before you begin?
- What is your understanding of the dependent older adult's environment and each player's roles and responsibilities?
- What site-specific documents and websites are important to review before you move forward?
- What existing professional and personal networks may be helpful to you?
- Who can help mentor you into this role?
- What degree of commitment is feasible for you; what are possible options for remuneration?

culture and values are inherent within the organization? Who are the decision-makers? What internal structural processes can be used to effectively implement change? How ready is the organization to accept change? Results of several studies emphasize the importance of partnering with an internal staff member to help increase the focus of daily mouth care and promote commitment among staff (Pronych *et al.,* 2010; Wardh *et al.,* 2003). Through shared leadership and collaboration with internal champions who have experience working within their organization, sustainable improvements can be made (MacEntee *et al.,* 2007; Weintraub 2011).

Getting to know the players
Many stakeholders are involved in the care of older adults, each with their own abilities, responsibilities, and priorities. In the home setting, family, friends, home care workers, and nurses serve as the primary caregivers. In LTC, there exists a hierarchy of caregivers, including:

- Administrators, who are responsible for meeting legislated requirements, managing finances, and overseeing a level of care that ensures low resident morbidity and mortality rates.
- Directors of Nursing and Unit Nurse Managers, who are concerned with staffing, supervising daily care, and liaising with physicians and family members or other decision-makers.
- Clinical Nurse Specialists or Nurse Educators, who are responsible for introducing new care programs and guidelines and providing ongoing staff education.

• Infection Control Nurses, who oversee wound management, ensure infection control standards are met, and manage infections and viral outbreaks among residents.

Managerial personnel can be powerful advocates and promoters for oral healthcare change; however, it is crucial to involve direct care staff and other health professionals involved in the individual's care. Certified Nursing Assistants (CNAs) or Residential Care Aides (RCAs) often possess the least amount of formalized education and training of all care staff, yet perform most of the day-to-day care for dependent older adults (Chalmers & Pearson, 2005a; Jablonski et al., 2005). These individuals are responsible for providing daily mouth care, among many other tasks. The literature consistently reports that direct care providers experience many conflicting demands and face numerous organizational, social, and practical barriers (McNally et al., 2012). It is important to take into consideration that their communication channels are typically more informal, relationship-based, and oral rather than written (Caspar, 2012). One must ensure that CNAs/RCAs are supported through effective two-way feedback loops that involve them in care plans and recognize their invaluable contribution. Thus, health promotion efforts must focus on empowering CNAs/RCAs through education, training, and administrative support.

Along with understanding the care environment, you may wonder how to identify the person with the authority to make decisions; whom to speak with first to gain commitment. Beginning the relationship with a LTC facility by meeting with administration provides a connection with key decision-makers who have the power to support your efforts through leadership, funding, policy enforcement, and opportunities for caregiver education. Administrators can identify the facility's primary oral health concerns, and guide you toward realistic, culturally appropriate interventions. Establishing a high level of commitment from nursing staff is also paramount as these individuals can work to address barriers faced by direct care providers, monitor the quality of mouth care provided, and liaise with families. The OHP champion also needs to establish and maintain a strong commitment from CNAs/RCAs by serving as their educator, mentor, ally, and advocate. You may also find strong supporters among dietitians, speech language pathologists, physiotherapists, occupational therapists, and caring family members. A social worker partner can help identify financial resources for needed care and become an advocate to help reduce costly treatment needs. The topic of oral healthcare holds importance to every individual involved in an older adult's care; the challenge is to make a meaningful connection.

Collaborating and partnering for a common ground approach

Oral health programs must be built on the connectivity of trusting relationships that promote involvement, collaboration, and empowerment of all stakeholders. A sense of partnership can be fostered using a "common ground, common language" approach. By highlighting the overlapping health concerns that OHPs share with other health professionals in relation to an older adult's health and quality of life, and tailoring the message to each staff member's role and responsibilities, the issue of poor oral health and the need for change become more tangible and realistic for everyone involved (Fig. 19.2). For speech language pathologists, it may be our shared concern over aspiration pneumonia; for a direct care provider, it may be resident comfort and maintaining a person's quality of life. The ability to "talk the same talk" and contextualize oral diseases, with phrases like "mouth care is infection control" and "gum disease is equal in size to a bed sore the size of the palm of your hand" translates oral health concerns into terms that are common to everyone (Figs 19.3 & 19.4). Avoiding blame and recognizing everyone's important contributions are additional important strategies for OHPs who wish to transformationally champion change.

Listening to learn and build trust

A good understanding of the environment is vital prior to strategizing ways to build capacity and plan for change. It is crucial to recognize that caregivers are experiencing increasingly heavier demands on their time and skill level as the resident population continues to become more frail, dependent, and medically compromised (McGregor & Ronald, 2011). This begins with asking the right questions, actively listening, and adopting a "move forward" attitude that supports and celebrates even small improvements.

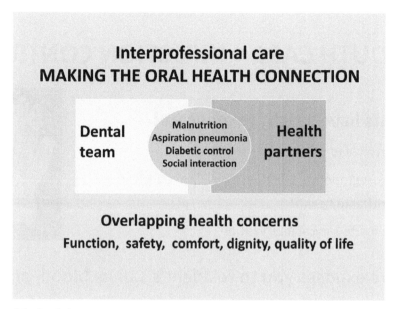

Figure 19.2 Training slide that helps to establish "common ground." Created by Wener, Bertone, and Yakiwchuk, 2012.

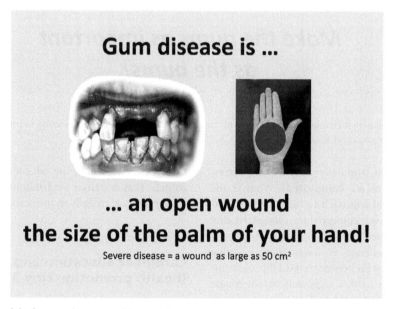

Figure 19.3 Training slide that translates "invisible" oral disease into a visible wound to which caregivers can relate. Reference: Slade *et al.* (2000). Intraoral photograph permission from J. Morreale. Created by Wener, Bertone, and Yakiwchuk, 2012.

Who is serving as the primary caregiver for those living at home? Are they following a mouth care protocol? Is the older adult able to cooperate? Observing in an open-minded nonjudgmental manner that avoids blaming, and openly exploring these questions with the family and caregivers provides a springboard for change. Similarly, within a facility, listening to their challenges and learning about their practices are crucial steps. What processes are in place for assessment,

MOUTH CARE = INFECTION CONTROL

Residents have a right to oral care!

- Neglect can lead to serious health risks
- It's not just grooming … it's an "Activity of Daily Living" that's critical to health!
- It's a 2-minute clinical intervention

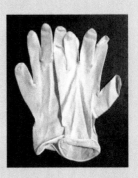

Oral care exposes you to resident's saliva, blood, and germs!

- Wear a new pair of clean, well-fitting gloves for each resident
- Use mask and eyewear if risk of splatter

Make the gums as important as the bums!

Figure 19.4 Training slide that changes the perception of daily mouth care from that of grooming to preventing infection. Created by Wener, Bertone, and Yakiwchuk, 2012.

screening, treatment, and daily care? What policies, protocols, and forms are being used? What is the overall philosophical approach to care? What licensure or accreditation requirements related to oral health need to be met?

The greatest challenge is maintaining ongoing commitment from stakeholders, especially of frontline caregivers who have a high staff turnover rate (Chalmers & Pearson, 2005a; Harrington & Swan, 2003; Jablonski *et al.*, 2005; National Centre for Assisted Living, 2011). Maintaining visibility, keeping everyone informed, and continuing to boost and sustain a commitment to quality oral health care is essential. When an OHP champion visits the unit to help caregivers solve mouth care challenges, this communicates interest and a willingness to sincerely work together toward a common goal, further deepening the level of commitment by everyone involved. The

next section describes the educational strategies and content that is crucial for commitment, in particular for the support of daily mouth care.

Caregiver education and training (health promotion ring 3)

The mouth … it's personal … I don't feel comfortable doing it. If a resident refuses to let me brush … I need to respect his or her rights.
Really … taking care of someone's mouth is not part of nursing. You mean you're going to teach me how to brush!
Caregiver quotes

Caregiver education on its own has not consistently resulted in sustainable oral health improvements for older adults, leading many to question its value and importance in supporting oral healthcare change (Gammack & Pulisetty, 2009; MacEntee *et al.*, 2007; McKelvey *et al.*, 2003; Munoz *et al.*, 2009; Peltola *et al.*, 2007; Simons *et al.*, 2000). Yet, there is no denying that education and training is an important part of the solution, based on extensive feedback from caregivers of their need for additional oral health knowledge, training, and skill (Coleman & Watson, 2006; Dharamsi *et al.*, 2009; McKelvey *et al.*, 2003; McNally *et al.*, 2012; Peltola *et al.*, 2007; Unfer *et al.*, 2011). Ageism prejudice, reportedly common among the health professions, also impacts caregivers' perceptions of this population's oral healthcare needs (Giles *et al.*, 2002; Larsen & Lubkin, 2009; Whitman & Whitman, 2006) (see also Chapter 4, Palmore's Facts on Aging Quiz). **Caregiver education and training**, the third ring of the model, plays a pivotal role in transforming people's attitudes and beliefs towards oral healthcare when opportunities for discussion, reflection, and feedback are included (Apte, 2009; Mezirow, 2009). Education and training provides caregivers with evidence-based information, tools, and skills that can help strengthen their commitment toward oral healthcare improvements.

Almost everyone involved in an older adult's circle of care needs education and training. Family members in the home setting may never have brushed another person's teeth, and be unaware of the impact of prescription medications on one's comfort and health (McNally *et al.*, 2012). Nurses involved in performing oral screenings may be unprepared to recognize normal versus abnormal findings or how to systematically examine the mouth. RCAs/CNAs may not know why mouth care needs to be provided several times a day, or why they should continue brushing when gums bleed. Oral health content and training is reportedly sparse and out-dated in nursing and other health professions curricula worldwide; hence, most care staff will benefit from initial and ongoing oral health education and training (Hahn *et al.*, 2012; Hein *et al.*, 2011; Jablonski, 2012). Even within the OHPs, there is an urgent need to more adequately prepare individuals to interact and work with geriatric populations and their caregivers through enhanced curricula, experiential learning opportunities, and mentorship (Bardach & Rowles, 2012; National Seniors' Task Force, 2008).

When planning training, there are many considerations. What format works best for your target audience? Are there other programs that can be used to model or piggy-back training sessions onto? What costs are involved? Where and when should training take place? How will administrative support be communicated? How will the schedule of sessions be publicized? Will this be required of staff, or voluntary, and if required, how will that be conveyed to staff members?

Venues and timing

Caregiver education and training can take place in a number of environments using a variety of approaches. Delivering a seminar to CNA/RNA students, offering a workshop at a local caregiver conference, manning a display in a facility, or even writing newsletter articles for LTC all represent excellent ways to share information. LTC facilities will have established structures and processes for how and when caregivers receive other types of education and training that are important to consider. What classroom facilities are on-site? What time of day and length of session will encourage attendance? Since time away from the unit is time away from caregiving responsibilities, a KISS approach works best: **K**eep **I**t **S**hort and **S**uccinct. For efficiency, offer one session to both the day and evening shift staff by scheduling the session mid-afternoon and asking those on the evening shift to arrive early. Bedside hands-on training and support, small group learning on-unit, and having staff access online resources (podcasts, blogs, fact sheets), or view videotaped training sessions are other workable strategies. Caregiver training held in preclinical dental education laboratories offers excellent hands-on learning opportunities for both caregivers and OHP students. It is a valuable learning experience for students as they coach caregivers while they practice positioning, opening a closed mouth, or using specialized products on realistic compliant "elders" (Fig. 19.5).

The train-the-trainer (TTT) model is particularly suitable when implementing caregiver education and training at larger facilities or across health regions, given its cost-effective collaborative approach that can serve to establish numerous champions and partners. Speech language pathologists in

Mouth care training for direct care providers
Adapt based on available time: 30, 60, 90, or 120 minutes

- Welcome and introduction
- Getting to know the participants: Their roles? Issues? Barriers? Questions?
- Research: Caregiver barriers and issues
- Research: Oral health barriers for older adults
- Plaque bacteria, tooth decay, and periodontal disease
- Mouth-body-health connections
- Caregiver and older adult positioning
- Inspections, screening assessments, and dental exams
- Strategies for care-resistant behavior
- Basic care for natural teeth
- Basic care for dentures
- Mouth care products that work
- Special considerations: swallowing issues; palliative care
- Professional dental care
- Hands-on practice
- Wrap-up: What did they learn? How will they use this information? What's the next step ...?

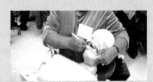
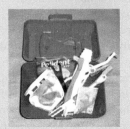

Figure 19.5 Tailor content to participants needs based on their role in supporting oral health in long-term care. Photographs depict training using a preclinical dental laboratory and reusable product kits. Created by Wener, Bertone, and Yakiwchuk, 2012.

our region attended our 2-hour TTT didactic and hands-on practice session then proceeded to train caregivers at each of the personal care homes where they worked, using a simplified training CD we provided. On-going involvement from an OHP expert as the trainer or a consultant is essential to ensure disseminated information is up-to-date and trainers remain mindful to avoid decision making beyond their knowledge base and scope of practice.

Content

Passionate OHPs can often overload caregivers by providing too much information, while neglecting to incorporate interactive learning activities that help facilitate knowledge translation, trust, and commitment. Avoid this pitfall by clearly identifying the target group's oral healthcare role, what key pieces

of information and skills they will need to do their job better, and how to engage them in meaningful dialogue before developing your presentation. For a family member, include a discussion on the importance of mouth care based on the individual's medical conditions and risk factors. Support their daily efforts by providing them with an individualized mouth care plan that identifies helpful products, and coaching them as they practice this new skill.

For LTC stakeholders, begin with a strong introduction about the silent oral disease epidemic in care facilities. Highlight some of the issues and barriers faced by caregivers, residents, and others. Provide the "why" before the "how to" of mouth care to raise awareness of how effective daily care can help prevent dental diseases, infections, pain, and systemic illness such as pneumonia. This information serves to "reconnect the mouth to the body" and provides concrete evidence to support a comprehensive oral healthcare program.

For administrators and others not involved in daily mouth care, add information on existing oral health guidelines and standards, the role OHPs and other champions can play, accessing professional dental care, and ordering effective oral health products. Drawing parallels between an oral care program and other successfully integrated programs, such as wound care, could provide the vision and push needed to operationalize oral healthcare (McNally et al., 2012). Regardless of the stakeholder's role, everyone should be aware of the key components of a comprehensive oral care program, such as the need for regular caregiver education and training, having oral care supplies on hand, oral screening, daily oral care, and on-site professional dental and dental hygiene care. Where there is no on-site OHP, it is also helpful to have a "go-to" OHP who can be contacted by phone or email if they have questions.

RCAs/CNAs perhaps have the greatest education and training needs. Information needs to be comprehensive yet practical, and include realistic time-saving strategies and hands-on practice. (Figure 19.6) Including tips on caregiver positioning that promote efficacy, safety, and good ergonomics; resident positioning for those with dysphagia; addressing care resistant behavior (CRB), gaining access when teeth are clenched; and caring for natural teeth and dentures can enable caregivers to become more effective and confident (Chalmers & Pearson, 2005b; Jablonski et al., 2011b; McNally et al., 2012). Strategies such as restraining an elder's hands that may be misconstrued as restraint must be discussed at the administrative level to ensure they blend with the organization's philosophy of care and recognize residents' rights. Again, an OHP resource whom the RCAs/CNAs can work with is especially important; these individuals may be reluctant to ask questions in a public/classroom setting or to provide candid insights about common on-unit practices. They should be encouraged to contact the OHP as part of the caregiving team and vice versa.

Start-up and on-going plans need to consider that adequate time and resources are set aside for sourcing out or creating new educational resources, regularly updating existing materials, and tailoring materials to best meet each group's needs. The importance of relevant and engaging materials and handouts that contain current information and evidence that align with your message/session cannot be understated.

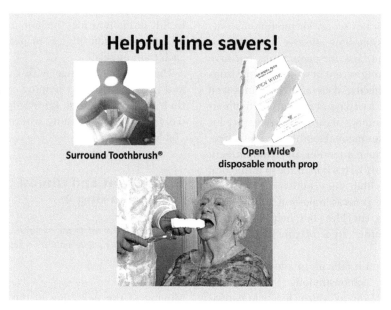

Figure 19.6 Training slide that introduces caregivers to new products helpful for dependent older adults. Photographs courtesy of Specializedcare.com. Created by Wener, Bertone, and Yakiwchuk, 2012.

Strategies that work

While there is no one set recipe for success, there are a number of effective strategies to enhance knowledge transfer, caregiver buy-in and commitment, and inter-professional collaboration. The importance of preassessing participants' knowledge and communicating an understanding of their role in oral health care early on in the presentation cannot be overemphasized. What successes and challenges have they experienced when providing mouth care? Is there a burning question they'd like addressed? Sharing evidence from the literature about caregivers' work ethic and the challenges they face affirms their voiced concerns and recognizes that they truly care, yet face many barriers in their oral care roles. This communicates empathy and a clear understanding by the OHP champion. An important strategy is to avoid blaming ("Why hasn't Mrs. Jones' denture been cleaned?") or assuming that their issues are our issues ("This is really important for you to do every day" – not appreciating that they are already operating at their maximum effort). Make the mouth care issue real by discussing their problems, such as bleeding gums, a lack of cooperation, and a bad smell on the unit, and how daily brushing can lead to a more pleasant work environment. Sharing a personal story about a specific resident's oral health makes these issues come alive. Whenever possible, use their statistics, such as quality indicator scores for pneumonia outcomes when discussing how effective oral care can not only reduce one's risk for pneumonia, but save lives too! Highlighting recent research on the connection between effective daily oral care, improved oral health, and reduced days of residents with pneumonia, or sharing findings of caregiver preference for using a suction versus manual toothbrush is an effective way to gain their attention and commitment (Yakiwchuk *et al.*, 2013). It's important to frame oral health messages within the context of LTC; for example, "Make the gums as important as the bums" not only results in chuckles, but helps caregivers draw parallels to other areas of care that receive more attention.

Caregivers will find it difficult to adopt new skills without viewing demonstrations and having hands-on practice. "How-to" video clips help participants observe a new technique before practicing. While caregivers can partner to practice positioning; intraoral techniques, such as inserting a mouth rest

and toothbrushing, are often done more comfortably on a typodont model rather than on a peer who may be embarrassed by their own oral condition. Integrating these activities within the presentation offers variety and keeps everyone's attention. Ending by reinforcing key messages or posing the question, "What's your next step?" are strategies that encourage participants to apply what they've learned by thinking of a small change they can personally implement right away, or possibly a larger change that needs to occur to support mouth care. Formalizing their action plan on paper is also an effective practice that has demonstrated success in other areas of caregiver practice (Rodriguez *et al.*, 2010). A "true and false" group activity is a fun way to debunk commonly held myths, while an effective visual can help summarize important information (Fig. 19.7). Use anonymous participant feedback to assess participants' knowledge, shape future training efforts, and generate data to share with stakeholders.

Serving as an OHP champion encompasses far more than caregiver education. Arranging to have recommended products on hand, getting involved in research projects that seek answers to practical oral care issues, and even securing financial remuneration for the OHP champion all bolster the ability of staff to translate education into positive practice. Funding options for an OHP position to support health promotion may include negotiating a salary or a per bed monthly fee, or just simply billing for each training session.

The biggest challenge with caregiver education and training is in fact helping caregivers translate their newly acquired knowledge into improved daily oral care, beginning with an oral assessment (Table 19.5).

Assessment and clinical care: health promotion ring 4

After being trained to use our oral assessment form, I am more comfortable and confident when looking in someone's mouth.

Nurse

Moving to the next ring of the health promotion model, a proper assessment of an older adult's oral health status is crucial to ensuring appropriate clinical and daily oral care, and thus promoting better

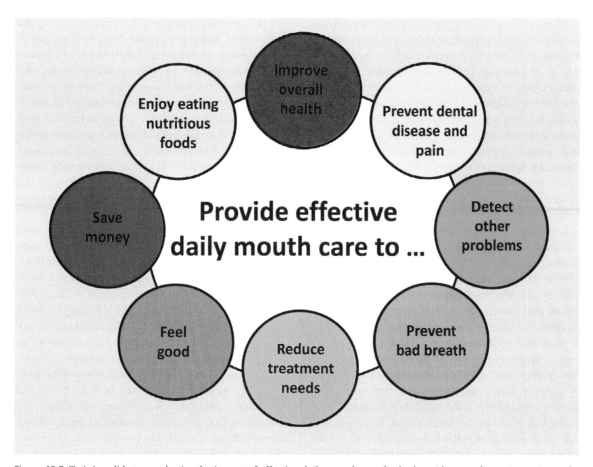

Figure 19.7 Training slide to emphasize the impact of effective daily mouth care for both residents and caregivers. Created by Wener, Bertone, and Yakiwchuk, 2012.

Table 19.5 Training lessons learned

- Facilitators need to be credible and experienced working with dependent older adults
- Plan to make it realistic, interesting, simple, visual and fun
- Participants need to have their voices and issues heard to move forward
- Demonstrations and hands-on practice are critical
- Recognize and communicate that as a facilitator you are also learning from them
- Ask "how can you help" instead of "you must do this"
- End on a message focused on change or a next step
- One dose isn't enough … keep reconnecting
- Use and adapt existing materials (see Appendix 19.1)

Table 19.6 Oral assessments in long-term care (LTC)*

Oral assessments in LTC
- *Inspection:* a cursory look with a specific purpose; can occur daily, weekly, or as needed
- *Screening assessment:* a snapshot of overall oral health; conducted upon admission and quarterly
- *Examination:* an assessment by an oral health professional (OHP) of the oral cavity, including all hard and soft tissues; recommended upon admission, annually, or to investigate symptoms

From Raghoonandan *et al.* (2013).

oral health and quality of life. Assessments vary depending on the desired outcome, staffing levels, and available resources; and can have many uses, such as to identify urgent needs, plan for needed treatment, develop daily oral care plans, and prompt collaboration and referrals. Oral health assessments may take the form of an inspection, a screening or an examination (Table 19.6). The differences in these terms will be described next.

An *inspection* is a cursory investigation, often relying heavily on self-reporting, and focused on a specific purpose (Chalmers & Pearson, 2005a; Kayser-Jones *et al.*, 1995). An inspection could determine if an individual's pain is due to a broken denture or if daily oral care is adequate. A dental *screening assessment* is broader than an inspection as it looks at an individual's overall oral health to identify oral concerns and prompt referral to the appropriate health professional (Chalmers & Pearson, 2005a, 2005b). A dental *examination* is more rigorous and detailed than a screening as it assesses all of the oral features including examination of the hard tissues, each individual tooth and all of the surrounding soft tissues, using intraoral and extraoral clinical examinations as well as radiographic examination. (Chalmers & Pearson, 2005a, 2005b). Dental exams are conducted to assess tooth function and diagnose dental decay, gum disease, and lesions that could be oral cancer. Dental exams can be "regular," conducted based on timing, i.e., annually, or "specific," performed to investigate known symptoms. Caregivers need to be aware of the need for both regular and specific professional examinations by a dentist, particularly as they are erroneously considered unnecessary if the individual no longer has teeth. An examination by a dental hygienist also assesses the oral hard and soft tissues and serves as the basis for developing a care plan, which would include referral to a dentist for oral issues outside a dental hygienist's scope of practice, i.e., surgical, endodontic, or prosthodontic concerns.

In the LTC environment, many health professionals may be involved in a resident's care, each with their own discipline-based understanding of what constitutes an oral assessment. The type of assessment chosen is influenced by the health professional's scope of practice and how the resident's oral health status relates to their discipline (Chalmers *et al.*, 2005). For example, a speech language pathologist and a dental hygienist may both indicate that they have performed an assessment, but they may have looked for different findings based on their training. It is important to determine which health providers will conduct oral assessments (Chalmers *et al.*, 2005) and ensure that the individual is qualified. When feasible, oral health assessments should ideally be performed by OHPs (Kayser-Jones *et al.*, 1995; Pronych *et al.*, 2010).

It is imperative that the individuals performing the assessments, whether they are OHPs or other health professionals, are properly trained to use the tool to record findings and to identify the resident's oral health needs (Kayser-Jones *et al.*, 1995; Lin *et al.*, 1999). OHPs will be comfortable and skilled in assessing oral conditions, but may not be as familiar with the resident's cognitive and physical abilities as the nondental caregivers who spend more time with them (Kayser-Jones *et al.*, 1996). Conversely, those same nondental caregivers may not possess the training needed to perform the oral assessments (Kayser-Jones *et al.*, 1995). OHPs and nondental caregivers should adopt a collaborative team approach to ensure the resident's oral health concerns are being addressed and that the assessments are done properly and meet agreed upon criteria (Chalmers *et al.*, 2005; Kayser-Jones *et al.*, 1995; McNally *et al.*, 2012; Pace & McCullough, 2010; Pronych *et al.*, 2010). With an individual's oral health well-documented, collaboration can continue to occur at scheduled care planning meetings.

There are well-researched oral assessment tools available that are suitable for use by both dental and nondental professionals. When choosing an assessment tool, care must be taken to ensure that it captures the data needed to provide an accurate picture of an individual's oral care needs (Berry *et al.*, 2011; Chalmers *et al.*, 2005), and also fits the needs of the setting. When examining many of the available tools, it is evident that they have their roots in the Kayser-Jones *et al.*'s (1995) Brief Oral Health Status Examination (BOHSE) and its subsequent adaptation by Chalmers *et al.*'s (2004) Oral Health Assessment Tool (OHAT). The OHAT is a one-page tool for assessing a resident's oral health status that has been proven to be both valid and reliable (Chalmers *et al.*, 2005). The 2004 version of the OHAT (Chalmers *et al.*, 2004) includes assessment of the lips, tongue, gums, and tissues, saliva, natural teeth (yes/no), dentures (yes/no), oral cleanliness, and dental pain. Each of these is scored as healthy (0), with changes (1), or unhealthy (2); all factors are then totalled to obtain an overall oral health status score. The Registered Nurses of Ontario (RNAO) and the University of Manitoba Centre for Community Oral Health have created modified versions of the OHAT for their own specific uses. See Appendix 19.3 for the University of Manitoba adaptation that adds swallowing and cognitive status as assessed factors. A simple user-friendly screening tool that directs caregivers to draw symbols representing concerns on an intraoral diagram was developed as part of the Brushing Up project (see Appendix 19.1, Resources for Promoting Oral Health in Long-Term Care). This useful visual tool can be used daily, weekly, or as needed according to the setting and protocols to identify findings that require follow-up.

The Minimum Data Set (MDS) is a computerized resident assessment instrument (RAI) widely used by LTC facilities to identify overall healthcare needs and provide standardized summary assessments for each individual (Sales *et al.*, 2011). As data can be aggregated to generate facility-wide quality indicators (QIs), this can help facilities identify, prioritize, and improve standards of care and meet government certification and accreditation requirements (Castle & Ferguson, 2010; Johnson & Chalmers, 2011; Sales *et al.*, 2011). There are two versions of the MDS in current use, 2.0 and 3.0, each with its own inherent abilities and limitations. The oral and dental status sections have been criticized as not providing a complete picture of the resident's oral health, including neglecting the health of the soft tissues and saliva, and stimulating little connection between assessment and actual referrals (Guay, 2005; Johnson & Chalmers, 2011; Thai *et al.*, 1997). To optimize the effectiveness of the MDS in triggering appropriate oral health care, it is not sufficient simply to ask the questions; an actual screening of the resident's oral health must also be performed, as was intended under the OBRA regulations (Nunez *et al.*, 2011).

Timing

An initial oral health assessment should be performed upon, or very soon after, an older adult has been admitted to a facility or begun receiving home care. This assessment, most likely in the form of an inspection and performed by a non-OHP, will confirm the presence of natural teeth, partial or full dentures, and any obvious oral health concerns, and helps establish preliminary oral healthcare goals. A common mistake by many nondental health professionals is to assume that this initial inspection is sufficient. It is not; a proper screening assessment using an appropriate tool should be performed within 6 weeks of admission. If the inspection or

screening uncovers dental concerns in need of attention, referrals should be made to the appropriate OHP or other health professionals. Oral screening results can then be used to create individualized daily care plans, which provide instruction to caregivers on each person's specific mouth care needs (Chalmers & Pearson 2005a; McConnell *et al.*, 2007; McNally *et al.*, 2012). Information gathered during an assessment also establishes a baseline from which to measure progress or deterioration of a resident's oral health status.

Given that physical and cognitive abilities among this population can deteriorate rapidly, re-evaluations should be conducted periodically to support the resident's oral health and dignity. In so doing, health professionals will be able to recognize and act on these changes well before significant oral health damage has occurred. LTC facilities typically schedule quarterly physical and cognitive re-evaluations; thus it may be easier for both the health providers and the residents to include oral health screenings with these regularly scheduled assessments. If oral health issues are discovered, daily mouth care plans can be modified and appropriate referrals to dentists, denturists, and dental hygienists made.

OHP champions need to establish and promote protocols whereby families are made aware of screening outcomes, educated on care plans and their impact upon overall health, and encouraged to support both these routines and regular visits to OHPs. As a result, families will be more aware of their loved one's oral healthcare needs, including what oral hygiene products they are responsible for providing, and necessary dental treatment that must be addressed. Treatment options may include traveling to a dental clinic in the community; on-site care with fixed, mobile, or other specialized equipment such as wheelchairs that recline for dental treatment; or even providing some care bedside.

Once the assessment has been conducted, results properly documented, and any urgent needs addressed, the OHP clinician may provide preventive/therapeutic clinical care and recommend products or strategies as needed. For example, the clinician may recommend 3–4 fluoride varnish treatment applications yearly, for prevention of root caries (Innes & Evans, 2009). Examples of some preventive strategies to reduce the risk of dental caries, improve gingival

Table 19.7 Preventive oral health strategies for dependent older adults

Fluoride varnish (Gibson *et al.*, 2011; Innes & Evans, 2009; Raghoonandan *et al.*, 2013)
- Optimal fluoride product for medically compromised or frail elderly due to difficulties with rinsing and swallowing risks with fluoride rinses

Fluoride rinses and gels (Chalmers & Pearson, 2005b; Gibson *et al.*, 2011)
- Significant effect when used with at-risk older adults

5000 ppm toothpaste (Gibson *et al.*, 2011)
- For best results from the extra fluoride, spit out excess, and avoid rinsing after use

MI paste (Chalmers & Pearson, 2005b)
- A mild, derived protein that has been shown to remineralize tooth structure

Chlorhexidine mouth rinse (Chalmers & Pearson, 2005b; El-Solh, 2011; Pace & McCullough, 2010)
- Bactericidal, fungicidal, and limited virus killing properties; variety of methods for application; gel, spray, swab, are application options for those with swallowing challenges

Saliva substitutes (Chalmers & Pearson, 2005b)
- Treatment for dry mouth in the form of gels or sprays; can be used on oral soft tissues on an as-needed basis

health, and reduce the risk of further tooth structure breakdown are given in Table 19.7.

Regardless of the professionals involved, expectations for the oral assessment should be determined, and used to choose the appropriate tool: an inspection, a screening, or an exam. With proper assessment, the foundation is laid for needed clinical care, collaborative referrals, and individualized daily mouth care plans, the focus of the next section.

Daily mouth care: health promotion ring 5

My grandmother had all her own teeth at the age of 92 when she moved to a care home. She needed help with her own mouth care, but whether it was provided, I don't know. What I do know is, that within 2 years her teeth were rotten, many broken off to just the roots. As a family, we were asked to consider having all her teeth extracted. How could this have happened?

Family member

Daily mouth care, the fifth and final ring in the model, perhaps is the most essential component of oral health care to protect the older adult from infections, pain, and tooth loss. Having a clean mouth also contributes to an elder's increased comfort, confidence, socialization and quality of life. As an OHP champion, understanding LTC facility or home-care-agency processes

for promoting oral health and integrating them into interactions with older adults, families, and caregivers helps reinforce expectations. To provide effective, consistent mouth care to residents, it is imperative that caregivers understand what needs to be done, why it needs to be done, and how to perform the care. Best practice guidelines for routine mouth care should include performing a proper assessment, and using the assessment findings to develop an individualized daily mouth care plan that serves as a procedural guide for caregivers (Chalmers *et al.*, 2004; Coleman, 2002; McConnell *et al.*, 2007).

Individualized daily mouth care plans

The protocol should require an individualized plan that outlines specific daily mouth care needs, and how to address them. Consider the following suggestions:
- Include, where possible, evidence-based procedures and practices.
- Keep the care plan simple, straightforward, prescriptive, and individualized so that caregivers understand clearly how to proceed. Mouth care is often an afterthought for some residents and even for some caregivers; a good plan can assist in keeping proper mouth care a priority.
- Include an alert on the plan for those with dementia or dysphagia.
- Mouth care may need to be performed completely by the caregiver, while other times the caregiver may

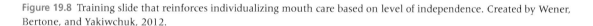

ORAL ASSESSMENT AND PLANNING

- **Assess all oral tissues**
- **Assess LEVEL of mouth care needed:**
  - REMIND – capable, sometimes forgetful
  - ASSIST – unable to do totally independently
  - PROVIDE – dependent for care
  - PALLIATIVE – requires end-of-life comfort and care
- **Develop a daily mouth care plan**

Assess + Observe + Decide + Record

Those who require help with feeding generally can not manage tooth brushing

Figure 19.8 Training slide that reinforces individualizing mouth care based on level of independence. Created by Wener, Bertone, and Yakiwchuk, 2012.

only need to assist the resident or simply remind the resident to perform the task. The plan should clearly indicate whether the caregiver reminds (independent, but forgetful), assists (partially dependent), provides (completely dependent), or is in palliative care (focused on comfort) (Fig. 19.8).

- Proper universal infection control precautions should be followed at all times. Reinforce

that new clean gloves should be worn when providing oral care (Stein & Henry, 2009) and hands washed between providing care for each resident.

Daily mouth care tip 1

If the resident is not capable of determining whether a product can be ingested, all oral health-related products should be stored securely, out of the resident's reach. Denture tablets have been mistakenly dissolved in water and swallowed like an antacid.

Daily mouth care tip 2

Collaborate with the speech language pathologist when dysphagia/swallowing issues are noted. Options: (i) use half a pea-sized amount of a nonfoaming toothpaste (without sodium lauryl sulphate) to brush the top teeth, and then the other half when brushing the bottom teeth. Wipe as you go with a clean face cloth or gauze to reduce the amount of toothpaste in the resident's mouth at any given time; (ii) if a suction unit is available, consider a commercially available suction toothbrush to reduce ingestion of bacteria and toothpaste; (iii) if toothpaste is not tolerated, dip toothbrush in fluoridated mouth rinse or brush with water.

- Outline the necessary mouth care basics: how often to brush, when to brush, the appropriate type of toothbrush to use, whether to use fluoridated or specialized toothpaste, and how much toothpaste to use. Interdental cleaning devices may be feasible to use for some individuals. A proxa-brush (i.e., GUM® Sunstar-Butler) requires less skill and dexterity than flossing; and can be successfully used even when teeth are clenched.
- Identify mouth care products that need to be provided, including any specialty products such as toothbrushes that clean three surfaces at once, that have handles that are suitable for mouth propping or can be attached to a suction unit (Stein & Henry, 2009). Ensure appropriate products are readily available either at the facility or through a local drug store. If not, advocate for a pharmacist to stock select products, or speak to the administration about options such as bulk purchasing. All mouth care products must be clearly labeled with the individual's name.

Daily mouth care tip 3

For those being treated for a fungal infection (candidiasis), the denture must also be treated to prevent reoccurrence.

- Dentures and denture care are of particular importance; label dentures; brush with liquid soap, not toothpaste. Keep out overnight to rest tissues and to disinfect the denture either in a bath of denture cleanser or air dry. Denture disinfection is particularly important for those susceptible to oral infections.
- Mouth care products need to be thoroughly rinsed after use and air dried, not placed in closed plastic containers or in a drawer where bacteria can grow (Berry *et al.*, 2011).

Daily mouth care strategies

- Document strategies that are known to work successfully for the individual. This will assist the caregiver and provide continuity of care between different caregivers. For example, is there a time of day that seems to work best, or a preferred location? Some individuals are more willing to accept mouth care while watching television or taking a bath.

- Indicate if resident cooperation or CRB is an issue. If so, identify strategies to try or that have been previously successful. Using a secure "head hug" position, cuing by putting the toothpaste on the toothbrush and handing it to the individual, or in more challenging circumstances, having two caregivers work together so that one can distract the individual and gently hold their hands, while the other is able to provide mouth care may work best for the individual (Stein & Henry, 2009). It is important that caregivers be educated about client safety. If faced with a particularly challenging scenario, it is best to wait until assistance is available to partner for mouth care, ensuring both the caregiver and elder are safely positioned.
- Indicate whether the mouth needs to be propped open to provide mouth care when the individual is unable to, or unwilling to, remain open. Caregivers can use a disposable mouth rest, the handle of a second toothbrush, or a clean rolled up face cloth.

Daily mouth care tip 4

Never place the prop on front teeth; use the back teeth to support the prop. When using the handle of a second toothbrush as a prop ensure it is fat, round, and sufficiently padded to prevent injury.

- When communicating with the older adult, the caregiver should maintain a very calm, reassuring demeanor, and, whenever possible, provide cues to the resident on what is to be done (Kayser-Jones *et al.*, 1996; Stein & Henry, 2009). Equally important is the communication between the caregiver and supervisory nursing staff. The caregiver should be diligent about reporting any changes in the elder's oral health, cognitive status, or abilities as this could impact upon the daily care plan or trigger a needed referral.

For detailed step-by-step instructions and strategies for daily mouth care for both natural teeth and dentures, refer to University of Manitoba Fact Sheets: Basic Mouth Care (Appendices 19.4 & 19.5). Also see Appendix 19.1 (Resources for Promoting Oral Health in Long-Term Care) for other helpful resources.

Supporting front-line caregivers

Ensuring elders receive effective mouth care does not end with the development of individualized daily mouth care plans. To be effective, the plan must of course be implemented and evaluated, and the reality is that the person who creates the daily care plan is seldom the person who implements it. Check that effective two-way communication is in place for feedback between direct caregivers and others as discontinuity can create challenges and barriers to proper implementation of the plan (Chalmers & Pearson, 2005b). The greatest barrier is often the caregiver's attitude towards providing mouth care, particularly if they do not understand or appreciate how important it is to the resident's quality of life (Forsell et al., 2010). The effects of daily mouth care are less visible than many of the other ADLs that they have to attend to, so there is an inherent lack of accountability to those effects (Jablonski et al., 2005; Pronych et al., 2010; Sumi et al., 2002). Avoiding daily mouth care may be due to caregiver uneasiness caused by issues such as unpleasant odors associated with halitosis, bleeding gums, or dental decay (McConnell et al., 2007). OHP champions and partners should implement a quality assurance program to routinely and randomly evaluate both caregiver compliance and resident oral health status. Resident charts can be audited, individuals randomly screened for oral health cleanliness, and interviews held with caregivers to gather data. Information collected can be useful to provide evidence of successes of the new oral healthcare program, and the need for further improvement.

COMMUNICATION TECHNIQUES TO BOOST COOPERATION

- **Rescuing:**
  Using the "good cop/bad cop" technique

- **Bridging:**
  Holding the same object as you, i.e. toothbrush

- **Distraction:**
  Using singing, music, holding items, rummage box, gentle touch, rubbing cheek, flowing conversation

- **Chaining:**
  You start the process, they finish it

- **Hand-over-hand:**
  Guiding them

- **Don't tower over the person:**
  Approach at eye level and in the field of vision

- **Avoid excessive noise:**
  Plan for a quiet environment and few people present

- **Gesture and pantomime:**
  Can minimize frustration and reduce threat perception

- **Use a gentle touch:**
  Reassures and reduces anxiety

- **Avoid "elderspeak":**
  Can trigger care-resistant behavior

Figure 19.9 Training slide that provides helpful strategies for individuals that exhibit care resistant behavior (CRB). From Jablonski et al. (2011a; 2011b). Created by Wener, Bertone, and Yakiwchuk, 2012.

The most noted concern expressed by caregivers is the significant challenge posed by working with an individual who is unable to cooperate due to cognitive impairments such as dementia or Alzheimer's disease (Brady *et al.*, 2006; McConnell *et al.*, 2007). They are fearful of being hit, bitten, or verbally abused (Pronych *et al.*, 2010). These barriers and concerns must be addressed through education and training sessions on how to manage challenges so that the caregiver can feel both safe and confident in providing effective daily mouth care (Forsell *et al.*, 2010; Jablonski *et al.*, 2011a; Pronych *et al.*, 2010). Care-resistive behavior requires not only strategy options, but patience and creativity (Fig. 19.9). OHP champions are advised to go on-unit to support and model daily mouth care with elders that present challenging behaviors.

It is the OHP's responsibility to stay current in best practices and current evidence regarding mouth care products, treatments, and procedures for this population; however, it is not reasonable to expect caregivers to possess this same level of knowledge and understanding. OHPs should be empathetic to the caregiver's situation, and understand that caregivers are not necessarily provided with appropriate mouth care products by the facility or by the family (Coleman & Watson, 2006; Gammack & Pulisetty, 2009); sometimes, suboptimal products are all they have to work with. For example, consider a caregiver who only has access to sponge swabs, an ineffective product for dental plaque removal (Pace & McCullough, 2010) in comparison to a soft bristled toothbrush, considered to be the gold standard (Berry *et al.*, 2011; Chalmers & Pearson, 2005a; Stein & Henry, 2009).

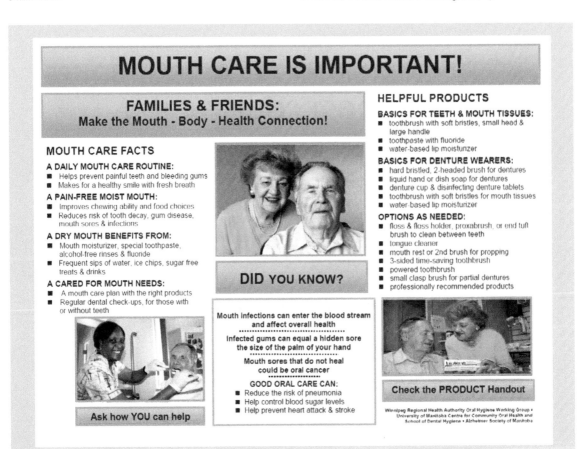

Figure 19.10 Poster providing the message that oral health is part of total health. Used with permission from the Winnipeg Regional Health Authority and the University of Manitoba Centre for Community Oral Health.

As oral health champions and interdisciplinary healthcare providers, OHPs should provide recommendations to LTC facilities, home care agencies, and families regarding appropriate daily mouth care strategies and products. Including oral health information in LTC new resident packages, on-line materials, publications and programs that support and train caregivers sends the important message that oral health **IS** part of total health (Fig. 19.10).

Case study

Mrs. Smith

Based on actual circumstances, this case study demonstrates the critical linkage between a detailed oral health screening/assessment, the individualized daily mouth care plan can, and the resident's quality of life. Names of those involved have been changed.

Daily mouth care plan for Mrs. Smith

Your new client, Mrs. Smith, is a 91-year-old widowed female who has been living at Sunset Personal Care Home for 8 months, where she has become reasonably acclimatized to her surroundings. She has diabetes mellitus, high blood pressure, mild to moderate dementia, and depends on caregivers for daily mouth care as her dexterity is too poor to care for herself.

Mrs. Smith has two sons and numerous grandchildren and great-grandchildren. You receive a call from Mrs. Smith's son indicating that his mother has been complaining that her tongue hurts. He also asks questions about her "burning mouth" and if she has a mouth infection. He would like you to visit her on-site at the facility, evaluate her situation, and provide advice. She recently had a dental examination by a dentist at the facility, who identified the need for several extractions and fillings. The dentist also indicated that he would confirm her treatment needs after she had her teeth cleaned. She is scheduled for an upcoming dental hygiene appointment.

The dental hygienist visits Mrs. Smith on unit at the LTC facility and performs a screening assessment using a modified OHAT tool. Mrs. Smith has been assessed as High Risk. She has urgent dental treatment needs and is dependent on caregivers for all of her daily mouth care needs. Dental hygiene clinical care was provided at bedside, including application of fluoride varnish, with a referral back to her dentist for follow-up. Findings from the assessment are as follows:

- Two anterior teeth remaining in upper arch; eight anterior teeth and one molar in the lower arch
- No partial dentures for the upper or lower arch
- Dry lips
- Swollen and coated tongue
- Generalized bleeding, swollen and red gums
- Very little saliva; resident reports that her mouth is dry
- Two broken teeth and two obviously decayed teeth
- Food debris, heavy plaque and tartar on all teeth
- Tongue thrusting
- Some difficulty swallowing
- Dental pain indicated by grimacing and verbal complaint of sore gums
- Dexterity problems requiring her to need assistance with mouth care
- Care resistant behavior (CRB) is not a concern, but she is very forgetful and repeats her conversations.

Based on this assessment information, a care plan was developed. Recommendations were discussed with the son and with the nurse-in-charge:

- Mouth–body–health connections were discussed regarding diabetes mellitus: oral infections can affect diabetic control; diabetes and dry mouth can predispose her to oral infections, including yeast/candidiasis; burning mouth syndrome (BMS) could be a complication from her diabetes (pamphlet provided regarding BMS).
- The importance of and protocol for good daily mouth care were emphasized and reviewed.
- To help with her dry mouth, caregivers are to moisturize Mrs. Smith's mouth with a water-based mouth moisturizer as needed. She is to use a water bottle with a straw, and to be encouraged to carry water around with her and sip frequently throughout the day to keep her mouth moist.
- Due to the unfortunate reality that her abilities may deteriorate, it is important to deal with dental issues now while she can tolerate the treatment. Treatment needs include:
  ○ Re-examination by dentist to determine treatment plan.
  ○ Dental hygiene recommendation for periodontal recall.
- She is fully dependent on caregivers for daily mouth care.
- Encouraged family to be involved in mouth care when they visit; discussed helping them learn how to provide mouth care. Discouraged family from providing sweets, particularly hard candies being used when mouth is dry.

- She was given a basic daily mouth care kit which included:
  - Soft bristled compact head toothbrush
  - End tuft brush for cleaning in between anterior teeth
  - Biotene nonfoaming dry mouth toothpaste
  - Water-based Oral Balance® mouth moisturizer
- Discontinue the use of a mouth rinse containing alcohol as it would contribute to the drying of her tongue and tissues; also, liquids may be difficult to manage with a swallowing issue.
- Follow-up regarding daily mouth care and burning tongue in 4 weeks by the dental hygienist.
- The screening assessment form and daily mouth care plan documents were added to the individual's chart, along with an entry documenting today's care.
- A reminder of her mouth care regimen will be posted in her bathroom.

Conclusion

Over the course of this chapter, you have learned more about promoting oral health in LTC facilities to protect and improve the oral health and overall health of this vulnerable population. Important and necessary steps to success have included: (1) advocating for, establishing, and enforcing standards; (2) acquiring and maintaining commitment; (3) providing engaging and appropriately timed education and training at all levels; (4) ensuring that initial and on-going assessments and professional care are provided; and (5) supporting the provision of quality daily mouth care. Remember to begin small, celebrate your accomplishments, and collaborate with many so that each older adult's oral health is included in their overall health care. With these thoughts in mind, what will your next step be?

DISCUSSION QUESTIONS

1 Think about each of the oral health promotion rings in the long-term care (LTC) model. Discuss why they are in that particular order. Would you change the order, and why?
2 LTC quality of life indicators for elders and their families include respect, a caring community and competent staff. Discuss how standards for oral health care can help contribute to the achievement of each of these indicators.

3 At a practical and personal level, what steps could you take to advocate for oral healthcare standards for dependent older adults?
4 What information do you require and what steps should you take to prepare yourself before contacting the LTC facility in your community?
5 Prepare a list of questions you might want to ask during your first meeting with the administrator at Happy Valley Nursing Home.
6 You have been asked to train all 70 caregivers (day, evening, and night shifts) in a small personal care home. How would you go about accomplishing this task?
7 Care resistant behavior (CRB) has been identified as the number one reason for noncompliance with caregivers at Seaside LTC facility. What must you consider before developing a training program? What might be the best way to support and enable caregivers to address CRB?
8 Explain the differences between an inspection, a screening, and an examination, and provide an example of when each would be the method of choice.
9 What are some advantages of using the computerized Minimum Data Set (MDS) instrument to assess the oral health of residents in LTC facilities? What are some of the disadvantages?
10 You have been asked to develop a user-friendly daily mouth care form to be used by caregivers in a home care agency. What information about the older adult is important to include? What mouth care basics should be included?

References

Abi-Nahed, J. (2007) *Legislative Review of Oral Health in Canada in Particular Long-Term Care Facilities.* Office of the Chief Dental Officer of Canada, Ottawa.

Apte, J. (2009) Facilitating transformative learning: a framework for practice. *Australian Journal of Adult Learning,* **49**(1), 169–89.

Bardach, S.H. & Rowles, G.D. (2012) Geriatric education in the health professions: are we making progress? *The Gerontologist,* **52**(5), 607–18.

Berry, A.M., Davidson, P.M., Nicholson, L., *et al.* (2011) Consensus based clinical guideline for oral hygiene in the critically ill. *Intensive and Critical Care Nursing,* **27**, 180–5.

Brady, M., Furlanetto, D., Hunter, R.V., *et al.* (2006) Staff-led interventions for improving oral hygiene in patients following stroke. *Cochrane Database Systematic Review,* **4**, 1–21.

Canadian Dental Association (2008) *Report On Seniors Oral Health Care.* Canadian Dental Association. From http://

www.cda-adc.ca/_files/members/news_publications/member/pdfs/cda_seniors_oral_health_report_may_2008.pdf. Accessed, April 14, 2014.

Canadian Dental Association (2009) *Optimal Health for Frail Older Adults: Best Practices Along the Continuum of Care.* Canadian Dental Association. From https://www.cda-adc.ca/_files/dental_profession/practising/best_practices_seniors/optimal_oral_health_older_adults_2009.pdf. Accessed April 14, 2014.

Canadian Healthcare Association (2009) *New Directions for Facility-Based Long Term Care.* From http://www.cmda.info/CHA_LTC_9-22-09_eng.pdf. Accessed April 14, 2014.

Canadian Interprofessional Health Collaborative (2007) *Interprofessional Education and Core Competencies: Literature Review.* http://www.cihc.ca/files/publications/CIHC_IPE-LitReview_May07.pdf. Accessed April 18, 2014.

Caspar, S. (2012) The influence of quality of work-place relationships on quality of care in LTC settings. Presentation at *Assessing and Taking Action on Oral Health for Older Adults in Canada.* Edmonton, AB.

Castle, N.G. & Ferguson, J.C. (2010) What is nursing home quality and how is it measured? *The Gerontologist,* **50**(4), 426–42.

Castle, N.G. (2012) Reviewing the evidence base for nurse staffing and quality of care in nursing homes. *Evidence Based Nursing,* **15**(2), 23–4.

Chalmers, J.M., Johnson, V., Tang, J.H. & Titler, M.G. (2004) Evidence-based protocol: oral hygiene care for functionally dependent and cognitively impaired older adults. *Journal of Gerontological Nursing,* **30**(11), 5–12.

Chalmers, J.M., King, P.L., Spencer, A.J., *et al.* (2005) The oral health assessment tool – validity and reliability. *Australian Dental Journal,* **50**(3), 191–9.

Chalmers, J.M. & Pearson, A. (2005a), A systematic review of oral health assessment by nurses and carers for residents with dementia in residential care facilities. *Special Care Dentistry,* **25**(5), 227–33.

Chalmers, J.M. & Pearson, A. (2005b) Oral hygiene care for residents with dementia: a literature review. *Journal of Advanced Nursing,* **52**(4), 410–19.

Chalmers, J.M., Spencer, A.J., Carter, K.D., *et al.* (2009) Caring for oral health in Australian residential care. Australian Institute of Health and Welfare, Canberra. From http://www.aihw.gov.au/publication-detail/?id=6442468243. Accessed April 14, 2014.

Coleman, P. & Watson, H.M. (2006) Oral care provided by certified nursing assistants in nursing homes. *Journal of American Geriatric Society,* **54**(1), 138–43.

Coleman, P., Hein, C. & Gurenlian, J.R. (2006) The promise of transdisciplinary nurse–dental hygienists collaboration in achieving health-related quality of life for elderly nursing home residents. *Grand Rounds in Oral-Systemic Medicine,* **1**(3), 40A–9A.

Coleman, P.R. (2002) Oral health care for the frail elderly: a review of widespread problems and best practices. *Geriatric Nursing,* **23**, 189–97.

Daft, M.L. (2008) *The Leadership Experience.* South-Western Publishing, Mason, OH.

De Visschere, L.M.J., van der Putten, G.-J., Vanobbergen, J.N.O., *et al.* (2011) An oral health care guideline for institutionalised older people. *Gerontology,* **28**, 307–10.

Dharamsi, S., Jivani, K., Dean, C. & Wyatt, C. (2009) Oral care for frail elders: knowledge, attitudes, and practices of long-term care staff. *Journal of Dental Education,* **73**(5), 581–8.

El-Sohl, A.A. (2011) Association between pneumonia and oral care in nursing home residents. *Lung,* **189**, 173–80.

Forsell, M., Kullberg, E., Hoogstraate, J., *et al.* (2010) A survey of attitudes and perceptions toward oral hygiene among staff at a geriatric nursing home. *Geriatric Nursing,* **31**, 435–40.

Forsell, M., Kullberg, E., Hoogstraate, J., *et al.* (2011) An evidence-based oral hygiene education program for nursing staff. *Nurse Education in Practice,* **11**, 256–9.

Forsell, M., Sjögren, P. & Johansson, O. (2009) Need of assistance with daily oral hygiene measures among nursing home resident elderly versus the actual assistance received from the staff. *The Open Dentistry Journal,* **3**, 241–4.

Frenkel, H., Harvey, I. & Newcombe, R.G. (2000) Oral health care among nursing home residents in Avon. *Gerodontology,* **17**(1), 33–8.

Gammack, J.K. & Pulisetty, S. (2009) Nursing education and improvement in oral care delivery in long-term care. *Journal of the American Medical Association,* **19**(9), 658–61.

Gibson, G., Jurasic, M.M., Wehler, C.J. & Jones, J.A. (2011) Supplemental fluoride use for moderate and high caries risk adults: a systematic review. *Journal of Public Health Dentistry,* **71**, 171–84.

Giles, L.C., Paterson, J.E., Butler, S.J. & Steward, J.J. (2002) Ageism among health professionals: a comparison of clinical educators and students in physical and occupational theory. *Physical & Occupational Therapy in Geriatrics,* **21**(2), 15–26.

Glasrud, P., Brickle, C., Jacobi, D. & Helgeson, M. (2005) Dental hygienists interest in community collaborative practice: results of a survey. *Northwest Dentistry,* **84**(6), 1e–10e.

Guay, A.H. (2005) The oral health status of nursing home residents: what do we know? *Journal of Dental Education,* **69**(9), 1015–17.

Hahn, J.E., FitzGerald, L., Markham, Y.K., *et al.* (2012) Infusing oral health care into nursing curriculum: addressing preventive health in aging and disability. Nursing Research and Practice. From http://www.hindawi.com/journals/nrp/2012/157874/. Accessed April 14, 2014.

Harrington, C. & Swan, J.H. (2003) Nursing home staffing, turnover, and case mix. *Medical Care Research and Review,* **60**, 366–92.

Haumschild, M.S. & Haumschild, R.J. 2009, The importance of oral health in long-term care, *Journal of the American Medical Directors Association,* **10**, 667–71.

Hein, C., Schonwetter, D.J. & Iacopino, A.M. (2011) Inclusion of oral-systemic health in predoctoral/undergraduate curricula of pharmacy, nursing, and medical schools around the world: a preliminary study, *Journal of Dental Education*, **75**(9), 1187–99.

Helgeson, M.J. & Smith, B.J. (1996) Dental care in nursing homes: guidelines for mobile and on-site care. *Special Care in Dentistry*, **16**(4), 153–63.

Henry, R.G. (2005) *Kentucky Elder Oral Health Survey: Executive Summary*. University of Kentucky College of Dentistry, Lexington, KY. From http://tinyurl.com/d4cfuk. Accessed April 14, 2014.

Innes, N. & Evans, D.I. (2009) Caries prevention for older people in residential care homes. *Evidence-Based Dentistry*, **10**, 83–7.

Institute for Oral Health (2008) *Oral Health Heeds For Seniors, Pt 2. Bringing Innovation to Dental Education, Care and Access for Aging Adults*. Institute for Oral Health, Denver, CO. From http://iohwa.org/2008fg/IOHJun08-FocusGroup-whitepaper.pdf. Accessed April 14, 2014.

Institute of Medicine (2011a) *Advancing Oral Health in America*. Institute of Medicine, Washington DC. From http://www.hrsa.gov/publichealth/clinical/oralhealth/advancingoralhealth.pdf. Accessed April 14, 2014.

Institute of Medicine (2011b) *Improving Access to Oral Health Care for Vulnerable and Underserved Populations*. Report Brief. Institute of Medicine, Washington DC. From http://www.iom.edu/~/media/Files/Report%20Files/2011/Improving-Access-to-Oral-Health-Care-for-Vulnerable-and-Underserved-Populations/oralhealthaccess2011 reportbrief.pdf. Accessed April 14, 2014.

Jablonski, R.A., Munro, C.L., Grap, M.J. & Elswick, R.K. (2005) The role of biobehavioral, environmental, and social forces on oral health disparities in frail and functionally dependent nursing home elders. *Biological Research for Nurses*, **7**(1), 75–82.

Jablonski, R.A. (2012) Oral health and hygiene content in nursing fundamentals textbooks. *Nursing Research and Practice*. From http://www.hindawi.com/journals/nrp/2012/372617/ref/. Accessed April 14, 2014.

Jablonski, R.A., Therrien, B. & Kolanowski, A. (2011a) No more fighting and biting during mouth care: applying the theoretical constructs of threat perception to clinical practice. *Research and Theory for Nursing Practice*, **25**(3), 163–75.

Jablonski, R.A., Therrien, B., Mahoney, E.K., *et al.* (2011b) An intervention to reduce care-resistant behavior in persons with dementia during oral hygiene: a pilot study. *Special Care in Dentistry*, **31**(3), 77–87.

Jackson, J. (2007) Nursing home fined $100,000 for death. *Argus-Courier*, July 11.

Jiang, Y.W. & MacEntee, M.I. (2013) Opinions of administrators and health authority inspectors on implementing and monitoring the oral health regulation in long-term care facilities in British Columbia. *The Canadian Journal of Dental Hygiene*, **47**(1), 15–23.

Johnson, V.B. & Chalmers, J. (2011) *Oral Hygiene Care for Functionally Dependent and Cognitively Impaired Older Adults*.

National Guideline Clearinghouse, US Dept. of Health and Human Services. From http://guidelines.gov/content.aspx?id=34447. Accessed April 14, 2014.

Katz, R.V., Smith, B.J., Berkey, D.B., *et al.* (2010) Defining oral neglect in institutionalized elderly – a consensus definition for the protection of vulnerable elderly people. *Journal of the American Dental Association*, **141**(4), 440–3.

Kayser-Jones, J., Bird, W.F., Redford, M., *et al.* (1996) Strategies for conducting dental examinations among cognitively impaired nursing home residents. *Special Care in Dentistry*, **1**(2), 46–52.

Kayser-Jones, J., Paul, S.M. & Schell, E.S. (1995) An instrument to assess the oral health status of nursing home residents. *The Gerontologist*, **35**(6), 814–24.

Larsen, P.D. & Lubkin, I.M. (2009) *Chronic Illness: Impact and Intervention*, 7th edn. Johnson and Bartlett Publishers, Sudbury, MA.

Lin, C.Y., Jones, D.B., Godwin, C., *et al.* (1999) Oral health assessment by nursing staff of Alzheimer's patients in a long-term-care facility. *Special Care Dentistry*, **19**(2), 64–71.

MacEntee, M.I. (2011) Muted dental voices on interprofessional healthcare teams. *Journal of Dentistry*, **2** (Suppl), s34–40.

MacEntee, M.I., Kazanjian, A., Kozak, J.-F., *et al.* (2012) A scoping review and research synthesis on financing and regulating oral care in long-term care facilities. *Gerodontology*, **29**, e41–e52.

MacEntee, M.I., Thorne, S. & Kazanjian, A. (1999) Conflicting priorities: oral health in long-term care. *Special Care in Dentistry*, **19**(4), 164–72.

MacEntee, M.I., Wyatt, C.C.L., Beattie, B.L., *et al.* (2007) Provision of mouth-care in long term care facilities: an educational trial. *Community Dentistry and Oral Epidemiology*, **35**, 25–34.

MacEntee, M.I., MacInnis, B., McKeown, L. & Sarrapuchiello, T. (2008) *Dignity With a Smile: Oral Healthcare for Elders in Residential Care: a Report for the Federal Dental Advisory Committee*. Federal Dental Care Advisory Committee. From http://www.fptdwg.ca/assets/PDF/0901-Dignity%20with%20a%20Smile%20Final.pdf. Accessed April 14, 2014.

Matthews, D.C., Clovis, J.B., Brillant, M.G., *et al.* (2012) Oral health status of long-term care residents – a vulnerable population. *Journal of the Canadian Dental Association*, **78**, c3.

McConnell, E.S., Lekan, D., Hebert, C. & Leatherwood, L. (2007) Academic practice partnerships to promote evidence-based practice in long term care: oral hygiene care practices as an exemplar. *Nursing Outlook*, **55**, 95–105.

McGregor, M.J. & Ronald, L.A. (2011) *Residential Long-Term Care for Canadian Seniors: Nonprofit, For-Profit or Does it Matter?* IRPP Study. Institute for Research on Public Policy, No. 14. From http://archive.irpp.org/pubs/IRPPstudy/2011/IRPP_Study_no1.pdf. Accessed April 14, 2014.

McKelvey, V.A., Thompson, W.M., Ayers, K.M.S. (2003) A qualitative study of oral health knowledge and attitudes among staff caring for older people in Dunedin long-term care facilities. *New Zealand Dental Journal,* **99**(4), 98–103.

McNally, M. & Lyons, R. (2004) *The Silent Epidemic of Oral Disease: Evaluating Continuity of Care and Policies for the Oral Health Care of Seniors.* Canadian Foundation for Health Care Improvement. From http://www.chsrf.ca/publicationsandresources/researchreports/opengrantscompetition/04-04-01/5f0a138b-6f9c-4f07-9a12-05f3510bd6be.aspx. Accessed April 14, 2014.

McNally, M.E., Martin-Misener, R., Wyatt, C.C.L., *et al.* (2012) Action planning for daily mouth care in long-term care: the brushing up on mouth care project. *Nursing Research and Practice.* From http://www.hindawi.com/journals/nrp/2012/368356/. Accessed April 14, 2014.

Mezirow, J. (2009) An overview on transformative learning. In: *Contemporary Theories of Learning: Learning Theorists in their Own Words* (ed. K. Illeris), pp. 90–105. Routledge, Taylor & Francis Group, Abingdon, Oxon, UK.

Minnesota Administrative Rules (1995) *Chapter 4658, Nursing Homes,* Minnesota Nursing Home Dental Regulations, Parts 4658.0720, .0725, .0730, effective Nov. 12, 1995. From https://www.revisor.mn.gov/rules/?id=4658. Accessed April 14, 2014.

Monajem, S. (2006) Integration of oral health into primary health care: the role of dental hygienists and the WHO stewardship. *International Journal of Dental Hygiene,* **4**, 47–51.

Munoz, N., Touger-Decker, R., Byham-Gray, L. & O'Sullivan, M.J. (2009) Effect of an oral health assessment education program on nurses' knowledge and patient care practices in skilled nursing facilities. *Special Care in Dentistry,* **29**(4), 179–85.

National Centre for Assisted Living (2011) *Findings Of The NCAL 2010 Assisted Living Staff Vacancy, Retention And Turnover Survey.* From http://www.ahcancal.org/ncal/resources/documents/2010%20vrt%20report-final.pdf. Accessed April 14, 2014.

National Seniors' Task Force (2008) *Report On Seniors' Oral Health Care.* Canadian Dental Association. From http://www.cda-adc.ca/_files/members/news_publications/member/pdfs/cda_seniors_oral_health_report_may_2008.pdf. Accessed April 14, 2014.

Nunez, B., Chalmers, J., Warren, J., *et al.* (2011) Opinions on the provision of dental care in Iowa nursing homes. *Special Care in Dentistry,* **31**(1), 33–40.

Pace, C.C. & McCullough, G.H. (2010) The association between oral microorganisms and aspiration pneumonia in the institutionalized elderly: review and recommendations. *Dysphagia,* **25**(4), 307–22.

Peltola, P., Vehkalahti, M.M., Simoila, R. (2007) Effects of 11-month interventions on oral cleanliness among the long-term care hospitalized elderly. *Gerodontology,* **24**, 14–21.

Petersen, P.E. & Yamamoto, T. (2005) Improving the oral health of older people: the approach of the WHO global oral health programme. *Community Dentistry and Oral Epidemiology,* **33**(2), 81–92.

Pronych, G.J., Brown, E.J., Horsch, K. & Mercer, K. (2010) Oral health coordinators in long-term care – a pilot study. *Special Care in Dentistry,* **30**(2), 59–65.

Raghoonandan, P., Cobban, S.J. & Compton, S.M. (2013) A scoping review of the use of fluoride varnish in elderly people living in long term care facilities. *The Canadian Journal of Dental Hygiene,* **45**(4), 217–22.

Rodriquez, E., Marquett, R., Hinton, L., *et al.* (2010) The impact of education on care practices: an exploratory study of whether "action plans" influence health professionals' behavior. *National Institutes of Health,* **22**(6), 897–908.

Sales, A.E., Bostrom, A.M., Bucknall, T., *et al.* (2011) The use of data for process and quality improvement in long-term care and home care: a systematic review of the literature. *Journal of the American Medical Directors Association,* **1**, 103–13.

Simons, D., Baker, P., Jones, B., *et al.* (2000) An evaluation of an oral health training programme for carers of the elderly in residential homes. *British Dental Journal,* **188**(4), 206–10.

Slade G, Offenbacher S, Beck J, Heiss G, Pankow J. Acute-phase inflammatory response to periodontal disease in the US population. *Journal of Dental Research,* 2000, **79,** 49–57.

Seniors' Oral Health Secretariat (SOHS) (2011) *Oral Health Care Delivery in Residential Care Facilities: a Report of the Seniors' Oral Health Secretariat.* British Columbia Dental Association. From http://www.bcdental.org/Dental_Health/Default.aspx?id=6202. Accessed April 14, 2014.

Stein, P.S. & Henry, R.G. (2009) Poor oral hygiene in long-term care. *American Journal of Nursing,* **109**(6), 44–50.

Stewart, S. (2013) Daily oral hygiene in residential care. *Canadian Journal of Dental Hygiene,* **47**(1), 25–30.

Sumi, Y., Nakamura, Y. & Michiwaki, Y. (2002) Development of a systematic oral care program for frail elderly persons. *Special Care Dentistry,* **22**, 151–5.

Thai, P.H., Shuman, S.K. & Davidson, G.B. (1997) Nurses' dental assessments and subsequent care in Minnesota nursing homes. *Special Care in Dentistry,* **17**, 13–18.

Thorne, S., Kazanjian, A. & MacEntee, M. (2001) Oral health in long-term care: the implications of organizational culture. *Journal of Aging Studies,* **15**, 271–83.

Unfer, B., Braun, K.O., de Oliveira Ferreira, A.C., *et al.* (2011) Challenges and barriers to quality oral care as perceived by caregivers in long-stay institutions in Brazil. *Gerodontology,* **29**(2), 324–30.

US Dept. of Health and Human Services (2009) *LongTermCare.gov.* The official US Government site for Medicare. From http://longtermcare.gov/medicare-medicaid-more/medicare/. Accessed April 14, 2014.

Wardh, I., Hallberg, L.R., Berggren, U., *et al.* (2003) Oral health education for nursing personnel; experiences among specially trained oral care aides: one-year follow-up interviews with oral care aides at a nursing facility. *Scandinavian Journal of Caring Science,* **17**, 250–6.

Way, D., Jones, L., Baskerville, B. & Busing, N. (2001) *Improving the Effectiveness of Primary Health Care Through*

Nurse Practitioner/Family Physician Structured Collaborative Practice. University of Ottawa, Toronto.

Weintraub, J.A. (2011) Sustainable oral health interventions, *Journal of Public Health Dentistry*, **71** (Suppl 1), S95–6.

Whitman, L.A. & Whitman, J.W. (2006) *Improving Dental and Oral Care Services for Nursing Facility Residents*. The TRECS Institute. From http://www.thetrecsinstitute.org/downloads/DentalCare.pdf. Accessed April 14, 2014.

World Health Organization (2010) *Framework for Action on Interprofessional Education and Collaborative Practice*. Health Professions Networks Nursing and Midwifery Human Resources for Health. From http://whqlibdoc.who.int/hq/2010/WHO_HRH_HPN_10.3_eng.pdf. Accessed April 14, 2014.

Yakiwchuk, C.P., Bertone, M., Ghiabi, E., *et al.* (2013) Suction toothbrush use for dependent adults with dysphagia: a pilot examiner blind randomized clinical trial. *Canadian Journal of Dental Hygiene*, **47**(1), 15–23.

Yoon, M.N. & Steele, C.M. (2012) Health care professionals' perspectives on oral care for long-term care residents: nursing staff, speech-language pathologists and dental hygienists. *Gerodontology*, **29**(2), 525–35.

Appendix 19.1

Resources for Promoting Oral Health in Long-Term Care*

Comprehensive oral care education and training programs and materials for caregivers

- Australian Government (2009) *Better Oral Health in Residential Care Professional Portfolio: Oral Health Assessment Toolkit for Older People*. From http://www.health.gov.au/internet/main/publishing.nsf/Content/2E625F7A23ED6F71CA257BF0001B5D73/$File/ProfessionalPortfolio.pdf. Accessed April 14, 2014.
- British Columbia Dental Association. *Seniors Oral Health Care*. From http://www.bcdental.org/caregiverresources/. Accessed April 14, 2014.
- Dalhousie University. *Brushing Up on Mouth Care*. From http://www.ahprc.dal.ca/projects/oral-care/default.asp. Accessed April 14, 2014.
- Iowa Geriatric Education Center, The University of Iowa. *Best Practice Geriatric Oral Health Training*. From http://www.healthcare.uiowa.edu/igec/resources-educators-professionals/. Accessed April 14, 2014.
- Regional Geriatric Program Central Hamilton. *Oral Health Best Practices and Resource Tools*. From http://www.rgpc.ca/resource/index.cfm. Accessed April 14, 2014.
- Registered Nurses Association of Ontario. *Best Practices Toolkit; Resources: Oral Health*. http://ltctoolkit.rnao.ca/resources/oralcare#Policies-and-Procedures. Accessed April 14, 2014.

Other educational materials

- Faculty of Dentistry, University of Manitoba. Centre for Community Oral Health. From http://umanitoba.ca/dentistry/ccoh/ccoh_longTermCareFacts.html. Accessed April 14, 2014.
- Ohio Dental Association. *Smiles for Seniors Program*. From http://oda.org/community-involvement/smiles-for-seniors/. Accessed April 14, 2014.
- Special Care Co., Inc. *Parents and Caregivers*. From http://www.specializedcare.com/shop/pc/viewCategories.asp?idCategory=33. Accessed April 14, 2014.
- University of Maryland. *Elder Health Care*. From http://www.videopress.umaryland.edu/careelderly/mouthcare_CE606.html. Accessed April 14, 2014.

Geriatric textbooks

- Lamster, I.B. & Northridge, M.E. (eds.) (2008) *Improving Oral Health for the Elderly: An Interdisciplinary Approach*, Springer, New York.
- MacEntee, M.I. (ed.) (2011) *Oral Healthcare and the Frail Elder: A Clinical Perspective*, Blackwell Publishing Ltd., Ames, IA.
- Van der Horst, M.L. & Bowes, D. (2012) High-risk patients: the frail older adult living in long term care homes. In: *Comprehensive Preventive Dentistry* (ed. H. Limeback), pp. 330–57. Wiley-Blackwell Publishing, Ames, IA.

Continuing education training program for oral health professionals

- School of Dentistry, University of Minnesota. *Miniresidency in Nursing Home and Long-Term Care for the Dental Team*. From http://www.dentistry.umn.edu/dentalce/courses/nursing-home/index.htm. Accessed April 14, 2014.

Documents for oral health promotion guidelines in LTC

Australia

- Carter, K.D., Spencer, A.J., Wright, C., *et al.* (2009) *Caring for Oral Health in Australian Residential Care.* Dental Statistics And Research Series No. 48. Cat. No. DEN 193. AIHW, Canberra. From http://www.aihw.gov.au/publication-detail/?id=6442468243. Accessed April 14, 2014.

Canada

- British Columbia Dental Association (2011) *Oral Health Care Delivery in Residential Care Facilities: A Report of the Seniors' Oral Health Secretariat.* From http://www.bcdental.org/Dental_Health/Default.aspx?id=6202. Accessed April 14, 2014.
- Canadian Dental Association (2009) *Optimal Oral Health for Frail Older Adults: Best Practices along the Continuum of Care.* From https://www.cda-adc.ca/_files/dental_profession/practising/best_practices_seniors/optimal_oral_health_older_adults_2009.pdf. Accessed April 14, 2014.
- Registered Nurses Association of Ontario (2008) *Oral Health: Nursing Assessment and Interventions, Nursing Best Practice Guideline.* From http://rnao.ca/sites/rnao-ca/files/Oral_Health_-_Nursing_Assessment_and_Interventions.pdf. Accessed April 14, 2014.

UK

- British Society for Disability and Oral Health. Unlocking Barriers to Care. From http://bsdhwebsite.co.uk/index.php. Accessed April 14, 2014.
- Department of Health (2011) *Promoting Older People's Oral Health.* From http://rcnpublishing.com/userimages/ContentEditor/1373368451935/Promoting-older-peoples-oral-health.pdf. Accessed April 14, 2014.
- The Relatives and Residents Association (2009) *Keep Smiling: Dental Care and Oral Health for Older People in Care Homes.* From http://www.relres.org/products-resources/keep-smiling.html. Accessed April 14, 2014.

USA

- Johnson, V.B. & Chalmers, J. (2011) *Oral Hygiene Care for Functionally Dependent and Cognitively Impaired Older Adults.* University of Iowa College of Nursing, Iowa City, IA. Guideline Summary No. NGC-8700. From US Dept. of Health & Human Services, National Guideline Clearinghouse, http://guidelines.gov/content.aspx?id=34447. Accessed April 14, 2014.
- **TIP:** For US federal and state legislation, including dental service requirements, search the University of Minnesota Nursing Home Regulations website www.hpm.umn.edu/nhregsplus/. Search Justia.com to locate specific US legislation by topic.

Continuous care community examples

- Eden Alternative®: http://www.edenalt.org/. Accessed April 14, 2014.
- Schlegel Villages: http://schlegelvillages.com/node/395. Accessed April 14, 2014.
- The Greenhouse Project: http://thegreenhouseproject.org/. Accessed April 14, 2014.

*Web addresses current at time of publication.

Appendix 19.2

An Example of Oral Health Promotion Guidelines for a Long-Term Care Facility

Purpose

1 To promote and ensure resident-centred oral care for all.
2 To promote best practices in attaining optimal oral healthcare outcomes for long-term care (LTC) residents.
3 To support residents' health and quality of life by reducing negative health outcomes associated with compromised oral and overall health

Policy

1 The facility will ensure that all residents receive an oral health assessment on admission, quarterly, and with any change in oral health status or abilities.
2 All residents will have an individualized oral care plan in place based on the assessment.
3 Findings will be documented according to facility protocol using standardized oral assessment and planning tools.
4 Oral care will occur morning and evening, and more frequently if necessary.
5 Oral care will include: cleaning of any teeth present, any dentures and/or partials, gums, roof of the mouth, cheeks and tongue; and mouth moisturizing as needed.
6 Oral care products will be chosen based on assessment and best practice.
7 The facility will designate an oral health coordinator, preferably an oral health professional.
8 The facility will make arrangements to access oral health professionals for examinations, and oral care planning and treatment.
9 Caregiver training will be provided by or in consultation with oral health professionals.

Operational procedures

1 All residents will have an initial assessment of their immediate oral health needs completed within 24 hours of admission, followed by a complete oral health assessment prior to the initial care conference. Assessment will continue quarterly and with any changes in oral health status or abilities.
2 An oral care plan will be developed based on the assessment and will be easily accessible for staff reference.
3 The assessment will include the degree of independence regarding ability to perform daily mouth care.
4 The oral care plan will be reviewed and revised as needed, minimally on a quarterly basis, based on the current oral assessment.
5 The nurse will discuss on an on-going basis the purchase of recommended supplies and will document this discussion in the progress notes. Oral hygiene products will be replaced as needed due to loss, wear or illness.
6 Any concerns identified during the assessment or the revision to the care plan will be discussed collaboratively by the appropriate members of the Interprofessional Team.
7 Staff will support independent oral care for residents who are able. Staff will supervise the resident if the resident is able to complete oral care independently but is assessed as being at risk for aspiration.
8 Staff will assist with oral care as needed at a minimum of twice daily for residents who need cuing and/or some assistance.
9 Staff will complete all aspects of oral care (cleaning of the gums, teeth, dentures and partials, roof of the mouth, cheeks and tongue; and mouth moisturizing as needed) at a minimum of twice daily for residents who need total assistance with oral care.
10 Staff will conduct a weekly visual oral inspection as a resident's oral health status and abilities can change over a short period of time.
11 Prior to initiating oral care, staff will be familiar with the current care plan, and be aware of the resident's cognitive status, any responsive behaviors, communication needs, sensory and functional impairments and dysphagia.
12 New gloves will be worn for each resident when providing or assisting with routine oral care. Other personal protective equipment will be used as needed.
13 Cleaned and rinsed oral hygiene tools, especially toothbrushes, will be stored open to the air.
14 Dentures (full and partial) and other oral hygiene tools will be labeled for identification.

Education

1 Facilities will offer education on oral health, common oral concerns, and daily mouth care during orientation and at a minimum of every 2 years to staff who are providing oral care to residents.

2 Common oral concerns to be addressed include: pain/discomfort, dental caries, gingivitis and periodontal disease, soft tissue lesions of the lips and oral cavity that do not heal, broken or ill-fitting dentures, xerostomia, halitosis, and oral infections such as candidiasis.

Professional dental care

1 Routine and emergent dental care will be provided in consultation with the resident and their family/guardian.
2 Residents will be assisted in obtaining dental assessments and treatment from oral health professionals on-site or through a community dental office.
3 Facilities will ensure that staff are aware of the process for consulting oral health professionals.

Modified with permission from Winnipeg Regional Health Authority Oral Care Directives Draft 2012, MB, Canada.

Appendix 19.3

University of Manitoba Oral Health Assessment Worksheet

UM CCOH Oral Health Assessment Worksheet

Client name:

Completed by: Date:

Natural Teeth Circle or highlight all that apply	Upper	All teeth Some missing Root tips No teeth
	Lower	All teeth Some missing Root tips No teeth

Dentures Circle or highlight all that apply	Upper	Full Partial Not worn No denture Name on denture
	Lower	Full Partial Not worn No denture Name on denture

Factors Affecting Daily Mouth Care

☐ ADL: independent

☐ ADL: some assistance

☐ ADL: fully dependent

☐ Physical issues (i.e. mobility, balance, dexterity, facial paralysis)

☐ Responsive behaviours (i.e. refusal, biting, grabbing, pushing)

Circle or mark any areas of concern

Oral Assessment Timing: Admission   Quarterly Assessment   1   2   3   4   Other: _____

Use the highest # recorded to score each category

Instructions: Circle or highlight all conditions that apply in all categories; A-H findings of 'Moderate' and 'High Oral Health Risk' require follow-up; I and J impact upon oral care and health.

Category	Low Oral Health Risk = 0	Moderate Oral Health Risk = 1	High Oral Health Risk = 2	Score
A. Lips	Smooth, pink, moist	Dry, chapped, or red at corners	White/red/ulcerated patch; swelling or lump; bleeding/ulcerated at corners	0 - 1 - 2
B. Tongue	Normal texture, pink, moist	Patchy, fissured, red, lightly coated	White/red/ulcerated area; smooth, swelling/lump; heavily coated	0 - 1 - 2
C. Gums and Tissues	Pink, moist, no bleeding	Localized: 1-2 areas with red, swollen or bleeding gums, one mouth ulcer, one sore spot under denture	Generalized: red, swollen, bleeding gums, loose teeth, abscess on gum; white/red/ulcerated area; red/sores under dentures	0 - 1 - 2
D. Saliva	Moist tissues; watery, free flowing saliva	Dry, sticky tissues; saliva reduced/thick	Tissues parched and red; very little/no saliva present	0 - 1 - 2
E. Natural Teeth	No decayed or broken teeth/roots	1-2 decayed or broken teeth/roots	3+ decayed or broken teeth/roots, very worn down teeth; fewer than 10 teeth and no dentures	0 - 1 - 2
F. Dentures	Dentures have no broken areas or teeth; worn regularly; removed daily	Denture has 1 broken area/tooth; worn 1-2 hours/day	Denture has more than 1 broken area/tooth; poor fit/worn with adhesive, never worn or missing	0 - 1 - 2
G. Oral Cleanliness	Clean, no food particles/plaque/tartar in mouth/on teeth or on dentures	Localized: food particles/plaque/tartar in 1-2 areas in mouth/on teeth or 1-2 areas on dentures; bad breath	Generalized: food particles/plaque/tartar in most areas in mouth/on teeth or on most of dentures; severe bad breath	0 - 1 - 2
H. Dental Pain	No verbal, behavioral, or physical signs of oral pain	Reports or shows signs of pain such as pulling at face, chewing lips, not eating, aggression	Reports or shows signs of pain; physical signs present such as abscess on gum, facial swelling, broken teeth, large ulcers	0 - 1 - 2
I. Swallowing	No swallowing problems	Some choking, pain or difficulty on swallowing	Unable to swallow	0 - 1 - 2
J. Cognitive Status	No cognitive impairment; able to communicate; typically able to do mouth care independently	Early to mid stage of dementia; some difficulty communicating; typically requires prompting and cuing for mouth care	End stage dementia; significant difficulty communicating; typically requires provision of mouth care	0 - 1 - 2

Follow-up:	Completed		Level of Mouth Care Assistance Required	Score Total
☐ Complete oral hygiene daily care plan and begin daily mouth care	☐		☐ Remind and encourage—prompt & cue	/20
☐ Refer for dental consult to: _____	☐		☐ Assist—help as needed	
☐ Refer to _____ for: _____	☐		☐ Provide—total mouth and denture care	
☐ Discuss concerns with: _____	☐		☐ Palliative—oral comfort measures	
☐ Review client's oral health again on (date): _____	☐			

FACULTY OF DENTISTRY
SCHOOL OF DENTAL HYGIENE
Centre for Community Oral Health
Adapted from Chalmers 2004 OHAT
Version: September 2013

Appendix 19.4

University of Manitoba Fact Sheet: Basic Mouth Care: Caring for Those With Natural Teeth

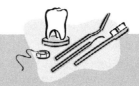

BASIC MOUTH CARE
Caring for those with natural teeth

Daily mouth care:
- Moisturize lips
- Do visual mouth check
- Brush teeth and gums for 2 minutes am & pm, especially before bed
- Clean between the teeth if resident is able to cooperate
- Clean tongue and all mouth tissues

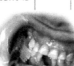

You will need:
- Gloves, cup & water
- Towel & face cloth or 4x4 gauze
- Water-based lip lubricant
- Soft small-headed toothbrush with large rubberized handle (option: two brushes, one to brush, one to prop using handle)
- Toothpaste or gel with fluoride
- Other *helpers*: proxabrush, end tuft brush, suction brush, floss, floss-piks, tongue cleaner, disposable mouth prop, professionally recommended products

Label all supplies with resident's name

Step-by-step brushing
- **Individualize mouth care.** Consider the resident's medical (e.g. dementia), oral (e.g. dry mouth), positioning (e.g. dysphagia), and mobility (e.g. in wheelchair) issues.
- **Wear well-fitting new gloves for mouth care.** Wear a mask and protective eyewear if there is a risk of splatter. Place a towel under the resident's chin.
- **Lubricate lips** before and after for comfort and to prevent cracking.
  Note: petroleum-based products increase the risk of aspiration pneumonia, and weaken the gloves.
- **Retract lips & cheeks** with toothbrush for initial look; never place fingers between teeth.
  If needed for access, use a mouth prop or handle of second toothbrush.
- **Remove any pocketed food and look for any obvious problems.** Record any findings.
- **Brush at gumline in small circles using a pea-size of toothpaste.** Moisten brush in water. Aim bristles where the teeth and gums meet and follow a routine that includes all surfaces.
  For those with swallowing issues, use 1/2 a pea-size of non-foaming toothpaste or gel with fluoride.
- **Encourage resident to spit or use gauze or a clean moist cloth to wipe tissues/teeth.**
  'Mopping as you go' and no rinsing decreases aspiration risks and increases contact with fluoride. Suction toothbrushes are very effective in controlling fluids and debris.
- **Clean all mouth tissues** with toothbrush. Clean tongue—start at the back & move forward.
  Bacteria on the tongue is the major cause of BAD BREATH. Try a tongue cleaner.
- **Rinse toothbrush, tap to remove excess water, and store standing up to dry.**
  Storing in a closed space/container encourages bacterial growth.
- **Replace toothbrush** when bristles are worn/splayed or if resident is ill *(virus, herpes, candidiasis/thrush, etc.)*. *Immunocompromised individuals should have their toothbrushes replaced more frequently (cancer care, HIV, transplant, dialysis, etc.).*

Cleaning between for residents able to cooperate
- Use a *proxabrush* in spaces/gaps between teeth. Insert the small cone-shaped brush and use an in-and-out horizontal motion to remove plaque & food debris. An *end-tuft brush is* good for cleaning around the gum line and between. Disposable *floss-piks* are a good alternative to finger flossing.
- For dental implants—ask an oral health professional for cleaning tips.

If gums bleed... they are infected & need your help!
With effective daily mouth care, bleeding gums should heal within 2 weeks;
if still bleeding, refer.

Revised September 2013
M Bertone, ME Wener, CP Yakiwchuk

FACULTY OF
DENTISTRY
SCHOOL OF
DENTAL HYGIENE

Centre for Community Oral Health

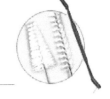

Appendix 19.5

University of Manitoba Fact Sheet: Basic Mouth Care – Caring For Those With Dentures/False Teeth/No Teeth

BASIC MOUTH CARE
Caring for those with dentures / false teeth / no teeth

Daily mouth care:

- Moisturize lips
- Do visual mouth & denture check
- Remove & clean dentures am & pm
- Clean mouth tissues and tongue
- Soak dentures in disinfectant daily
- Keep dentures out at night or 4-6 hours/day

Denture adhesives: use zinc-free products; powdered adhesives are preferred; avoid oozing creams for those with swallowing issues.

Denture tablets: have caused allergic reaction.

For safety, store tablets out of resident's reach!

You will need:

- Gloves, towel, cup & water
- Water-based lip lubricant
- 4x4 gauze or face cloth
- Soft toothbrush
- Denture brush (2 headed) & denture cup
- Liquid soap for dentures or denture paste
- Commercial disinfecting denture cleaner
- *Other options:* tongue cleaner, clasp brush for partials

Label all supplies & dentures with resident's name

Step-by-step denture care

- **Individualize mouth care.** Consider the resident's medical (e.g. dementia), oral (e.g. dry mouth), positioning (e.g. dysphagia), and mobility (e.g. in wheelchair) issues
- **Wear new gloves.** Wear a mask and protective eyewear if risk of splatter. Place towel under chin.
- **Lubricate lips** before and after for comfort and to prevent cracking. *Note: petroleum-based products increase the risk of aspiration pneumonia and weaken gloves.*
- **Line the sink** with a towel to prevent breakage if dropped.
- **Remove complete denture.** Ask resident to remove, or use a rocking motion to break the seal. *Tip: ask resident to blow with lips closed to help break suction.* **Remove partial denture.** Place thumbnails under clasps and carefully lift out so as not to bend the clasps or injure tissues.
- **Rinse dentures with cool water** to remove debris. *Hot water can warp dentures.*
- **Thoroughly brush all surfaces** using liquid soap or denture paste and a denture brush; rinse well after. Remove adhesives daily to prevent infection. *Note: use the small brush to clean the tissue side of the denture. Clean metal clasps gently with soft toothbrush or by twirling clasp brush.*
- **Disinfect dentures** daily by soaking in a commercial denture cleaner, preferably at night after brushing to remove stain, bacteria and prevent infection. After disinfecting, rinse thoroughly under running water for 1 minute before replacing. *When placing dentures in mouth, tissues should be wet for retention; replace the upper denture before the lower one. Although not ideal, if using denture cleaners is a safety issue, following cleaning, dentures may be soaked in cool water or air dried over night. Note that water does not reduce bacteria and if air drying, any remaining debris will become hard and difficult to remove.*

Mouth tissue care

- **Retract lips & cheeks** with gloved fingers or toothbrush; never place fingers between teeth.
- **Clean and massage all mouth tissues**–cheeks, gums, roof & floor of mouth–using gauze, face cloth or soft toothbrush.
- **Clean tongue** with soft toothbrush from the back to the tip using large, sweeping strokes. *Bacteria on the tongue is the major cause of BAD BREATH. Try a tongue cleaner.*
- **Rinse brushes with warm water, tap to remove excess water, and stand up to dry.** *Don't store used brushes in a closed space or container as they will grow bacteria. Clean & air dry denture cup daily.*
- **Replace brushes** when bristles are worn and splayed or if resident is ill (virus, herpes, candidiasis/thrush, etc.). *Immuno-compromised individuals should have their brushes replaced more frequently (cancer care, HIV, transplant, dialysis, etc.)*

Note:

- For a poorly fitting denture or one with heavy deposits, make a dental referral.
- Dry mouth will make denture retention more difficult. Try a mouth moisturizer.

FACULTY OF
DENTISTRY
SCHOOL OF
DENTAL HYGIENE
Centre for Community Oral Health

Revised September 2013
M Bertone, ME Wener, CP Yakiwchuk

CHAPTER 20

Dental Professionals as Part of an Interdisciplinary Team

Teresa E. Johnson[1], Jayne E. Cernohous[2], Paul Mulhausen[3], and Deborah A. Jacobi[4]

[1]Apple Tree Dental, Minneapolis, MN, USA
[2]Department of Dental Hygiene, Metropolitan State University, St. Paul, MN, USA
[3]Telligen, West Des Moines, IA, USA
[4]Helping Services for Northeast Iowa, Decorah, IA, USA

Introduction

This chapter is divided into three sections. The first reviews the relationship between oral health and systemic health starting with a brief history of the focal infection theory of disease and then addressing our current understanding of the oral health–overall health connection in older adults, including an overview of a number of oral and medical conditions that have the potential for interaction and association. There is a growing body of literature supporting this important linkage, which emphasizes the importance of an interprofessional healthcare approach to caring for our aging population. The second section addresses the value of an interprofessional team approach to address the physical, medical, dental, psychologic, social, and nutritional needs of older adults. In addition, strategies and opportunities for dental professionals (DPs) to collaborate and engage others in interprofessional care for their elderly patients are included, as well as suggestions for enhancing effective consultations between DPs and other health professionals. The third section of this chapter will present the growing interest in exploring workforce solutions to improve access to care and help meet the dental care needs of the elderly and other age groups. New mid-level providers, with expanded clinical skill sets, can expand the available dental workforce and also participate on the interprofessional care team.

THE ORAL HEALTH–OVERALL HEALTH RELATIONSHIP

Historical retrospective: focal infection theory of disease

The relationship between oral health and overall health is not a new concept. In fact, the relationship between oral and systemic disease has been discussed for more than a century. In an 1891 *Dental Cosmos* report, American physician and dentist Willoughby D. Miller, who at the time was working in Robert Koch's laboratory in Berlin, coined the term "focus of infection" and implicated oral microorganisms in the etiology of systemic diseases such as brain abscesses, gastric disorders, and pulmonary diseases (Miller, 1891). Similarly, in 1900, British physician William Hunter published a report attributing oral infections to several systemic diseases such as obscure fevers, anemia, numerous nervous system disturbances, gastritis, colitis, chronic rheumatic infections, and kidney diseases. Later, in 1911, he gave a speech implicating poor dental health and oral infections, brought on by poorly made or ill-fitting dental prostheses, to systemic disease (Barnett, 2006; Pallasch & Wah, 2003; Reimann & Havens, 1940; Rhein, 1912). In the USA, American physician Frank Billings promoted his own theories regarding focus of infection and systemic health affects. In 1909 he reported that 4 of 12 patients with infective endocarditis (IE),

Geriatric Dentistry: Caring for Our Aging Population, First Edition. Edited by Paula K. Friedman.
© 2014 John Wiley & Sons, Inc. Published 2014 by John Wiley & Sons, Inc.
Companion website: www.wiley.com/go/friedman/geriatricdentistry

whose blood cultures yielded streptococci, had a history of tonsillitis or alveolar abscesses shortly before cardiac symptoms began. He proposed a relationship between endocarditis, bacteremia, and oral focal infections (Gibbons, 1998).

Billings introduced the focal infection theory in 1912. He explained that systemic diseases occurred when bacteria from a focus of infection disseminate through the blood stream or lymphatic system to distant organs. Billings proposed that foci of infection usually occur in the head, with tonsils and teeth particularly vulnerable, since the mouth and airways are subject to frequent microbial exposure (Gibbons, 1998). He attributed oropharyngeal foci of infection to pathologies such as arthritis and nephritis, and advocated tonsillectomies and the extraction of teeth to cure those maladies. With the support of prominent physicians of the time and acceptance within the dental community, the focal infection theory of disease (FITD) lead to the removal of millions of tonsils, adenoids, and teeth over the ensuing years (Pallasch & Wahl, 2003).

This dramatic approach to managing mouth and pharyngeal infections to prevent systemic diseases wasn't without its detractors in the scientific community. By the 1930s, the popularity of the FITD waned. An influential publication in 1940 questioned the FITD-driven removal of tonsils and teeth, citing several concerns – namely, that the FITD had not been proven and its infectious etiology remained unknown; that individuals often continued to experience symptoms of the original diseases for which their teeth and or tonsils were removed; and that large numbers of individuals having had tonsils removed, were no better off than individuals who retained their tonsils (Pallasch & Wahl, 2003; Reimann & Havens, 1940). In addition to the lack of scientific support for the removal of teeth based on the influences of the FITD, a number of other factors contributed to a decrease in performing extraction of teeth in the second half of the 20th century. These factors included the discovery of penicillin and other antibiotics; advances in diagnosis, treatment and management of periodontal disease as well as increasingly predictable endodontic techniques; improved and expanded restorative options; growing personal preferences to retain teeth; and dental insurance availability.

Despite the de-emphasis of the FITD by the mid-1900s, advances in scientific inquiry and clinical research methods acknowledged situations where oral bacteria could affect distant organs and tissue, such as IE in susceptible individuals (Barnett, 2006). Similar examples would be streptococcal pharyngitis and acute rheumatic fever and in rare cases, orthopedic prosthetic joint infections (OPJIs) or brain abscesses with oral bacteria isolates. A 2003 review of focal infection described IE, brain abscess, and OPJI as the three most documented, publicized, and litigated examples of focal infection (Pallasch & Wahl, 2003).

Current understanding: the mouth–body connection

In recent years there has been renewed interest in the associations between oral and systemic health, which justifies continued advocacy for expanded interprofessional health collaboration among the various health disciplines. Dr. David Satcher, 16th US Surgeon General, when announcing the release of *Oral Health In America: A Report of the Surgeon General*, said: "In the past half-century, we have come to recognize that the mouth is a mirror of the body, it is a sentinel of disease, and it is critical to overall health and well-being" (US Department of Health and Human Services, 2000). Several oral–systemic health interrelationships are relevant in the management of older adults' health. There are oral diseases and conditions that influence systemic health as well as systemic diseases and conditions that affect oral health (Griffin *et al.*, 2012). Likewise, treatments used to cure or manage various conditions can affect oral or systemic health, or both. Citing the example of chronic inflammatory diseases to other conditions, Iacopino wrote, "The human body is a single unit composed of related biologic processes such that abnormalities of almost any of its parts have profound effects on other body parts and processes" (Iacopino, 2009).

Oral diseases and conditions known to affect overall health include periodontal disease, poor oral hygiene, tooth loss, and untreated intraoral infections. Intraoral infections can lead to facial and periorbital cellulitis and subsequent brain abscesses, cellulitis within facial planes of the neck compromising the airway, sinusitis, and bacteremia capable of harm at distant sites. The consequences of untreated or poorly managed oral conditions such as dental decay, oral pain, tooth loss, loss of oral function, oral malodor, and esthetically compromised dentition can affect the elderly by way of social stigma, decreased self-confidence, isolation, and depression. The following paragraphs describe a number of conditions that reflect the relationship between oral health and systemic health. These examples illustrate the importance of interprofessional education and collaboration in working to improve the health of our aging population.

Oral and system conditions – interrelationships

Periodontal disease

Periodontal disease has received considerable attention the past two decades as a possible contributing factor to, or as having some association with the following systemic conditions: diabetes, metabolic syndrome, coronary artery disease and atherosclerosis, stroke, and chronic obstructive pulmonary disease. The proposed mechanisms for these associations are complex and beyond the scope of this chapter. (See Chapter 11 for further discussion of periodontal disease.) Yet, it is appreciated that periodontal diseases and systemic conditions share similar risk or modifying factors such as smoking, stress, aging, race or ethnicity, male gender (Li *et al.*, 2000), chronic inflammation, and genetics. Diabetics with periodontal disease have greater difficulty with glycemic control, further complicating the management of this metabolic disease.

Current knowledge suggests that oral inflammatory processes and inflammatory mediators produced in response to periodontal infections are significantly involved in the associations between periodontal disease and cardiovascular disease (CVD), atherosclerosis and stroke. Periodontal bacteria, such as *Porphyromonas gingivalis,* and bacterial byproducts, such as lipopolysaccharides, travel hematologically and cause harmful effects to heart and blood vessels (Babu & Gomes, 2011). According to the American Dental Association (ADA), investigations have demonstrated an association between periodontal

disease, atherosclerotic vascular disease, heart disease, and stroke, but they have not demonstrated a periodontal disease causal relationship for CVD (Lockart *et al.*, 2012). While supporting the ADA's position, the American Academy of Periodontology (AAP) suggests that this should not decrease concerns about the impact of periodontal diseases on cardiovascular health (AAP, 2012).

Tooth loss and edentulism

While complete edentulism (the loss of all natural teeth) has declined across US age groups over the past several decades, there are socioeconomic, ethnic, age, and state of residence differences in edentulous rates (CDC, 2003; Wu *et al.*, 2012; and see Chapter 1, Aging). In the USA, approximately 25% of adults aged over 65 are edentulous (CDC, 2011). Tooth loss has been linked to heart disease, stroke-related and CVD deaths, atherosclerotic plaque formation in carotid arteries, and angina pectoris; in addition to higher fasting plasma glucose, cholesterol, and blood pressure (Holmlund & Lind, 2012; Lee *et al.*, 2010; Okoro *et al.*, 2005; Watt *et al.*, 2012; Ylöstalo *et al.*, 2006).

Other reported associations between tooth loss and poorer general health include nephropathy, poor oral hygiene, cancer, and neurologic diseases (Tramini *et al.*, 2007). Ten years of longitudinal data of 144 elderly religious women of the School Sisters of Notre Dame, Milwaukee, Wisconsin, ranging in age from 75 to 98 years, demonstrated that those with the fewest teeth had the highest risk of dementia prevalence and incidence (Stein *et al.*, 2007). These religious women belonged to a much larger and still ongoing "Nun Study," a longitudinal study of Alzheimer's disease and aging involving 678 American members of the School Sisters of Notre Dame religious congregation.

Associations between edentulism and health outcomes such as malnutrition, poor quality of life, and mortality necessitate interprofessional collaboration. Tooth loss negatively impacts nutrition as fewer natural teeth coincide with decreasing fruit, fiber, dark green and orange vegetable intake, and lower serum levels of beta carotene, folate, and vitamin C (Nowjack-Raymer & Shelham, 2003; Savoca *et al.*, 2010). Persistent vitamin B complex and vitamin C deficiencies result in oral soft tissue changes. Multiple US and international studies have shown a relationship between tooth loss and early mortality while controlling for confounding factors (Anasi *et al.*, 2010; Brown, 2009; Padilha *et al.*, 2008).

Aspiration pneumonia

Aspiration of oropharyngeal bacteria has been shown to cause nosocomial pneumonia in older adults (Russell *et al.*, 1999). Frail elderly residing in long-term care facilities or admitted to the hospital are at considerable risk for aspiration pneumonia (AP) (Pace & McCullough, 2010). El-Solh and colleagues investigated the association between dental plaque colonization and lower respiratory tract infection in hospitalized long-term care elders. For some who developed pneumonia, their dental plaque pathogens matched those isolated from their lungs, implicating dental plaque bacteria and poor oral hygiene to cases of AP (El-Solh *et al.*, 2004). Since AP is a significant cause of morbidity and death in frail elderly (Tada & Miura, 2012), improved oral hygiene may be protective and play an important preventive role (van der Maarel-Wierink *et al.*, 2013). (Editorial Comment: This reinforces the importance of the discussion of oral health care in long-term care facilities, discussed in Chapters 17 and 19.) The use of oral antiseptic agents such as chlorhexidine or povidone-iodine has shown beneficial effects in the prevention of ventilator-associated pneumonia (Labeau *et al.*, 2011). Scannapieco reported that in two studies using either 0.12% chlorhexidine rinses or 0.2% chlorhexidine gel applications twice daily on patients in hospital intensive care units, the incidence of pneumonia was 60% lower than control groups. Scannapieco noted that the association of poor oral health and periodontal disease to community-acquired pneumonia appears to be minimal (Scannapieco, 2006).

Peptic ulcer disease

Oral health status has been linked to peptic ulcer disease. *Helicobacter pylori*, a spiral gram-negative organism, is involved in the pathogenesis of gastritis as well as peptic and duodenal ulcer disease; however, only a small percentage of persons infected by *H. pylori* develop gastrointestinal ulcers (Namiot, *et al.*, 2006). The observation of *H. pylori* in association with dental plaque has implicated the oral environment as one of many potential pathways for *H. pylori* transmission (Eskandari *et al.*, 2010). There have been conflicting

results worldwide as to the relationship between *H. pylori* found in dental plaque with gastric *H. pylori* infection, and the uncertainties continue. Navabi *et al.* (2011) evaluated all published papers since 2000 found through international databases and narrowed the eligible papers to 23 that met specific quality requirements. A meta-analysis of those reports, involving 1861 patients, found that the prevalence of co-infection with gastric and dental plaque *H. pylori* was 50%; however, the authors conclude insufficient evidence exists to suggest the efficacy of dental treatment and dental plaque control to the prevention of recurrent gastric *H. pylori* infection (Navabi, *et al.*, 2011). Gebrara *et al.* (2006) looked for the persistence of *H. pylori* in the oral cavity after systemic eradication using triple systemic antibiotic therapy in patients positive for gastric *H. pylori*. They reported that 18 (60%) of the 30 patients with gingivitis or chronic periodontitis who received the antibiotic therapy continued to harbor *H. pylori* in their mouths. The authors concluded that the mouths of patients with gingivitis or chronic periodontitis who have *H. pylori* in their stomachs may be reservoirs for the bacteria (Gebrara *et al.*, 2006).

Therapeutics and treatments affecting oral health, systemic health, or both

Unintended adverse drug reactions (ADRs) are known to occur in every organ system in the body and are often mistaken for objective signs of underlying disease (Abdollahi *et al.*, 2008). Dentists administering or prescribing medications should be mindful of ADRs. Drugs interacting with drugs can enhance or diminish the effects of drugs taken alone, thereby causing potential harmful effects. A discussion about the ADRs of most concern in dentistry is available in a recently published review (Becker, 2011). Drug-related problems are common in older adults and cause considerable morbidity (Hajjar *et al.*, 2011), including oral reactions such as xerostomia, opportunistic infections such as *Candida albicans*, stomatitis, dysgeusia, glossitis, gingival hyperplasia, discolored teeth (Smith & Burtner, 1994), and osteonecrosis of the jaw (Pazianas *et al.*, 2007). Two recent publications provide a comprehensive discussion and listing of drug-induced oral reactions and side effects. Table 20.1 provides an abbreviated summary (Abdollahi *et al.*, 2008; Kalmar *et al.*, 2012). Drug-related oral problems impact seniors' quality of life, cause pain and discomfort,

Table 20.1 Common oral side effects associated with drugs or drug classes

Oral manifestations	Drugs/classes of drugs
Ulceration and mucositis	NSAIDs (naproxen, salicylates, indomethacin, etc.)
	Antineoplastics (doxorubicin, methotrexate, 5-fluorouracil, etc.)
	Propranolol, spironolactone, thiazides, alendronate, phenytoin, captopril, methyldopa, barbiturates, sulfonamides, tetracyclines, etc.
Xerostomia	Antidepressants, antipsychotics, anticholinergics, antihypertensives, antihistamines, decongestants
Gingival enlargement	Calcium channel blockers (diltiazem, amlodipine, bepridil, nifedipine, verapamil, etc.)
	Dihydropyridines (bleomycin)
	Cyclosporine, sodium valproate, phenytoin
Pigmenation	Antimalarials (chloroquine, hydrochloroquine, quinidine, etc.)
	Tranquilizers (chlorpromazine)
	Amiodarone, busulfan, clofazimine, estrogen, ketoconazole, minocycline, zidovudine, etc.
Swelling	Ace inhibitors, penicillins, sulfa drugs, aspirin
Vesiculobullus or ulcerative lesions	*Lichen planus-like:*
	Antimalarials, arsenicals, beta-blockers
	Several other drugs such as: allopurinol, furosemide, chlorothiazide, methyldopa, lorazepam, cimetidine, dapsone, propranolol, phenothiazines, spironolactone, sulfonylureas, tetracycline, tolbutamide, lithium, and many more
	Erythema multiforme-like:
	Antibiotics (antimalarials, penicillins, sulfonamides, tetracyclines)
	Other drugs: allopurinol, NSAIDS, barbiturates, protease inhibitors
	Lupus erythematosus-like:
	Hydantoins, thiouracils
	Other drugs: isoniazid, lithium, methyldopa, quinidine, reserpine, trimethodone, carbamazepine, griseofulvin, hydralazine, etc.
	Pemphigoid-like:
	Antirheumatics (ibuprofen, penicillamine, phenacetin)
	Antibiotics (penicillins, sulfonamides)
	Cardiovascular drugs (furosemide, captopril, clonidine)
	Antimicrobials
	Thiol-containing drugs and sulfonamide derivatives
	Pemphigus-like:
	Several drugs such as: ibuprofen, phenobarbital, propranolol, rifampin, ampicillin, cephalexin, captopril, heroin, etc.

*Table created from information provided by Kalmar *et al.*, 2012.
NSAIDs, nonsterodial anti-inflammatory drugs.

affect chewing, swallowing and nutritional intake, and diminish oral hygiene efficacy.

Drug-induced salivary hypofunction

Salivary hypofunction resulting in dry mouth or "xerostomia" is not caused by aging per se; rather, it is an age-associated acquired oral phenomena. Xerostomia in older adults is attributed primarily to the effects of polypharmacy associated with the management of multiple chronic illnesses, and attributed less so,

to various systemic diseases. There are more than 500 medications associated with xerostomia (Kalmar *et al.*, 2012). In addition to the subjective symptom of dry mouth, xerostomia negatively impacts oral health and increases oral disease risks (Moore & Guggenheimer, 2008). As discussed elsewhere in this book (Chapter 14, Xerostomia), problems associated with xerostomia in the elderly include root and coronal caries, periodontal disease, gingival inflammation, decreased debris clearance, difficulties with food bolus preparation and

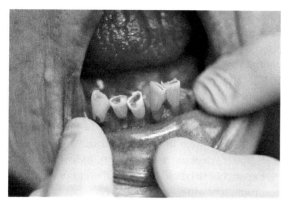

Figure 20.1 Clinical manifestations of xerostomia. Rampant root caries and coronal caries resulting in unsupported and fractured enamel of mandibular anterior teeth. Note the dry, fissured tongue in the background. Photograph courtesy of Teresa E. Johnson, DDS.

swallowing, susceptibility to denture sores and stomatitis, among others. Figure 20.1 illustrates dry mouth in an elderly woman with concomitant coronal and root caries.

Herbal supplements

While not considered drugs by the US Food and Drug Administration (Meredith, 2001), herbal supplements, such as St. John's wort, are associated with xerostomia. Other oral manifestations attributed to various herbs include gingival bleeding (feverfew, ginkgo); aphthous ulcers, lip and tongue irritation, and swelling (feverfew); oral and lingual dyskinesia (kava); numbness of tongue (echinacea); and hypersalivation (yohimbe) (Abebe, 2003). Herbal supplements interact with other drugs by altering inflammatory and immune responses, interacting with blood clotting processes and altering enzymatic drug metabolizing activities (Meredith, 2001).

Zinc-containing denture adhesives

Dental professionals should educate their denture-wearing patients about the potential problems associated with zinc-containing denture adhesives, and remind patients to avoid or minimize their use. Excessive zinc is known to cause copper deficiency myelopathy affecting walking and balance, widespread sensory and motor neuropathies, anemia, and

bone marrow depression (Crown & May, 2012; Doherty *et al.*, 2011; Nations *et al.*, 2008; Tezvergil-Mutluay *et al.*, 2010). The effects of zinc in denture adhesives should be communicated to other health professionals so that, if denture-wearing patients present to healthcare providers with these symptoms and conditions, the possibility of zinc toxicity from denture adhesives can be considered among differential diagnoses.

Head and neck radiation therapy

Radiation therapy to treat head and neck cancer can result in limited mouth opening and reduced oral motor function, diminished salivary gland function, and subsequent xerostomia and oral mucositis. Mucositis, consisting of erythematous and ulcerative lesions, is an unavoidable and undesirable effect of radiotherapy, and causes pain, dysphasia and decreased oral intake that adversely affects nutrition and quality of life, and contributes to local and systemic infections. The most severe cases of radiation-induced oral mucositis are associated with radiation to primary tumors in the oral cavity and oro- or nasopharynx. It can manifest with concomitant radiation and chemotherapy, or when the total radiation dose is greater than 5000 centigray (Kumar *et al.*, 2009).

Antiresorptive drugs and osteonecrosis of the jaw

Antiresorptive agents, such as bisphosphonates, and denosumab, a nonbisphosphonate antiresorptive agent, are prescribed to strengthen bones and prevent bone fractures in susceptible individuals, especially those with osteoporosis. Long-term use of bisphosphonates is associated with diminished blood supply to the jaw and subsequent development of osteonecrosis of the jaw (ONJ). It has also been called "bisphosphonate-associated osteonecrosis" or "bisphosphonate-related ONJ." A 2010 report described a 65-year-old woman who developed ONJ while receiving denosumab for the management of a giant cell tumor (Aghaloo *et al.*, 2010). Subsequently, the ADA Council on Scientific Affairs recommended the term "antiresorptive agent-induced osteonecrosis of the jaw" (ARONJ) since it encompasses both bisphosphonate and denosumab-associated ONJ (Hellstein *et al.*, 2011).

Bisphosphonates are prescribed to prevent and treat conditions associated with bone fragility such as osteoporosis, osteitis deformans (Paget's disease), bone metastasis, and multiple myeloma. Given to arrest bone loss, increase bone density and decrease the risk of pathologic fracture resulting from progressive bone loss, bisphosphonates prevent or slow the loss of bone mass by inhibiting osteoclasts, the bone destroying cells (Little *et al.*, 2008). Denosumab, a human monoclonal antibody, interferes with osteoclast activation and diminishes osteoclast activity. Unlike bisphosphonates, which accumulate in the mineralized bone matrix to an extent reflective of the duration and type of therapy, denosumab does not incorporate into bone and has a substantially lower terminal half-life (Adler & Gill, 2011). Denosumab is administered to treat osteoporosis in postmenopausal women at high risk of bone fractures and to prevent skeletal fractures in persons with bone metastases (Hellstein *et al.*, 2011).

Agent-induced osteonecrosis of the jaw may occur spontaneously or develop when dental conditions or procedures likely to cause trauma to alveolar bone occur. Most commonly, ARONJ is associated with invasive procedures affecting the alveolar bone such as tooth extractions (Hellstein *et al.*, 2011). The exact mechanisms leading to ARONJ remains unknown, but seem to result from the interchange of bone metabolism, local trauma, heightened demand for bone repair, infection, and hypovascularity (Little *et al.*, 2008). ARONJ is associated with discomfort, local inflammation, and possible infection, including a potentially deleterious impact on quality of life. In most cases it never resolves and is managed palliatively or with antimicrobial therapy. In severe cases, jaw fractures occur or jaw resection may be indicated. Therefore, DPs must encourage older adults to achieve optimal oral health before starting antiresorptive therapy whenever possible through patient education and interprofessional communication with physicians, geriatricians and oncologists. It is imperative that DPs' health history forms include questions on antiresorptive drug use to identify patients at risk for ARONJ.

Systemic diseases affecting oral health

Systemic conditions of the elderly that purportedly influence oral health status include diabetes, neurodegenerative diseases, osteoporosis, acquired autoimmune diseases, and depression. Uncontrolled diabetes affects oral health by exacerbating periodontal infections, interfering with wound healing, and diminishing intraoral pain perception (Saini *et al.*, 2011). The neuromuscular deficits associated with neurodegenerative diseases such as Parkinson's disease (PD) and multiple sclerosis make it difficult to maintain plaque control and oral health; and the medications to treat them diminish saliva flow (Fiske *et al.*, 2002; Friedlander *et al.*, 2009). Individuals with PD experience decreased oral proprioception affecting occlusion, chewing, and food clearance as well as adaptability to removable prostheses (Friedlander *et al.*, 2009).

Osteoporosis is known to affect alveolar bone height in edentulous patients (Hildebolt, 1997; Kossioni & Dontas, 2007). Autoimmune diseases such as lupus erythematosus and Sjögren's syndrome are associated with dry mouth, oral mucosal lesions, and dental caries (Brennan *et al.*, 2005; Nazmul-Hossain *et al.*, 2011). Depression can result in poorer oral health due to lack of motivation to carry out routine and effective oral hygiene care, and medications to treat depression are known to cause dry mouth (McFarland, 2010). Gastroesophageal reflux disease is associated with dental caries and tooth erosion due to repeated exposure to acidic gastric contents. Erosion over time can result in poor esthetics, sharp teeth likely to cause mucosal ulcerations, dentinal hypersensitivity, and changes in occlusion and vertical dimension (Barron *et al.*, 2003; Lackey & Barth, 2003; Ranijitkar *et al.*, 2012).

Diagnostic uses of oral fluids

This discussion of the mouth–body connection would not be complete without some attention to "the mouth as a window to general health," and the known diagnostic capabilities the secretions of the mouth offer for systemic as well as oral disease detection. Currently available and highly accurate salivary diagnostic tests include various hormonal, human immunodeficiency virus (HIV), and alcohol tests. Studies are underway on salivary biomarkers for early oral cancer detection and salivary proteomic and genomic biomarkers for primary Sjögren's syndrome (National Institute of Health, 2010). Even hepatitis B surface antigen (HBsAg) is detectable in the saliva of hepatitis B-infected individuals with approximately a 75% level of sensitivity (Arora *et al.*, 2012). Gingival crevicular fluid is found to contain diagnostic markers for active periodontal disease (Koregol *et al.*, 2011). The endless possibilities the future holds for saliva and gingival crevicular fluids as widely used tools for systemic disease diagnosis provides optimism that one day innumerable diseases will be diagnosed in an efficient and noninvasive way through easily obtained saliva and crevicular fluid sampling. Certainly, the less invasive the testing, the less stress and risk is placed upon older adults – in particular, the most vulnerable, frail elderly.

Case study 1

Ms. Joanne W.

Ms. Joanne W., a 67-year-old single White female with no children, resides in a nursing facility. She has advanced dementia and is verbally noncommunicative. She is spoon-fed and able to sit in a wheelchair. Nursing assistants complain that Ms. W. has foul bad breath, drools, and noisily grinds her teeth. She has not received routine preventive dental care since her admission several years ago. Two months earlier, Ms. W.'s physician examined her and found no general health changes except that she had an infected mouth, but the physician did not initiate a dental referral at that time.

A dentist is called by a concerned nursing facility nurse to examine Ms. W.'s mouth on a Thursday afternoon. The dentist confirms the presence of repugnant oral malodor and observes purulent suppuration exuding from the gingival sulcus with pooling of suppurative fluids in the buccal vestibules. Upon gentle pressure, purulent exudate is easily expressed from the gingival sulci. Ms. W. has a full dentition, with generalized gingival inflammation with localized areas of intense erythema and edema. Her teeth have predominantly Class II–III mobility and flare buccally and facially under the pressure of grinding compounded by her moderate-to-advanced periodontal disease. There is no visual evidence of tooth decay or fractured teeth and no detectable intraoral or extraoral swelling (Figs 20.2 & 20.3). The nursing staff denies changes in Ms. W.'s behavior. Radiographs are not taken due to lack of equipment and periodontal probing is bypassed given the limited scope of the dentist's after-hours visit. To address Ms. W.'s septic periodontal condition in a definitive and immediate way, the dentist, in consultation with an oral surgeon, advises Ms. W.'s healthcare proxy to consent to the extraction of all Ms. W.'s teeth under general anesthesia in a hospital setting. Informed consent is obtained.

Case study 1 resolution

Ms. W. is immediately started on a 300 mg clindamycin every 8 hours. On Friday morning, a panoramic radiograph taken at the oral surgeon's office confirms the presence of generalized moderate-to-advanced adult periodontitis and several periapical abscesses. The Director of Nursing and Ms. W.'s physician are informed and consulted. On Saturday morning, Ms. W. is admitted to the hospital, prepped and administered intravenous antibiotics and transferred to the operating room. Neither the nurse anesthetist nor the anesthesiologist succeeded in nasopharyngeal intubation, purportedly because of pharyngeal swelling; they therefore resort to oropharyngeal intubation. Ms. W.'s teeth are removed, alveoloplasty done where indicated and ample sutures placed for proper closure and bleeding control (Figs 20.4 & 20.5). Presumably because of the extent of swelling and related breathing difficulties, Ms. W. is not extubated until 2 days later, and discharged to the nursing facility the following day (Tuesday). The dentist provided post-operative follow-up for Ms. W. at the nursing home. She healed very well but no dentures were made.

Ms. W.'s case highlights the need for routine and regular dental and preventive care, as well as timely treatment to decrease the extent of disease severity, treatment complications, the cost of care, and, as in this case, the need for and the number of hospitalization days. The value of patient advocacy, especially for those patients who cannot express themselves or act in their own interest, is also illustrated. The evidence in the operating room that Ms. W.'s infection had in some way prevented nasopharyngeal intubation is a noteworthy example of the oral–systemic health link. Fortunately for Ms. W., her oral infection did not lead to a catastrophic adverse health outcome. The importance of timely referrals between members of the interprofessional healthcare team and a coordinated approach to patient care cannot be overstated. Ms. W.'s case provides a fitting transition to the next section addressing interprofessional care.

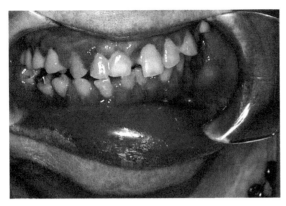

Figure 20.2 The dentition of Ms. W. Note the severity of the gingival inflammation and the supperative fluids accumulating in the buccal vestibules, as well as the flaring teeth. Photograph courtesy of Teresa E. Johnson, DDS.

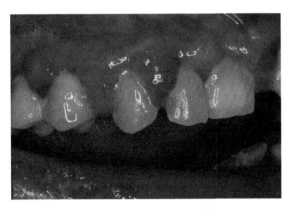

Figure 20.3 A close up of Ms. W.'s marginal gingiva and the purulent suppuration from the gingival sulci. Photograph courtesy of Teresa E. Johnson, DDS.

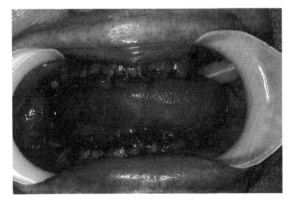

Figure 20.4 Ms. W.'s mouth after extractions, alveoloplasty, and suture placement. Photograph courtesy of Teresa E. Johnson, DDS.

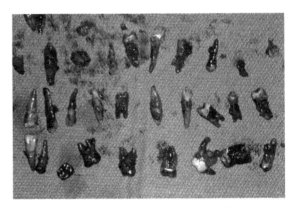

Figure 20.5 Ms. W.'s extracted teeth. Observe the many granulomas clinging to several of the teeth roots. Photograph courtesy of Teresa E. Johnson, DDS.

INTERPROFESSIONAL CARE

Dental professionals best serve their older patients when they provide dental care as part of a comprehensive healthcare strategy. This care should be patient-centered (Hellyer, 2011) and delivered in partnership with a collaborative interprofessional healthcare team across the healthcare system (Reuben, 2009). Interprofessional teams are widely considered to be essential to the delivery of quality geriatric care (Tsukuda, 1990; Ham, 2002). Well-functioning team care has been shown to have positive effects on patients' health and it results in better clinical outcomes, higher patient satisfaction, and enhanced delivery of care (Grumbach & Bodenheimer, 2004).

In the care of the older patient, the DP has the greatest impact when working with an expanded interprofessional team that may include physicians, nurse practitioners, physician assistants, nurses, social workers, pharmacists, rehabilitation specialists, and nursing assistants (Coleman, 2005; Polverini, 2012). Additionally, the now-established relationship between oral health and systemic health highlights the need for integrating oral health care into the management of general health care by multiple healthcare providers (Albert *et al.*, 2012; Allen *et al.*, 2008; Iacopino, 2008). While the model of interprofessional care may not be necessary for all geriatric patients, the frequent visits they make to other practitioners present opportunities for promoting oral health (Mouradian & Corbin, 2003). Because oral and systemic health are so closely intertwined in old age, and barriers to dental care are common among the elderly, interprofessional, team-based approaches to care can improve oral health and general well-being. Working as a member of an interprofessional team, DPs maximize their ability to work with other health professionals to assess, diagnose, coordinate, and deliver care to their older patients (Institute of Medicine and National Research Council, 2011).

Because many older patients have a complex set of dental, medical, and social needs, the DP must be able to coordinate their care, respond to these multiple patient needs, and deliver care across many different settings. Providing this care requires effective communication across the locations of care and the disciplines that make up the interprofessional team (Dyer *et al.*, 2004; Institute of Medicine, 2003; Keough *et al.*, 2002; Williams *et al.*, 2002). For example, implementation of a dental treatment plan for a nursing home resident may require coordination with the patient's medical provider to adjust and manage medications; communication with a licensed nurse to provide treatments, monitoring, and assessment; and delivery of basic oral care by a direct care worker. A social worker may help the patient with transportation needs and payment mechanisms, a pharmacist may provide consultative input into the medication regimen, and family members will have an interest in recommended interventions. By understanding other disciplines and interprofessional collaboration, the DP maximizes the potential to successfully optimize the oral health and well-being of the patient. Table 20.2 lists various patient conditions and the interprofessional care members DPs can collaborate with.

Dental–medical collaboration

DPs can establish successful collaborations with medical colleagues to provide higher quality treatment and better oral health care to their shared patients.

Table 20.2 Potential interprofessional collaboration for dental professionals

Condition	Association	Potential collaborations with other health professionals	
A1C control	Important element of diabetes management	• Dieticians • Care coordinators • Pharmacists • Primary care providers	• Adjusting and managing medications • Dietary controls • Preventing and treating mouth infections
Loss of fine motor skills	Arthritis, stroke, neurodegenerative diseases, trauma, etc.	• Occupational therapists • Physical therapists • Social workers	• Practicing fine motor skills using the affected side • Supporting/assisting with Activities of Daily Living • Providing adaptive devices • Coordination of transportation needs and payment mechanisms
Dysphagia	Stroke, Parkinson's, cancer treatment, etc.	• Dietician • Primary care providers • Speech therapists	• Diagnosis of condition/cause • Guidance to prevent aspiration • Recommendations for oral intake, diet texture
Edentulism	Compromised ability to chew, inadequate nutrition	• Dieticians • Long-term care staff	• Recommendations for oral intake, diet texture • Monitoring fit and function of dentures • Oral cancer screening
Mucositis / glossitis	Erythematous and ulcerative lesions secondary to cancer tx, drug reactions, etc.	• Radiologists • Oncologists • Dieticians • Direct care staff	• Diagnosis of condition • Avoidance of spicy, acidic, hard, and hot foods and beverages • Minimization with appropriate products and oral hygiene practices
Xerostomia	Increased susceptibility to tooth decay, swallowing difficulties	• Dieticians • Long-term care staff • Pharmacists • Primary care providers	• Alerting patient and caregiver to potential side effects • Prescribing saliva substitutes, fluoride, and other antimicrobial agents

Since older patients are more likely to see a primary care medical provider (physicians, physician assistants, and nurse practitioners) than a DP, a more effective integration of medical colleagues into the spectrum of oral health care could have a large impact (Institute of Medicine and National Research Council, 2011). A number of successful dental–medical collaborations have been described in both the dental and the medical literature (Mouradian et al., 2004; Rozier et al., 2003). Interprofessional collaboration implies a higher degree of interaction and coordination than a typical consultation. In the collaborative model, the DP and medical provider integrate their observations, fields of expertise and areas of decision-making in a collaborative and coordinated way to optimize care (Institute of Medicine, 2003). Fundamental to an effective working collaboration, both DPs and medical providers must commit to a shared responsibility for patient care in a climate of mutual respect and trust (Williams et al., 2006; Xyrichis & Lowton, 2008). They should also have knowledge of, and respect for the competences, roles and contributions of other professionals on the team, without any prejudice or stereotyped perceptions (Vyt, 2008).

The ability to communicate and share information efficiently is also essential to successful collaboration. The DP may find that modern communication technology and the use of shared electronic health records facilitate collaboration. Unfortunately, both DPs and medical providers work in fast-paced, interruptive healthcare settings where face-to-face interprofessional collaboration is rare and the absence of this personal contact may prove to be a barrier to effective communication and establishing effective interprofessional relationships (Rice et al., 2010). Perceived busyness is often reported as a barrier to interprofessional collaboration. In the absence of programmatic linkages between providers, clinicians often work in parallel, rather than collaboratively (Stille et al., 2005).

Dental–rehabilitation collaboration

With age, many persons neglect their oral hygiene because of diminished motivation and/or impaired function. The elderly suffer from a heavy burden of chronic medical problems, including dementia, arthritis, paralysis due to stroke, and Parkinson's disease. They may have impaired vision, diminished sense of touch, or poor hand function (Bellomo et al., 2005; Padilha et al., 2007). In these circumstances, the DP should seek productive collaboration with members of the rehabilitation disciplines. It is important to know that if the individual does not provide his or her own oral hygiene care, the likelihood that caregivers or family members will provide it is small. Despite best professional intentions, as described in greater detail below, multiple factors contribute to the difficulty of others providing oral hygiene, especially in chronic care facility settings. The longer that an individual can retain autonomy in providing his or her oral hygiene care, the better the outcome will be. In that context, the effectiveness of rehabilitation team members will be described.

Occupational therapists (OTs), physical therapists (PTs), and speech-language pathologists (SLPs) are particularly effective at improving oral care and dental hygiene for the elderly with functional impairment. OTs are trained to recognize patient strengths and limitations and to teach patients how to adapt to functional loss. Adapting to loss of function may require the use of specially designed, adaptive equipment to allow independent self-care as long as possible. OTs can help patients improve their oral care by exploring adaptive devices, such as modified toothbrush handles or wrist-cuff adapted toothbrushes, to improve mouth care, implement programs to promote recall, and teach caregivers adaptive tooth and denture brushing techniques (Bellomo et al., 2005).

PTs are trained to diagnose, prevent, and treat conditions that limit the body's ability to move and function in daily life. DPs will often encounter patient immobility constraints when providing accessible dental care to older adults with arthritis, Parkinson's disease, and other neuromuscular disorders, or cerebral vascular accidents (Walsh et al., 1999). Poor oral health has been associated with both physical disability and limited mobility (Hanada & Tada, 2001; Avcu et al., 2005; Sumi et al., 2009). Through collaboration between DPs and PTs, patients with physical limitations and dexterity problems can receive physical therapy intended to gain functional abilities sufficient to perform their own oral care. Such collaboration can foster and promote the importance of quality oral care to maintain well-being while educating PTs to recognize oral conditions that require the attention of a dental provider (Yoon & Steele, 2007).

SLPs specialize in communication and swallowing disorders. They are trained to evaluate and treat speech, language, and cognitive disorders of communication and swallowing. As experts on dysphagia, SLPs are especially concerned about oral health, both because of its link to AP and how it affects their recommendations for oral intake, diet texture, and allowance for oral intake of water. DPs and other interprofessional team members will find SLPs to be effective advocates and educators for oral health and experts in oral hygiene techniques for those at risk for aspiration (Yoon & Steele, 2012).

Dental–nursing collaboration

Nurses and nursing assistants provide essential direct care support for many older patients and patients with disabilities. In institutional settings, they are the interprofessional team members best positioned to provide frequent assessment of oral health problems and daily oral care to patients requiring functional support (Yoon & Steele, 2012). Many successful programs to improve the oral health of institutionalized elderly have targeted nurses to improve their knowledge of and commitment to oral health care (Frenkel *et al.*, 2001; Coleman, 2005; Chalmers & Ettinger, 2008). A number of these initiatives demonstrate that, with adequate training, nurses can identify oral health problems, make appropriate referrals to DPs, and minimize the significant morbidity associated with poor oral health (Kayser-Jones, *et al.*, 1995; Arvidson-Bufano *et al.*, 1996). Unfortunately, nursing personnel face many barriers to the delivery of effective oral care in geriatric care settings. These include low staffing, lack of time and organizational support, resident behaviors resistive to oral care, and fear of being hurt while providing the care (Chalmers *et al.*, 1996; Coleman & Watson, 2006). Many nursing caregivers report the provision of oral care to be a lonely and isolated experience which inhibits them from sharing the unique challenges of oral care with others (Wårdh *et al.*, 2000). These challenges and the unique position of nurses in the care of the elderly present a great interprofessional opportunity for DPs working to improve the oral health of their older patients. Although the healthcare community has yet to develop "best practices" for a collaborative approach to care between dentistry and nursing, working together will benefit the older patient because any dental treatment will ultimately fail if it is not maintained through preventive and regular oral care provided by nursing (Coleman, 2005).

Dental–pharmacy collaboration

Pharmacists focus on safe and effective medication use. The role of the pharmacist has expanded from the classic compounding and dispensing of medications to include being an integrated member of the healthcare team. As members of interprofessional teams, pharmacists have been shown to improve health-related outcomes (Koshman *et al.*, 2008; McLean *et al.*, 2008; Murray *et al.*, 2009). Many patients may seek advice and consultation from pharmacists regarding tooth pain relief, oral ulcers, sore mouth, bleeding gums, teething, dentures or product advice. (Gilbert, 1998). Pharmacists are frequently asked what medications can be used for oral symptoms and how to treat their oral health problems themselves (Cohen, 2009). Because of these frequent requests, pharmacists often express a desire for closer collaborations with the interdisciplinary team and have key contacts with local DPs (Maunder & Landes, 2005). Pharmacists also act as counselors to patients and DPs about safety, drug interactions, and potential drug problems (Jacobsen & Lofholm, 2008). Over-the-counter and prescription drugs are used frequently by older adults. By working with the pharmacist in collaborative drug therapy management, the DP can more effectively identify potential problems in patient drug regimens (Schmader *et al.*, 2004), provide more effective implementation of treatment plans (Bluml *et al.*, 2000), and reduce ADRs (Hanlon *et al.*, 1996).

Case study 2

Mr. John S.

Mr. John S. is a 93-year-old man with intact dentition, residing in an assisted living center. He has moderate problems with forgetfulness. He receives assistance with his daily medications (aspirin, calcium carbonate, vitamin D, furosemide, finasteride, tamsulosin, solifenacin, and docusate) with the help of the nursing staff. Mr. S. presents to his dentist after a single choking episode, reporting great difficulty swallowing a piece of meat while at a restaurant, because his "mouth is so dry." Mr. S.'s other medical problems include severe osteoarthritis, spinal stenosis, obstructive sleep apnea, benign prostatic hyperplasia, and urge urinary incontinence.

Case study 2: resolution

Mr. S.'s dentist is concerned that one of his medications may be causing xerostomia and subsequent swallowing problems. He contacts Mr. S.'s primary physician who notes that the solifenacin is a likely culprit, but that Mr. S. may also have a swallowing disorder. Mr. S. is seen by a speech-language pathologist who conducts and evaluates a video-fluoroscopic swallowing study. No oro-motor dysphagia is found in this evaluation. Mr. S.'s dentist and physician discuss a trial without the solifenacin, and Mr. S. agrees to this intervention. His nurses at the assisted living center suggest a trial of a saliva substitute to manage his xerostomia, which is prescribed by his dentist. His xerostomia and swallowing dysfunction subsequently improve.

Dental–dietician collaboration

Registered dietitians (RDs) are food and nutrition experts who work to treat and prevent disease by providing medical nutrition therapy as part of the interprofessional healthcare team. Poor oral health may lead, both indirectly and directly, to malnutrition (Steele & Walls, 1997), and poor nutrition can contribute to problems with oral health (Ritchie & Kinane, 2003). Because oral health and nutrition have this synergistic, bidirectional relationship, DPs and RDs can work together to provide screening, education, and referral to each other as part of a comprehensive care plan (Touger-Decker *et al.*, 2007). DPs can also educate RDs on the probable dental caries risk of various liquid dietary supplements that are often added to boost caloric, fiber, and protein intake and provide important nutrients that may otherwise be lacking.

Dental–social worker collaboration

Social workers (SWs) are trained to help patients and their families enhance or restore their capacity for social functioning. Healthcare SWs help their clients understand their health problems and make the necessary adjustments to their lifestyle, housing, or health care. They may help older clients find services such as programs that provide transportation, meals, or home health care. SWs help their clients and families make plans for possible health complications or where they will live if they can no longer care for themselves (Bureau of Labor Statistics, 2012). They have historically been a core discipline on the geriatric interprofessional team because of their leadership role in the identification of psychosocial issues (Dyer *et al.*, 2004). The SW's knowledge about service delivery systems in both public and private sectors enables him or her to facilitate the coordination of services and assume a lead role in the interprofessional team (Dobrof, 1999).

There are few "best practice" models of social work integration into the dental health team, but models of this collaboration have demonstrated their value (Levy *et al.*, 1979; Petrosky *et al.*, 2000; Zittel-Palamara *et al.*, 2005). Common problems referred to social work by DPs include poor adherence to treatment, inadequate resources, family issues, systems issues, and barriers to care, including unreliable transportation and cultural or language differences (Petrosky *et al.*, 2009). Given the great impact of psychosocial determinants on general and oral health (Dobrof, 1999; Watt & Sheiham, 1999), there are numerous opportunities for DPs to improve the health of their older patients by working with SWs (Petrosky *et al.*, 2009).

Interprofessional geriatric dental care

In its groundbreaking study, *Improving Access to Oral Health Care for Vulnerable and Underserved Populations*, the Institute of Medicine called for a greater role in oral health for all nondental members of the inter-professional healthcare team (Institute of Medicine and National Research Council, 2011). DPs working with older patients have a unique opportunity to collaborate fully with their nondental colleagues to address the oral health needs of their patients (Mouradian *et al.*, 2004). Each member of the inter-professional team brings their own unique motivators to improve oral health and their unique areas of expertise to the care of the DP's geriatric patients (Yoon & Steele, 2012). Institutional organizations can play an important role in promoting effective communication and collaboration (MacEntee, 2006), but without the commitment of the DP to the workings of the interprofessional health team, the team will be without the necessary knowledge and expertise to provide required oral hygiene, needed regular assessment, and timely referral for dental care. A successful strategy for the DP treating older patients requires: (i) an oral healthcare plan that is clear to all members of the interprofessional team; (ii) a commitment from team members to implement the plan; and (iii) an awareness of the individual and shared responsibilities brought by team members to the care of the geriatric patient (MacEntee, 2006).

Strategies for successful interprofessional consultations

A healthcare consultation is communication between healthcare or other service professionals to seek guidance and clarification, share relevant information and clinical findings, alert interprofessional team members of discipline-specific concerns, and discuss diagnosis, prognosis, as well as treatment and patient management options for a particular patient. The overall goals of a healthcare consultation are to achieve optimal interprofessional dialogue and awareness, and to gain sufficient information about a patient's health and well-being to ensure the best possible outcome in the delivery of patient care while minimizing iatrogenic risks for medical or other unintended events. Consultation is not about receiving "clearance" to proceed with dental care (Brown *et al.*, 2007)

Traditionally, the majority of dentists have practiced in isolation from other healthcare disciplines. As a result, interprofessional consultations have primarily been written or by telephone; however, these methods have inherent limitations. Telephone consultations are sought during the workday and often met with mixed results. For those concerned about interrupting another provider's workday with a phone call, a written consultation may be preferred. While the potential for a direct conversation with the targeted provider exists, a timely discussion between the DP and other healthcare professional may be unsuccessful due to provider unavailability, delays due to patient record retrieval, being placed on-hold while waiting for a busy provider, resorting to voice messages that may not be promptly returned, or having to make several call-back attempts. Even when successful and timely, phone consultations necessitate a written follow-up letter, email, or fax and a returned reply from the consulted provider to avoid misunderstandings.

Written consultation letters and faxes are not conducive for same-day patient care in most instances. Written correspondences may not be reviewed or responded to by other health professionals in a timely manner; and without actual dialogue between providers, the responses may lack the information being sought. To be effective, consultation letters by DPs should include relevant medical and dental health status information and a summary of the planned dental treatment. A succinct statement of concerns and clearly worded questions are ideal. DPs should, whenever possible, provide enough patient information to the intended healthcare professional to facilitate a complete response to the questions. By including published guidelines, (for example, the AHA guidelines for the prevention of IE), a DP can enhance the exchange of information, foster collegiality, and avoid conflicting views regarding appropriate patient management. Table 20.3 provides an outline of appropriate steps to take for achieving successful consultations.

Tips for optimizing the outcomes of a request for a medical consultation

One strategy that DPs may find helpful when a written medical consultation is needed is the use of a custom-designed form that has space reserved for individualized patient information, check boxes of the medical conditions being inquired about, space to express various concerns or customize questions as needed, as well as space for the physician to reply and relay directives and opinions. A website where a sample form can be accessed is listed in Table 20.4. In addition,

Brown *et al.* (2007) provide a comprehensive table of suggested scripts one may use, depending upon the circumstances and the medical information being sought. These are succinct and to the point and include referral narratives that request patient evaluation for conditions such as hypertension or diabetes.

To manage frail older adult dental patients appropriately and successfully, it is imperative that DP's receive sufficient training and updates on the management of medically compromised patients. This includes identifying the "red flags" that should trigger a consultation, know what to ask, understand the consulted provider's guidance, and execute them

Table 20.3 Dental professionals' guide to interprofessional consultation

Considerations for optimal consultations

Information gathering
(a) Thorough health and dental history
  (i) Careful review of over-the-counter and prescription drugs (what, why)
  (ii) Further patient interviewing is indicated if conflicting information or inconsistencies exist, or the patient information is vague or questionable
(b) Discuss socioeconomic supports and resources
(c) Discuss the patient's chief complaint and his or her goals for resolution
(d) Provide a problem-focused or comprehensive dental exam (depending on the nature of the visit)
(e) Develop a problem-focused or comprehensive care plan that reflects the patient's treatment goals
(f) Provide patient education (findings, diagnosis, prognosis, treatment options, preventive care plan and home care, indications for consultation or referral, etc.)
(g) Identify any need for interprofessional consultation

Preparing for a consultation
(a) Gather all pertinent patient information and carefully review
(b) Identify the concerns that warrant consultation and prepare a list of questions to be asked
(c) Identify the pertinent dental health status information, including the preliminary dental care plan, and the patient information deemed important to share
(d) Identify which interprofessional care member (ICM) or members to consult
(e) Identify which consultation method to use: phone, letter (mail, fax, electronic), in person

Phone consultations
(a) Be prepared! Have the list of information (b & c in previous section) and the patient record
(b) Initiate the consultation. The ICM may not be reached on the first try, if so, leave a message
(c) Be cordial, yet succinct and to the point; ask questions as needed to ensure accuracy
(d) Take notes during the conversation and plan for a written follow-up to the phone consultation

Written consultations
(a) Prepare a written draft:
  (i) Identify yourself and introduce the patient of concern at the outset
  (ii) Include information using b & c in the "*Preparing for a consultation*" section above
  (iii) Prepare a succinct statement of concerns and clearly worded questions
  (iv) Provide enough information to help guide the ICM in his/her decisions and recommendations
  (v) Include a statement (if applicable) about what published guidelines will be followed
  (vi) Provide directions to the ICM about returning the reply (fax, email, mail, phone, etc.)
(b) Refer to Table 20.4 "Written consultations content and example"
(c) Have an established process for storing both written requests for consultation and the responses

Additional considerations
(d) Insure HIPAA compliance when sharing and seeking protected information
(e) Document all consultations and any impact on the treatment plan in the patient's dental record
(f) Include reference materials, such as published guidelines, that can be helpful to the ICM
(g) Consultations should not be about receiving clearance to proceed with dental care, but rather obtaining the necessary medical information to adequately prepare for and manage the delivery of care based on each patient's unique situation and needs (Brown *et al.*, 2007)

during dental care delivery. DP's must know their own limitations and make referrals whenever necessary. Likewise, they must keep abreast of new medico-dental guidelines; renew their medical emergencies training on a regular basis as well as cardiopulmonary resuscitation techniques. When DPs encounter an older adult who appears in poor health and is in need of medical assessment and care, a medical referral is indicated before elective dental care is rendered. If that patient needs emergency dental intervention to address pain or infection and this need surpasses the expected medical needs, then rendering limited, problem-focused care is appropriate. This may only involve an analgesic or antibiotic prescription prior to the medical referral, or include initiation of limited dental treatment to ameliorate or eliminate the dental problem of concern. Similarly, if a DP encounters a patient who has not accessed routine healthcare services throughout adulthood, who does not have a regular physician, who presents with abnormal vital signs or other screening tests, or whose physical, social, or psychologic presentation is suspect, a medical referral is indicated. If, after patient education, he or she refuses a medical referral, it may not be prudent to proceed with dental care.

Communication technologies are expanding the alternatives for interprofessional consultation and collaboration. With the shift from paper-based patient records to electronic health records and electronic communication options such as email, webinars, webcams, and smartphone capabilities, there appears to be endless possibilities for much improved consultation processes that abide by HIPAA (Health Insurance Portability and Accountability Act of 1996) regulations. While the merging of traditional solo and group dental practices into interprofessional healthcare clinics may be a goal in professional circles, it seems that it may be several years until this is more fully utilized. In the meantime, the further development and widespread use of patient case-managers to coordinate care between the multiple disciplines, to remove communication barriers among providers, to monitor patient progress through the interprofessional system and to advocate for patients, hold promise for improving healthcare and health outcomes. Table 20.4 provides suggestions for content and an example consultation letter.

Table 20.5 lists several educational links and resources relevant to this chapter.

EXPANSION OF THE DENTAL WORKFORCE

Access to care for older adults

Approximately one-third of Americans, including many seniors and frail elders, struggle to access dental care due to a variety of barriers. Recent data from the National Health Interview Study show that in 2010, 40% of adults did not have a visit to any DP (Schiller *et al.*, 2012). Obstacles to care include lack of transportation, cost and financial limitations, lack of perceived need, and inability to locate providers that are comfortable and competent treating medically, physically and/or mentally challenged patients. In 2004, Manski *et al.* reported that approximately 28% of Americans between the ages of 65 and 74 had private dental insurance, which decreased to 16% for those aged 75 and older. Data showed that 36% of Americans aged 65–74 had a household income that is less than 200% of the federal poverty level, while 49% of those aged 75 and older had a household income of less than 200% of the federal poverty level (Manski *et al.*, 2004). People who do not have dental insurance are less likely to seek regular care than those with insurance (Wall & Brown, 2003). An increasing number of people in the USA are keeping all or most of their teeth into old age. It is important for seniors to have access to regular preventive and restorative care to maintain their oral and general health.

The impetus behind the initiative to expand the dental workforce

In 2000 Dr. David Satcher released the first ever Surgeon General's report on oral health, stating "There are profound and consequential oral health disparities within the US population." He also reported that a "silent epidemic of oral diseases is affecting our most vulnerable citizens – poor children, the elderly, and many members of racial and ethnic minority groups." One of many action steps listed in the original report was to "build an effective health infrastructure that meets the oral health needs of all Americans" which includes a "diverse workforce of trained public health practitioners knowledgeable about oral health" (US Department

Table 20.4 Written consultation content and example

Contact information
- Interprofessional care member (ICM) name, address
- Dental professional's (DPs) name, address, phone, fax, email
- Re: Patient's full name, including identifiers such as date of birth (DOB), social security no. (SS#), address

Introductory paragraph: Setting the stage
- Describe the DP–ICM connection (mutual patient) and indicate the purpose of the letter

Paragraphs 2 and 3: What do you know
- Health information; dental status

Paragraph 4: What do you need and what do you have
- Need: Clarification of health information
- Need: ICM recommendations for patient management and approval to proceed with dental care
- Have: A plan for how the DP will proceed with care. Introduce any available dental or medical guidelines and indicate if DP plans to follow them (American Heart Association, American Academy of Orthopedic Surgeons, hypertension guidelines, etc.)

Paragraph 5: When and how
- Describe the timing for planned care
- Identify how the ICM can reply to the DP

Example consultation
Contact Information of DP & ICM (Typical of any business letter)
Re: Ms. XYZ (Address, DOB, SS#)

Dear <u>ICM</u>,

This letter concerns a mutual patient of ours, <u>Ms. XYZ</u> (DOB, SS#) who presented last week for a dental examination after a four-year absence. Because she reports a significant change in her medical history, I am seeking clarification about her health status and your input about my plan to manage her during dental care.

    Ms. XYZ indicated she had a "moderate" myocardial infarction six weeks ago and underwent successful emergency triple-bypass surgery. At last weeks visit, she appeared well and her vital signs were within normal limits. In addition to antihypertensive and cholesterol-lowering medications, nitroglycerin (prn) has been added to her prescription regime; although she stated she had not use it.

    Ms. XYZ's dental status has deteriorated significantly. She has advanced periodontal disease, severe generalized bone loss and gingival inflammation, along with poor plaque control. She has multiple decayed teeth, two of which are abscessed and increasingly symptomatic to chewing. She experiences intermittent spontaneous pain at night and takes analgesics. Her oral condition has become a relatively pressing problem for her and would be difficult to manage palliatively for any extended time period. Ms. XYZ's treatment goal is to have her 17 remaining teeth removed and complete dentures fabricated. She is very nervous about dental care.

    Please provide additional information about the nature of Ms. XYZ's heart condition and any other health problems identified and/or medications that were not reported to me. Is her cardiovascular status sufficiently stable to undergo the extraction of her teeth using Nitrous Oxide inhalation for anxiety control and 2% lidocaine with 1:100,000 epinephrine or 3% carbocaine without a vasoconstrictor? If not, do you recommend we postpone her care until such time as her cardiovascular status is stable?

    Thank you in advance for your time and expertise. The space below is reserved for your recommendations.

    I will not proceed with Ms. XYZ's care until I have heard from you; however, a timely response is appreciated. You may fax your comments at: _____, call me at: _____ or email me at: _____

Sincerely,

Physician's recommendations and comments

---

of Heath & Human Services, 2000). The next Surgeon General, Dr. Richard Carmona, issued a "National Call to Action To Promote Oral Health" in 2003 to further detail steps to address oral health disparities. These include "enhance oral health workforce capacity, moving society toward optimal use of its health professionals and state practice act changes that would permit alternative models of delivery of needed care" (US Department of Heath and Human Services, 2003).

Table 20.5 Links and resources

Educational resources

Overcoming Obstacles to Oral Health, 5th edn
- http://dental.pacific.edu/Community_Involvement/Pacific_Center_for_Special_Care_(PCSC)/Special_Care_Resources.html
- "The purpose of the *Overcoming Obstacles* training program is to provide a resource for caregivers and professionals training caregivers about oral health for people with disabilities and frail elders."

Smiles for Life: A National Oral Health Curriculum, 3rd edn
- http://smilesforlifeoralhealth.org/default.aspx?tut=555&pagekey=62948&s1=1823618
- "Designed to enhance the role of primary care clinicians in the promotion of oral health for all age groups through the development and dissemination of high-quality educational resources."

Working Together To Manage Diabetes: A guide for Pharmacy, Podiatry, Optometry, and Dental Professionals
- National Diabetes Education Program. In print: available for purchase through Amazon.com.
- "An course developed by the National Diabetes Education Program's Pharmacy, Podiatry, Optometry, and Dental Professionals' work group."

Oral Health for the Elderly – Evaluation and Care
- http://dynamicgrp.cm-hosting.com/catalog.php?item=73
- "Dysphagia Therapists, Speech-Language Pathologists, Occupational Therapists, Nurses, and Dietitians all play a role in the oral health of their patients, yet oral hygiene continues to be vastly neglected in nursing home residents."

Clinical Management Of Diabetes in the Elderly
- *Clinical Diabetes*, 2001, **19**(4), 172–5.
- "Understanding the special dynamics of geriatric patientswill aid in the optimum management of their diabetes."

Dignity with a Smile Oral Healthcare for Elders in Residential Care: A Report for the Federal Dental Advisory Committee 2008
- http://www.fptdwg.ca/assets/PDF/0901-Dignity%20with%20a%20Smile%20Final.pdf
- "Recommends collaboration between oral and other healthcare providers and placement of certified dental assistants and dental hygienists in every facility to co-ordinate oral healthcare."

Association websites/mission

Special Care Dentistry Association
- http://www.scdaonline.org/
- "To act as a central focus for diverse individuals and groups with a common interest in oral health for people with special needs and direct its resources accordingly."

The American Geriatrics Society
- http://www.americangeriatrics.org/
- "To improve the health, independence and quality of life of all older people."

Special Case Advocates in Dentistry
- saiddent.org
- "To improve the oral health of people with disabilities through service, education, and advocacy."

World Health Professionals Alliance
- http://www.whpa.org/
- "To improve global health and the quality of patient care and facilitate collaboration among the health professions and major stakeholders. Fact Sheets and links to other resources."

National Association of Professional Geriatric Care Managers
- http://www.caremanager.org/
- "To advance professional geriatric care management through education, collaboration, and leadership."

Historical perspective

Dental therapists (DTs) began providing oral health-care services in New Zealand in 1921 (Nash *et al.*, 2012). These practitioners, originally called "dental nurses," were dental mid-level providers that performed restorative procedures and extraction of primary teeth in government run school-based programs. This concept has expanded to 54 countries including the UK, Canada, Australia, and Thailand. In 2005, dental health aide therapists (DHATs) began bringing dental services in the USA to underserved Native Alaskan communities through the Alaska Native Tribal Health Consortium (Nash *et al.*, 2012).

From planning to action: Minnesota

In response to the Surgeon Generals' reports and action plans, the American Dental Hygienists' Association (ADHA) proposed the concept of a dental mid-level provider. In 2001, the ADHA convened a workgroup to develop competencies for a Master's level Advanced Dental Hygiene Practitioner to take an existing workforce of dental hygienists and expand their present scope of practice to include restorative dentistry and minor oral surgery in addition to their focus on prevention and health promotion (ADHA, 2012). At that time, Minnesota was already utilizing Restorative Functions legislation authorizing trained hygienists and dental assistants to place amalgam and composite resin restorations prescribed by the dentist. In addition, dental hygienists who had Collaborative Management Agreements with Minnesota dentists were authorized to provide community-based preventive services without a dentist on site, i.e., under General Supervision. The decline in the dentist to population ratio (Dolan *et al.*, 2005), with Minnesota having the greatest decline in the USA (ADA, 2001), provided some of the justification for legislative approval for a new mid-level oral health provider.

Normandale Community College at Bloomington, Minnesota and Metropolitan State University at St. Paul, Minnesota partnered to develop an educational program (approved in 2006) for dental hygienists with an Associate's Degree to obtain a Bachelor of Science in Dental Hygiene and a Master's Degree in Advanced Dental Therapy. The University

of Minnesota School of Dentistry in Minneapolis developed curriculum and received approval from the Minnesota Board of Dentistry for their own DT program with an initial focus on training nonhygienists to become DTs. Legislation authorizing both the dental therapist (DT) and advanced dental therapist (ADT) was passed in 2009. The education of Minnesota DTs provides the basis for competency in all aspects of their scope of practice. One requirement to obtain a DT license in Minnesota is successful completion of both the manikin and patient components of the Central Regional Dental Testing Service examination.

Minnesota DTs and ADTs are legislatively authorized to deliver services in hospitals, nursing homes, home health agencies, group homes, local public health facilities, community and tribal clinics, schools or Head Start programs, military and veterans' settings as well as in a patient's home. Many of these locations offer access to seniors. The legislation requires the majority of DT and ADT patients be uninsured or underinsured, in an attempt to provide greater access for those in need, including low-income seniors. These DTs and ADTs work as a member of the dental team within the guidelines of a written Collaborative Management Agreement (CMA) with a supervising dentist. A CMA established between a dentist and a DT or ADT practicing in Minnesota are individualized and tailored to reflect the needs of the collaborating parties, for example limiting the therapist's scope of practice if that were the preference of the dentist. Table 20.6 provides a list of the essential elements that must be included in a CMA, and Table 20.7 summarizes the dental services DTs and ADTs can provide and the level of supervision from the Collaborating Dentist.

Dental workforce expansion status in other states

Other states are exploring expanding the duties of their current dental workforce through development and implementation of mid-level providers. The scope of practice for dental hygienists varies from state to state. Some states continue a traditional work role for hygienists being limited to indirect supervision (dentist on site) within private practice settings. Some states allow hygienists to see patients

Table 20.6 Required content of a dental therapy CMA in Minnesota*

CMA required content	Description details
1 Practice settings where services may be provided and the populations to be served [by the DT or ADT]	• List practice settings by zip code and county • List the populations [to be served per defined categories] • At least 50% of the total patient base to be seen by the DT/ADT must consist of specific patient populations describe in the MN Statute
2 Description of any limitations on the services that may be provided by the DT/ADT, including the level of supervision by the collaborating dentist	• List limitations on the services that may be provided by the DT/ADT • List services within the Scope of Practice of the DT/ADT that are restricted or limited by the CMA
3 Age and procedure specific protocols, case selection criteria, assessment guidelines, and imaging frequency	• Description of: age specific protocols, procedure specific protocols, case selection criteria, assessment guidelines, and imaging frequency guidelines
4 Dental records management	• Procedures for creating and maintaining dental records for patients treated by the DT/ADT
5 Medical emergencies management	• Develop a plan to manage medical emergencies in each practice setting where the DT/ADT will provide care

6 Quality assurance plan	• Develop a quality assurance plan for monitoring care provided by the DT/ADT that provides a description of:
	  ○ the patient care review
	  ○ the plan for referral follow-up
	  ○ the quality assurance record review

7 Dispensing and administering medications protocols[†]	• Include specific conditions and circumstances under which authorized medications are to be dispensed and administered within the parameters of the CMA and Scope of Practice • Analgesics, anti-inflammatory and antibiotic medications • Describe the process whereby the dentist prescribes and the DT/ADT dispenses and administers these medications

8 Criteria for the provision of care to patients with various medical conditions	• Provision of care criteria for patient with:
	  ○ specific medical conditions
	  ○ complex medical histories
	• Outline requirements for medical consultation prior to the initiation of care by DT/ADT

9 Supervision criteria	• Either general supervision or indirect supervision by the CMA dentist as defined by the DT/ADT Scope of Practice, unless restricted or prohibited in the CMA
10 Provision of clinical resources and referrals	• A plan for situations that are beyond the DT/ADT capabilities

*From Minnesota Board of Dentistry (2014).
[†]DT/ADT are prohibited from dispensing or administering narcotic medications.
ADT, advanced dental therapist; DT, dental therapist; CMA, Collaborative Management Agreement; MN, Minnesota.

under general supervision, where a dentist authorizes the hygienist to perform procedures while the dentist is absent from the clinical facility where the care is being provided. As of 2009, 46 states and the District of Columbia allowed dental hygienists to perform services in at least one setting under general supervision (ADHA, 2014a). Hygienists delivering services closer to where patients reside may reduce

transportation barriers. Appropriate community sites for elder dental care may include workplaces, group homes, Community or Senior Centers, housing complexes, and long-term care facilities.

The scope of practice for allied DPs also varies from state to state and depends upon respective dental practice acts. As of June 2012, Minnesota is the only state to have passed legislation authorizing a mid-level

Table 20.7 Delegated duties of Minnesota dental therapists (DTs) and advanced dental therapists (ADTs)*

General supervision†		Indirect supervision‡	Clinical procedures
ADT	–	–	Limited and periodic oral evaluation and assessment
ADT	DT	–	Radiographs
ADT	DT	–	Application of fluoride, oral hygiene instruction, disease prevention education, nutritional counseling, Sealants
ADT	DT	–	Local anesthesia
ADT	–	DT	Amalgam and composite restorations Stainless steel crowns, re-cement crowns, temporary crowns, pulp cap, pulpotomy suture removal
ADT	–	DT	Extraction of deciduous teeth
ADT	–	–	Nonsurgical extraction of periodontally involved permanent teeth

*From Minnesota Board of Dentistry (2014). Approved 9/24/2010.
†General supervision: The dentist has prior knowledge and has given consent for the procedures being performed during which the dentist is not required to be present in the dental office or on the premises.
‡Indirect supervision: The dentist is in the office, authorizes the procedures, and remains in the office while the procedures are being performed by the allied dental professional.
This table highlights categories of clinical procedures performed by dental therapists and advanced dental therapists. A complete listing can be found at:
https://www.revisor.mn.gov/statutes/?id=150A.105 (DTs)
https://www.revisor.mn.gov/statutes/?id=150A.106 (ADTs)

dental provider. However, some states have introduced or are developing legislation to improve access to care via expanded scope of practice for existing dental team members or by creating new categories of dental team members. Illinois has proposed that a hygienist may be employed by a healthcare facility to provide services without a patient being seen by a dentist first. Nebraska, New Hampshire, Tennessee, Virginia, and West Virginia have proposed that hygienists be allowed to provide various preventive services in public health settings within the guidelines of a written agreement with a supervising dentist (collaborative agreement). New York has proposed the addition of a Registered Dental Hygienist – Collaborative Practice. Kansas has proposed the addition of a "registered dental practitioner," and Vermont and Washington have proposed a "dental therapist" with a scope of practice similar to that of Minnesota's ADT. Maine introduced a bill to establish "oral health practitioners," and Connecticut has introduced a bill to develop Advanced Dental Hygiene Practitioners (ADHA, 2014b).

Because the development and deployment of dental mid-level providers is recent in the USA, data is not yet available to show their impact on access to care and oral health disparities. The US Department of Health and Human Services Strategic Plan for financial years 2010–2015 lists many strategies to improve overall health, one of which is to: "Expand the primary oral healthcare team and promote models that incorporate new providers, expanded scope of existing providers, and utilization of medical providers to provide evidence-based oral health preventive services, where appropriate" (US Department of Health and Human Services, 2010). An increase in productivity leading to improved access to care is the intent of proposed dental therapist legislation. The Pew Center on the States developed a financial calculator to estimate the impact on productivity and profitability with the addition of one DT or ADT seeing either all private pay patients or seeing an 80% private pay, 20% Medical Assistance (Medicaid) patient mix. Estimates ranged from a small decrease in profit to an increase of 50% in both productivity and profit (Pew Center on the States, 2010).

Case study 3

Ms. Louise F.

Ms. Louise F. is a 73-year-old woman living independently. She has type 2 diabetes and osteoarthritis, managed by metformin and ibuprofen respectively. She has not had a dental visit in over 10 years. She has no dental insurance and lives on a fixed income. As an active woman, she enjoys gardening and daily walks, but is experiencing significant pain in her right knee. Her primary care physician referred her to an orthopedic surgeon for evaluation of her right knee pain. After evaluation and consultation, Ms. F. and her surgeon agreed that a prosthetic knee replacement was indicated; however, she had to have a dental examination and have any oral disease addressed before the surgery would be scheduled.

Case study 3: Resolution

Ms. F. found a dental clinic with a fee scale based upon her income. She had a comprehensive assessment and full mouth radiographs taken. Her treatment plan included four quadrants of scaling and root planning and placement of three restorations. A DT was able to complete all treatment and Ms. F was granted clearance to schedule her knee replacement.

Summary

Recognition of the negative impact of untreated oral disease on systemic health and vice versa warrants varied and innovative attempts to improve access to care for vulnerable and medically complex older adults. Advocacy among physicians, DPs, nurses and others on the interprofessional healthcare team regarding the importance of the mouth–systemic health connection is continually needed. The well-being and health of older adults goes beyond just the patient, just the dentist or just the physician … it requires collaborative efforts between dedicated interprofessional care members and elderly patients desiring improved health. New educational models that encourage and enhance interprofessional training experiences and emphasize an interdisciplinary team approach in patient care will provide improved healthcare outcomes. Including oral health care in health professionals' curriculum will reinforce the interrelationship of oral health and overall health. Finally, workforce models may expand and change the roles of healthcare providers across the healthcare team spectrum. Physicians, nurses, physician assistants, nurse practitioners, social workers, and rehabilitation specialists must have increased knowledge of normal and abnormal oral conditions and know when to refer. It is expected that dental mid-level providers will significantly impact access to dental care, especially for the underserved elderly, in areas where current dental services are lacking. If adequately trained to collaborate with dental colleagues and other healthcare professionals as members of interprofessional healthcare teams, mid-level DPs can share in the responsibilities of improving the oral and general health of older adults.

DISCUSSION QUESTIONS

Answers are found at the end of the book.

1 Which one of the three cases presented in this chapter demonstrated a lack of interprofessional collaboration that adversely affected the patient?
2 In the case referred to in Question 1, what two interprofessional team members were most responsible for delays in the patient getting care?
3 These two types of drugs, when given to strengthen bone to prevent skeletal fractures, may result in antiresorptive therapy osteonecrosis of the jaw (ARONJ)?
4 Current scientific data reveals a direct cause and affect relationship between periodontal disease and cardiovascular disease:
   A Statement is true
   B Statement is false

5 Social workers are core interprofessional team members in the care of older adults because of which of the following observations? (Choose the single best answer.)

A Interprofessional communication is an essential competency for effective team function.

B Interprofessional collaboration requires a high degree of integration and coordination of care.

C Interprofessional care teams working with older adults frequently encounter psychosocial barriers to health.

D Interprofessional team care may not be necessary for all older adults encountered by the dental health professional.

6 Which member of the interprofessional care team is in the best position to provide frequent assessment of oral health problems in institutional settings? (Choose the single best answer.)

A Nursing

B Medical provider

C Speech-language pathologist

D Pharmacist

E Dental health professional

7 Which of the following features of healthcare in old age highlight the advantages of interprofessional team care? (Choose the best single answer.)

A Healthcare professionals working with older adults can provide optimal care by working in parallel with colleagues through consultation.

B Healthcare professionals working with older adults must frequently implement treatment programs that meet a complex set of needs.

C Healthcare professionals working with older adults must provide compassionate and competent consultation.

D Healthcare professionals working with older adults often find their patients' needs being met with their discipline's professional expertise.

8 *Statement A:* As people age, the likelihood of having private dental insurance increases. *Statement B:* People with dental insurance are more likely to seek regular dental care.

A Statements A & B are true

B Statement A is true, Statement B is false

C Statements A & B are false

D Statement A is false, Statement B is true

9 How is a mid-level dental provider authorized to practice?

A Independently

B In collaboration with a dentist

C Under the supervision of any doctor, ie, physician or dentist

D Employee of a health center

10 *Statement A:* The scope of practice for all mid-level dental providers includes adult prophylaxis and scaling and root planning. *Statement B:* The scope of practice for hygienists is uniform across the USA.

A Statements A & B are true

B Statement A is true, Statement B is false

C Statements A & B are false

D Statement A is false, Statement B is true

References

AAP (American Academy of Periodontology) (2012) *Periodontal Disease Linked To Cardiovascular Disease.* From http://www.perio.org/consumer/AHA-statement. Accessed April 16, 2014.

Abdollahi, M., Rahimi, R. & Radfar, M. (2008) Current opinion on drug-induced oral reactions: a comprehensive review. *Journal of Contemporary Dental Practice*, **9**(3), 1–15.

Abebe, W. (2003) An overview of herbal supplement utilization with particular emphasis on possible interactions with dental drugs and oral manifestations. *Journal of Dental Hygiene*, **77**(1), 37–46.

ADA (American Dental Association) (2001) *Future of Dentistry.* From http://www.ada.org/sections/professionalResources/pdfs/future_execsum_fullreport.pdf. Accessed April 16, 2014.

ADHA (American Dental Hygienists' Association) (2012) *Facts About the Dental Hygiene Workforce in the United States.* From https://www.adha.org/resources-docs/75118_Facts_About_the_Dental_Hygiene_Workforce.pdf. Accessed April 16, 2014.

ADHA (American Dental Hygienists' Association) (2014a). *Direct Access 2014*. From http://www.adha.org/resources-docs/7524_Direct_Access_Map.pdf. Accessed April 16, 2014.

ADHA (American Dental Hygienists' Association) (2014b) *Legislation by State*. From http://www.adha.org/legislation-by-state. Accessed April 18, 2014.

Adler, R.A. & Gill, R.S. (2011) Clinical utility of denosumab for treatment of bone loss in men and women. *Clinical Interventions in Aging*, **6**, 119–24.

Aghaloo, T.L., Felsenfeld, A.L. & Tetradis, S. (2010) Osteonecrosis of the jaw in a patient on denosumab. *Journal of Oral and Maxillofacial Surgery*, **68**(5), 959–63.

Albert, D.A., Ward, A., Allweiss, P., *et al.* (2012) Diabetes and oral disease: implications for health professionals. *Annals of the New York Academy of Sciences*, **1255**(1), 1–15.

Allen, E.M., Ziada, H.M., O'Halloran, D.O., *et al.* (2008) Attitudes, awareness, and oral health-related quality of life in patients with diabetes. *Journal of Oral Rehabilitation*, **35**, 218–23.

Ansai, T., Takata, Y., Soh, I., *et al.* (2010) Relationship between tooth loss and mortality in 80-year-old Japanese community-dwelling subjects. *BioMed Central Public Health*, **10**, 386–91.

Arora, G., Sheikh, S. & Pallagatti, S. (2012) Saliva as a tool in the detection of hepatitis B surface antigen in patients. *Compendium of Continuing Education in Dentistry*, **33**(3), 174–8.

Arvidson-Bufano, U.B., Blank, L.W. & Yellowitz, J.A. (1996) Nurses' oral health assessments of nursing home residents pre- and post-training: a pilot study. *Special Care in Dentistry*, **16**(2), 58–64.

Avcu, N., Ozbek, M., Kurtoglu, D., *et al.* (2005) Oral findings and health status among hospitalized patients with physical disabilities, aged 60 or above. *Archives of Gerontology and Geriatrics*, **41**, 69–79.

Babu, N.C. & Gomes, A.J. (2011) Systemic manifestations of oral disease. *Journal of Oral Maxillofacial Pathology*, **15**(2), 144–7.

Barnett, M.L. (2006) The oral–systemic disease connection – an update for the practicing dentist. *Journal of the American Dental Association*, **137**, S5–6.

Barron, R.P., Carmichael, R.P., Marcon, M.A., *et al.* (2003) Dental erosion in gastroesophageal reflux disease. *Journal of the Canadian Dental Association*, **69**(2), 84–89.

Becker, D.E. (2011) Adverse drug interactions. *Anesthesia Progress*, **58**(1), 31–41.

Bellomo, F., De Preux, F. & Müller, F. (2005) The advantages of occupational therapy in oral hygiene measures for institutionalized elderly adults. *Gerodontology*, **22**, 24–31.

Bluml, B.M., McKenney, J.M. & Cziraky, M.J. (2000) Pharmaceutical care services and results in project IMPACT: hyperlipidemia. *Journal of the American Pharmacists Association*, **40**(2), 157–65.

Brennan, MT, Valerin, M.A., Napeñas, J.J., *et al.* (2005) Oral manifestations of patients with lupus erythematosus. *Dental Clinics of North America*, **49**(1), 127–41.

Brown, D.W. (2009) Complete edentulism prior to age 65 years is associated with all-cause mortality. *Journal of Public Health Dentistry*, **69**(4), 260–6.

Brown, R.S., Farquharson, A.A. & Pallasch, T.M. (2007) Medical consultations for medically complex dental patients. *The Journal of the California Dental Association*, **35**(5), 343–9.

Bureau of Labor Statistics (2012) *Social Workers, Occupational Outlook Handbook, 2012–13 Edition*. From http://www.bls.gov/ooh/community-and-social-service/social-workers.htm. Accessed April 16, 2014.

CDC (Centers for Disease Control and Prevention) (2003) Retention of natural teeth among older adults – United States, 2002. *Morbidity and Mortality Weekly Report*, **52**(50), 1226–9.

CDC (Centers for Disease Control and Prevention) (2011) *Oral Health. Preventing Cavities, Gum Disease, Tooth Loss, and Oral Cancers*. From http://www.cdc.gov/chronicdisease/resources/publications/AAG/doh.htm. Accessed April 16, 2014.

Chalmers, J.M. & Ettinger, R.L. (2008) Public health issues in geriatric dentistry in the United States. *Dental Clinics of North America*, **52**, 423–46.

Chalmers, J.M., Levy, S., Buckwalter, K. *et al.* (1996) Factors influencing nurses' aides provision of oral care for nursing facility residents. *Special Care in Dentistry*, **16**, 71–9.

Cohen, L.A. (2009) The role of non-dental health professionals in providing access to dental care for low-income and minority patients. *Dental Clinics of North America*, **53**, 451–68.

Coleman, P. (2005) Opportunities for nursing–dental collaboration: addressing the oral health needs among the elderly. *Nursing Outlook*, **53**(1), 33–9.

Coleman, P. & Watson, N.M. (2006) Oral care provided by certified nursing assistants in nursing homes. *Journal of the American Geriatrics Society*, **54**, 138–43.

Crown, L.A. & May, J.A. (2012) Zinc toxicity: denture adhesives, bone marrow failure and polyneuropathy. *Tennessee Medicine*, **105**(2), 39–42.

Dobrof, R. (1999) From the editor. *Journal of Gerontological Social Work*, **30**(3–4), 1.

Doherty, K., Connor, M. & Cruickshank, R. (2011) Zinc-containing denture adhesives: a potential source of excess zinc resulting in copper deficiency myelopathy. *British Dental Journal*, **210**(11), 523–5.

Dolan, T., Atchison, K. & Huynh, T. (2005). Access to dental care among older adults in the United States. *Journal of Dental Education*, **69**(9), 961–74.

Dyer, C.B., Hyer, K., Feldt, K.S., *et al.* (2004) Frail older patient care by interdisciplinary teams: a primer for generalists. *Gerontology & Geriatrics Education*, **24**(2), 51–62.

El-Solh, A.A., Pietrantoni, C., Bhat, A. *et al.* (2004) Colonization of dental plaques: a reservoir of respiratory pathogens for hospital-acquired pneumonia in institutionalized elders. *Chest,* **126**(5), 1575–82.

Eskandari, A., Mahmoudpour, A., Abolfazli, N., *et al.* (2010). Detection of *Helicobacter pylori* using PCR in dental plaque of patients with and without gastritis. *Medicana Oral Patologia Oral y Ciugia Bucal,* **15**(1), e28–31.

Fiske, J., Griffiths, J. & Thompson, S. (2002) Multiple sclerosis and oral care. *Dental Update,* **29**(6), 273–83.

Frenkel, H., Harvey, I. & Newcombe, R.G. (2001) Improving oral health in institutionalized elderly people by educating caregivers: a randomized controlled trial. *Community Dentistry and Oral Epidemiology,* **29**(4), 289–97.

Friedlander, A.H., Mahler, M., Norman, K.M. *et al.* (2009) Parkinson disease: systemic and orofacial manifestations, medical and dental management. *Journal of the American Dental Association,* **140**(6), 658–69.

Gebrara, E.C., Faria, C.M., Pannuti, C., *et al.* (2006) Persistence of *Heliobactor pylori* in the oral cavity after systemic eradication therapy. *Journal of Clinical Periodontology,* **33**(5), 329–33.

Gibbons, R.V. (1998) Germs, Dr. Billings, and the theory of focal infection. *Clinical Infectious Diseases,* **27**, 627–33.

Gilbert, L. (1998) The role of the community pharmacist as an oral health adviser – an exploratory study of community pharmacists in Johannesburg, South Africa. *South African Dental Journal,* **53**(8), 439–43.

Griffin, S.O., Jones, J.A., Brunson D., *et al.* (2012) Burden of oral disease among older adults and implications for public health priorities. *American Journal of Public Health,* **102**(3), 411–18.

Grumbach, K. & Bodenheimer, T. (2004) Can health care teams improve primary care practice? *JAMA: the Journal of the American Medical Association,* **291**, 1246–51.

Hajjar E.R., Gray S.L., Guay D.R., *et al.* (2011) Geriatrics. In: *Pharmacotherapy: A Pathophysiologic Approach* (eds. R.L. Talbert, J.T. DiPiro, G.R. Matzke, *et al.*), 8th edn. McGraw-Hill, New York.

Ham, R.J. (2002) Assessment. In: *Primary Care Geriatrics: A Case-Based Approach* (eds. R.J. Ham, P.D. Sloane & G.A. Warshaw), 4th edn, pp. 51–78. Mosby, St. Louis, Mo.

Hanada, N. & Tada, A. (2001) The relationship between poor oral health status and biological and psychosocial function in the bedridden elderly. *Archives of Gerontology and Geriatrics,* **33**, 133–40.

Hanlon, J.T., Weinberger, M., Samsa, G.P., *et al.* (1996) A randomized, controlled trial of a clinical pharmacist intervention to improve inappropriate prescribing in elderly outpatients with polypharmacy. *American Journal of Medicine,* **100**(4), 428–37.

Hellstein, J.W., Adler, R.A., Edwards, B., *et al.* (2011) Managing the care of patients receiving antiresorptive therapy for prevention and treatment of osteoporosis: executive summary of recommendations from the American Dental Association Council on Scientific Affairs. *The Journal of the American Dental Association,* **142**(11), 1243–51.

Hellyer, P.H. (2011) The older dental patient – who cares? *British Dental Journal,* **211**(3), 109–11.

Hildebolt, C.F. (1997) Osteoporosis and oral bone loss. *Dentomaxillofacial Radiology,* **26**(1), 3–15.

Holmlund, A. & Lind, L. (2012) Number of teeth is related to atherosclerotic plaque in the carotid arteries in an elderly population. *Journal of Periodontology,* **83**(3), 287–91.

Iacopino, A.M. (2008) Practicing oral–systemic medicine: the need for interprofessional education. *Journal of the Canadian Dental Association,* **74**(10), 866–7.

Iacopino, A.M. (2009) Management of systemic inflammation by dentists and physicians: new guidelines. *Journal of the Canadian Dental Association,* **75**(8), 564–5.

Institute of Medicine (2003) *Health Professions Education: a Bridge to Quality* (eds. A.C. Greiner & E. Knebel). The National Academies Press, Washington, DC.

Institute of Medicine and National Research Council (2011) *Improving Access to Oral Health Care for Vulnerable and Underserved Populations.* The National Academies Press, Washington, DC.

Jacobsen, P.L. & Lofholm, P.W. (2008) Dentists/pharmacist relations: professional responsibility, scope of practice, and rational prescription wiring. Interview by Debra Belt. *Journal of the California Dental Association,* **36**(10), 781–9.

Kalmar, J., James, W.D., Fivenson, D.P. *et al.* (2012) Oral Manifestations of Drug Reactions. *Medscape Reference,* From http://emedicine.medscape.com/article/1080772-overview. Accessed April 16, 2014.

Kayser-Jones, J., Bird, W.F., Paul, S.M., *et al.* (1995) An instrument to assess the oral health status of nursing home residents. *Gerontologist,* **35**(6), 814–24.

Keough, M.E., Field, T.S. & Gurwitz, J.H. (2002) A model of community-based interdisciplinary team training. *Academic Medicine,* **77**(9), 936.

Koregol, A.C., More, S.P., Nainegali, S., *et al.* (2011) Analysis of inorganic ions in gingival crevicular fluid as indicators of periodontal disease activity: A clinico-biochemical study *Contemporary Clinical Dentistry,* **2**(4), 278–82.

Koshman, S.L., Charrois, T.L. & Simpson, S.H. (2008) Pharmacist care of patients with heart failure. *Archives of Internal Medicine,* **168**(7), 687–94.

Kossioni, A.E. & Dontas, A.S. (2007) The stomatognathic system in the elderly. Useful information for the medical practitioner. *Journal of Clinical Interventions in Aging,* **2**(4), 591–7.

Kumar, P.S., Balan, A., Sankar, A., *et al.* (2009) Radiation induced oral mucositis. *Indian Journal of Palliative Care,* **15**(2), 95–102.

Labeau, S.O., Van de Vyver, K., Brusselaers, N., *et al.* (2011). Prevention of ventilator-associated pneumonia with oral antiseptics: a systematic review and meta-analysis. *The Lancet Infectious Diseases*, **11**(11), 845–54.

Lackey, M.A. & Barth, J. (2003) Gastroesophageal reflux disease: a dental concern. *General Dentistry*, **51**(3), 250–4.

Lee, H.K., Lee, K.D., Merchant, A.T., *et al.* (2010) More missing teeth are associated with poorer general health in the rural Korean elder. *Archives of Gerontology and Geriatrics*, **50**(1), 30–3.

Levy, R.L., Lambert, R. & Davis, G. (1979) Social work and dentistry in clinical, training, and research collaboration, *Social Work in Health Care*, **5**(2), 177–85.

Li, X., Kolltveit, K.M., Tronstad, L., *et al.* (2000) Systemic diseases caused by oral infection. *Clinical Microbiology Reviews*, **13**(4), 547–58.

Little, J.W., Falace, D.A., Miller, C.S. *et al.* (2008). Cancer and oral care of the patient. In: *Dental Management of the Medically Compromised Patient* (eds. J. Dolan, C. Sprehe & J.Pendill), 7th edn, pp. 447–9. Mosby Inc., St. Louis, MO.

Lockart, P.B., Bolger, A.F., Papapanou, P.N., *et al.* (2012) Periodontal disease and atherosclerotic vascular disease: does the evidence support an independent association? A scientific statement from the American Heart Association. *Circulation*, **125**, 2520–44.

MacEntee, M.I. (2006) Missing links in oral health care for frail elderly people. *Journal of the Canadian Dental Association*, **72**(5), 421–5.

Manski, R., Goodman, H., Reid, B., & Macek, M. (2004). Dental insurance visits and expenditures among older adults. *American Journal of Public Health*, **94**(5), 759–64.

Maunder, P.E. & Landes, D.P. (2005) An evaluation of the role played by community pharmacies in oral healthcare situated in primary care trust in the north of England. *British Medical Journal*, **199**(4), 219–23.

McFarland, L. & Rhor Inglehart, M., (2010) Depression, self-efficacy, and oral health: an exploration. *Oral Health and Dental Management In the Black Sea Countries*, **9**(4), 214–22.

McLean, D.L., McAlister, F.A., Johnson, J.A., *et al.* (2008) A randomized trial of the effect of community pharmacist and nurse care on improving blood pressure management in patients with diabetes mellitus. *Archives of Internal Medicine*, **168**(21), 2355–61.

Meredith, M.J. (2001) Herbal nutriceuticals: a primer for dentists and dental hygienists. *Journal of Contemporary Dental Practice*, **2**(2), 1–24.

Miller, W.D. (1891) The human mouth as a focus of infection. *Dental Cosmos*, **33**, 689–713.

Minnesota Board of Dentistry (2014) *Dental Therapists: Background and Updates on Implementation.* From http://www.dentalboard.state.mn.us/Licensing/ProcessingandApplications/DentalTherapistsAdv-DentalTherapist/tabid/1165/Default.aspx. Accessed April 18, 2014.

Moore, P.A. & Guggenheimer, J. (2008) Medication-induced hyposalivation: etiology, diagnosis, and treatment. *Compendium of Continuing Education in Dentistry*, **29**(1), 50–5.

Mouradian, W.E. & Corbin, S.B. (2003) Addressing health disparities through dental–medical collaborations, part II: cross-cutting themes in the care of special populations. *Journal of Dental Education*, **67**(12), 1320–6.

Mouradian, W.E., Huebner, C. & DePaola, D. (2004) Addressing health disparities through dental–medical collaborations, part III: leadership for the public good. *Journal of Dental Education*, **68**(5), 505–12.

Murray, M.D., Ritchey, M.E., Wu, J., *et al.* (2009) Effect of a pharmacist on adverse drug events and medication errors in outpatients with cardiovascular disease. *Archives of Internal Medicine*, **169**(8), 757–63.

Namiot, D.B., Namiot, Z., Kemona, A., *et al.* (2006) Peptic ulcers and oral health status. *Advances in Medical Science*, **51**, 153–5.

Nash, D.A., Friedman, J.W., Mathu-Muju, K.R., *et al.* (2012) *A Review of the Global Literature on Dental Therapists.* W. K. Kellogg Foundation, Battle Creek, MI.

National Institutes of Health (2010) *Salivary Diagnostics. NIH Fact Sheet.* From http://report.nih.gov/nihfactsheets/ViewFactSheet.aspx?csid=65. Accessed April 16, 2014.

Nations, S.P., Boyer, P.J., Love, L.A., *et al.* (2008) Denture cream: an unusual source of excess zinc, leading to hypocupremia and neurologic disease. *Neurology*, **71**(9), 639–43.

Navabi, N., Aramon, M. & Mirzazadeh, A. (2011) Does the presence of the *Helicobacter pylori* in the dental plaque associate with its gastric infection? A meta-analysis and systematic review. *Dental Research Journal*, **8**(4), 178–82.

Nazmul-Hossain, A.N., Morarasu, G.M., Schmidt, S.K., *et al.* (2011) A current perspective on Sjögren's syndrome. *Journal of the California Dental Association*, **39**(9), 631–7.

Nowjack-Raymer, R.E. & Sheiham, A. (2003) Association of edentulism and diet and nutrition in US adults. *Journal of Dental Research*, **82**(12), 123–6.

Okoro, C.A., Balluz, L.S., Eke, P.I., *et al.* (2005) Tooth loss and heart disease: findings from the Behavioral Risk Factor Surveillance System. *American Journal of Preventive Medicine*, **29**(5 Suppl 1), 50–6.

Pace, C.C. & McCullough, G.H. (2010) The association between oral microorganisms and aspiration pneumonia in the institutionalized elderly: review and recommendations. *Dysphagia*, **25**(4), 307–22.

Padilha, D.M., Hugo, F.N., Hilgert, J.B., *et al.* (2007) Hand function and oral hygiene in older institutionalized Brazilians. *Journal of the American Geriatrics Society*, **55**, 1333–8.

Padilha, D.M., Hilgert, J.B., Hugo, F.N., *et al.* (2008) Number of teeth and mortality risk in the Baltimore Longitudinal Study of Aging. *The Journal of Gerontology Series A: Biological Sciences and Medical Sciences*, **63**(7), 739–44.

Pallasch, T.J. & Wahl, M.J. (2003) Focal infection: new age or ancient history? *Endodontic Topics*, **4**, 32–45.

Pazianas, M., Miller, P., Blumentals, W.A., *et al.* (2007) A review of the literature on osteonecrosis of the jaw in patients with osteoporosis treated with oral bisphosphonates: prevalence, risk factors, and clinical characteristics. *Clinical Therapeutics*, **29**(8), 1548–58.

Petrosky, M., Shaffer, C.L, Devlin, L., *et al.* (2000) An on-site social work program in an urban academic dental center. *Journal of Dental Education*, **64**(5), 370–4.

Petrosky, M., Colaruotolo, L.A., Billings, R.J. *et al.* (2009) The integration of social work into a postgraduate dental training program: a 15 year perspective. *Journal of Dental Education*, **73**(6), 656–64.

Pew Center on the States (2010) *It Takes A Team: How New Dental Providers Can Benefit Patients And Practices.* From http://www.pewtrusts.org/uploadedFiles/wwwpewtrustsorg/Reports/State_policy/Report_It_Takes_a_Team_final.pdf. Accessed April 16, 2014.

Polverini, P.J. (2012) A curriculum for the new dental practitioner: preparing dentists for a prospective oral health care environment. *American Journal of Public Health*, **102**(2), e1–3.

Ranijitkar, S., Smales, R.J. & Kaidonis, J.A. (2012) Oral manifestations of gastroesophageal reflux disease. *Journal of Gastroenterology and Hepatology*, **27**(1), 21–7.

Reimann, H.A. & Havens, W.P. (1940) Focal infection and systemic disease: a critical appraisal. *Journal of the American Medical Association*, **114**(1), 1–6.

Reuben, D. (2009) Better ways to care for older persons: is anybody listening? *Journal of the American Geriatrics Society*, **57**, 2348–9.

Rhein, M.L. (1912). Oral sepsis. *Dental Cosmos*, **54**, 529–34.

Rice, K., Zwarenstein, M., Gotlib, L., *et al.* (2010) An intervention to improve interprofessional collaboration and communications: a comparative qualitative study. *Journal of Interprofessional Care*, **24**(4), 350–61.

Ritchie, C.S. & Kinane, D.F. (2003) Nutrition, inflammation, and periodontal disease. *Nutrition*, **19**, 475–6.

Rozier, R.G., Sutton, B.K., Bawden, J.W., *et al.* (2003) Prevention of early childhood caries in North Carolina medical practices: implications for research and practice. *Journal of Dental Education*, **67**(8), 876–85.

Russell, S.L., Boylan, R.J., Kaslick, R.S., *et al.* (1999) Respiratory pathogen colonization of the dental plaque of institutionalized elders. *Special Care Dentistry*, **19**(3), 128–34.

Saini, R., Saini, S. & Sugandha, R.S (2011) Periodontal disease: the sixth complication of diabetes. *Journal of Family and Community Medicine*, **18**(1), 31.

Savoca, M.R., Arcury, T.A., Leng, X. *et al.* (2010) Severe tooth loss in older adults as a key indicator of compromised dietary quality. *Public Health Nutrition*, **13**, 466–74.

Scannapieco, F.A. (2006) Pneumonia in nonambulatory patients. The role of oral bacteria and oral hygiene. *The Journal of the American Dental Association*, **137**, S21–5.

Schiller, J.S., Lucas, J.W., Ward, B.W., *et al.* (2012). Summary health statistics for US adults: National Health Interview Survey 2010. National Center for Health Statistics. *Vital and Health Statistics*, **10**(252), 1–252.

Schmader, K.E., Hanlon, J.T., Pieper, C.F., *et al.* (2004) Effects of geriatric evaluation and management on adverse drug reactions and suboptimal prescribing in the frail elderly. *American Journal of Medicine*, **116**(6), 394–401.

Smith, R.G. & Burtner, A.P. (1994) Oral side effects of the most frequently prescribed drugs. *Special Care Dentistry*, **14**(3), 96–102.

Steele, J.G. & Walls, A.W.G. (1997) Strategies to improve the quality of oral health care for frail and dependent older people. *Quality in Health Care*, **6**(3), 165–9.

Stein, P.S., Desrosiers, M., Donegan, S.J., *et al.* (2007) Tooth loss, dementia and neuropathology in the Nun study. *Journal of the American Dental Association*, **138**(10), 1314–22.

Stille, C.J., Jerant, A., Bell, D., *et al.* (2005) Coordinating care across diseases, settings, and clinicians: a key role for the generalist in practice. *Annals of Internal Medicine*, **142**, 700–8.

Sumi, Y., Miura, H., Nagaya, M., *et al.* (2009) Relationship between oral function and general condition among Japanese nursing home residents. *Archives of Gerontology and Geriatrics*, **48**, 100–5.

Tada, A. & Miura, H. (2012). Prevention of aspiration pneumonia (AP) with oral care. *Archives of Gerontology and Geriatrics*, **55**(1), 16–21.

Tezvergil-Mutluay, A., Carvalho, R.M. & Pashley, D.H. (2010) Hyperzincemia from injestion of denture adhesives. *Journal of Prosthetic Dentistry*, **103**(6), 380–3.

Touger-Decker, R., Mobley, C.C. & American Dietetic Association (2007) Position of the American Dietetic Association: oral health and nutrition. *Journal of the American Dietetic Association*, **107**(8), 1418–8.

Tramini, P., Montal, S. & Valcarcel, J. (2007) Tooth loss and associated factors in long-term institutionalized elderly patients. *Gerodontology*, **24**(4), 196–203.

Tsukuda, R.A. (1990) Interdisciplinary collaboration: teamwork in geriatrics. In: *Geriatric Medicine* (eds. C.K. Cassel, D.E. Reisenberg & L.B. Sorensen), 2nd edn, pp. 668–9. Springer-Verlag, New York.

US Department of Health and Human Services (2000) *Oral Health in America: A Report of the Surgeon General.* From http://profiles.nlm.nih.gov/ps/retrieve/ResourceMetadata/NNBBJT/. Accessed April 16, 2014.

US Department of Health and Human Services (2003) *National Call to Action to Promote Oral Health.* From http://www.ncbi.nlm.nih.gov/books/NBK47472/. Accessed April 16, 2014.

US Department of Health and Human Services (2010) *Strategic Plan. Fiscal Years 2010–2015.* From http://www.hhs.gov/strategic-plan/stratplan_fy2010-15.pdf. Accessed April 16, 2014.

van der Maarel-Wierink, C.D., Vanobbergen, J.N., Bronkhorst, E.M., *et al.* (2013) Oral health care and aspiration pneumonia in frail older people: a systematic literature review. *Gerodontology*, **30**(1), 3–9.

Vyt, A. (2008) Interprofessional and transdisciplinary teamwork in health care. *Diabetes/Metabolism Research and Reviews*, **24** (Suppl 1), S106–9.

Wall, T.P. & Brown, L.J. (2003). Recent trends in dental visits and private dental insurance, 1989 and 1999. *Journal of the American Dental Association*, **134**, 621–7.

Walsh, K., Roberts, J. & Bennett, G. (1999) Mobility in old age. *Gerodontology*, **16**(2), 69–74.

Wårdh, I., Hallberg, L.R., Berggren, U. *et al.* (2000) Oral health care – a low priority in nursing: in-depth interviews with nursing staff. *Scandinavian Journal of Caring Sciences*, **14**, 137–42.

Watt, R. & Sheiham, A. (1999) Health policy: inequalities in oral health. A review of the evidence and recommendations for action. *British Dental Journal*, **187**(6), 6–12.

Watt, R., Tsakos, G., de Oliveira, C., *et al.* (2012) Tooth loss and cardiovascular disease mortality risk – results from the Scottish Health Survey. *PLoS One*, **7**(2), e30797.

Williams, B.C., Remington, T. & Foulk, M. (2002) Teaching interdisciplinary geriatrics team care. *Academic Medicine*, **77**(9), 935.

Williams, B.C., Remington, T.L., Foulk, M.A., *et al.* (2006) Teaching interdisciplinary geriatrics ambulatory care: a case study. *Gerontology & Geriatrics Education*, **26**(3), 29–45.

Wu, B., Liang, J., Plassman, B.L., *et al.* (2012) Edentulism trends among middle-aged and older adults in the United States: comparison of five racial/ethnic groups. *Community Dentistry and Oral Epidemiology*, **40**(2), 145–53.

Xyrichis, A. & Lowton, K. (2008) What fosters or prevents interprofessional teamworking in primary and community care? *International Journal of Nursing Studies*, **45**, 140–53.

Ylöstalo, P.V., Järvelin, M.R., Laitinen, J., *et al.* (2006) Gingivitis, dental caries and tooth loss: risk factors for cardiovascular diseases or indicators of elevated health risks. *Journal of Clinical Periodontology*, **33**(2), 92–101.

Yoon, M.N. & Steele, C.M. (2007) The oral care imperative: the link between oral hygiene and aspiration pneumonia. *Topics in Geriatric Rehabilitation*, **23**(3), 280–8.

Yoon, M.N. & Steele, C.M. (2012) Health professionals' perspectives on oral care for long-term care residents: nursing staff, speech-language pathologists and dental hygienists. *Gerodontology*, **29**(2), e525–35.

Zittel-Palamara, K., Fabiano, J.A., Davis, E.L., *et al.* (2005) Improving patient retention and access to oral health care: the CARES program. *Journal of Dental Education*, **69**(8), 912–18.

PART 6

Future Vision

CHAPTER 21

Planning for the Future

Teresa A. Dolan[1] and Douglas Berkey[2]

[1]DENTSPLY International, York, PA, USA; University of Florida College of Dentistry, Gainesville, FL, USA
[2]University of Colorado School of Dental Medicine, Aurora, CO, USA

Introduction

The aging of America is often referred to as the demographic imperative, or perhaps more dramatically, as a tsunami or the "Age Wave"(Dychtwald & Flower, 1989). These terms refer to the dramatic shift in the age composition of the USA. Never before in human history have so many people lived beyond the age of 65 years. For example, as seen in Fig. 21.1, in 1900 only 4.1% of the US population was over the age of 65 years as compared to 13% in 2010 and a projected 20.2% in 2050. The USA is projected to experience rapid growth in its older population as baby boomers or those born between the years 1946 and 1964 begin crossing into the category of older adults, which can be chronologically defined as those over the age of 65. By the year 2030, the US Census Bureau estimates that there will be 57.8 million baby boomers aged between 66 and 84 (US Census Bureau, 2006). This shift has profound social, political, healthcare, business, financial, workforce, and cultural implications.

Policy implications of the aging US population include the impact on federal spending, as well as on our healthcare, long-term care and social service systems. The USA is challenged to ensure appropriate access to necessary healthcare services, and doing so within constrained resources to achieve the best possible health outcomes. From an oral health perspective, we are challenged to ensure that the dental workforce is well prepared to serve the needs of older adults and that dental care is organized and delivered in a way that meets the needs of older patients.

The purpose of this chapter is to explore the impact of the aging population on US health policies, the preparation of health professionals, and delivery of oral health services. In thinking towards the future, how can we anticipate the healthcare needs of all older adults, and particularly vulnerable elders? Can we ensure that our public policies, care delivery, reimbursement systems, and health professionals are aligned and prepared to meet the dental needs of the growing number of elders? Case studies will be used to illustrate some key concepts in geriatric dentistry including innovative models of care delivery, and the development of public policies that are sensitive to the needs of older adults.

The continuum of aging

Because of the great variability in physical, social, medical, oral and mental health status among people over the age of 65 years (Dychtwald & Flower, 1989; Dolan *et al.*, 2005), it is overly simplistic to use a chronological definition of aging. It is more appropriate to discuss the needs of older adults according to their health and functional status, rather than by their age alone (Dychtwald & Flower, 1989). A broader definition offered by the Bureau of Health Professions described "elderly" to mean "a population with healthcare conditions and needs which differ significantly from those of younger people, which are often complicated by the physical, behavioral, and social changes associated with aging. This would include all persons over sixty, but may include slightly younger people who are subject to similar

Geriatric Dentistry: Caring for Our Aging Population, First Edition. Edited by Paula K. Friedman.
© 2014 John Wiley & Sons, Inc. Published 2014 by John Wiley & Sons, Inc.
Companion website: www.wiley.com/go/friedman/geriatricdentistry

physical and/or mental conditions" (Bureau of Health Professions, 1993).

Ettinger and Beck classified elders as being independent, frail, or functionally dependent (Ettinger & Beck, 1984). While the majority of older adults live independently in the community, a smaller proportion of elders are frail and need some assistance, while others with significant functional dependence require assistance in their "activities of daily living" or ADLs. ADLs refer to the basic tasks of

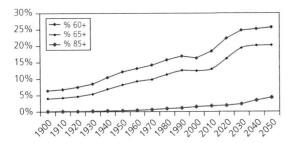

Figure 21.1 Older population by age from 1900 and projected through 2050. Projections for 2010 through 2050 are from US Census Bureau (2008), Table 12. The source of the data for 1900–2000 is US Census Bureau (2002), Table 5. This table was compiled by the US Administration on Aging using the Census data noted.

everyday life, such as eating, bathing, dressing, toileting, mobility, and transferring from a chair to a bed, for example. When people are unable to perform these activities, they need help from other people, from mechanical assistive devices or from both (Katz *et al.*, 1963).

Although persons of all ages may have problems performing their ADLs, prevalence rates of people with these limitations are much higher for the elderly than for the nonelderly. The prevalence of a condition is defined as the number of persons in a certain population who have a specific disease or condition at a designated point in time. A prevalence rate is the proportion of persons with a defined disease or condition at the time they were studied (Katz, 1997). As seen in Table 21.1, the prevalence of chronic diseases as well as disabilities and limitations increases with advancing age and is especially high for persons aged 75 years and over (IOM, 2008). For example, about half of adults ages 75 years and older have trouble hearing as compared to only about 16.8% of adults ages 18 years and over. These prevalence estimates do not include adults living in long-term care and other institutional settings. Thus, the prevalence is most likely an underestimate and the number of adults affected by chronic diseases and related

Table 21.1 Prevalence of chronic diseases and disability or limitations by age group, 2006*

	Ages 18+(%)	64–74(%)	Ages 75+(%)
Prevalence of chronic disease			
Hypertension	22.9	52.9	53.8
Chronic joint symptoms	25.2	42.7	44.2
Heart disease	10.9	26.2	36.6
Any cancer	7.1	17.2	25.7
Diabetes	7.7	18.6	18.3
Stroke	2.6	7.6	11.2
Asthma	7.3	7.8	6.1
Chronic bronchitis	4.2	5.6	6.7
Prevalence of disability/limitations			
Trouble hearing	16.8	31.9	50.4
Vision limitations, even with glasses or contacts	9.5	13.6	21.7
Absence of all natural teeth	8.0	22.8	29.4
Any physical difficulty	14.6	30.2	48.1

Note: Does not contain information on the institutionalized adult population.

*Adapted from IOM (2008), Table 2.1, p. 42.

limitations is probably higher than reported in the table. These changes in health status with age impacts oral health as well. As people age and become more vulnerable and functionally impaired, they are less likely to have regular dental visits and are more likely to have oral health problems (Dolan *et al.*, 1998).

A person's health status can be dynamic, and older persons may be independent at one point in time and then become frail or functionally dependent after suffering an acute ailment or the exacerbation of a chronic condition. Likewise, an older person can recover from an acute illness and regain functional independence (Dolan & Atchison, 1993). Thus, organizing and providing health services for older patients can be more complex than for the healthy adult patient. The American Dental Association has been engaged in several national initiatives focused on "vulnerable elders," defined as patients over the age of 65 who have any or all of the following: limited mobility, limited resources, or complex health status (ADA, 2009). This focus recognizes some of the unique challenges in providing care to older patients who have limitations in their functional abilities and may be homebound or living in long-term care facilities. Regardless of the location of the care being provided, the astute clinician needs to be aware of possible variations in health status, frequently review the health status of the patient, "check in" with how the patient may be feeling during a particular visit, and be willing to adjust the daily care plan accordingly.

Health professionals as well as policy makers should also reflect on their personal beliefs and opinions about the aging process and older adults, and how this could potentially impact the approach to patient care. Our attitudes, beliefs, and conceptions of the characteristics of older persons, termed ageism, may be prejudicial and distorted (Hooyman & Kiyak, 2010). (See Chapter 4 on Palmore's Facts on Aging Quiz to learn more about facts and myths of aging.) While some may have negative views of older adults, others may hold compassionate stereotypes about older adults in which they assume that most older people are poor, frail, ill-housed, and deserving and/or in need of public or government assistance. We must guard against ageism and both positive and negative stereotypes in our care of older patients. Patient-centered care recognizes and acknowledges

the uniqueness of each person as we plan for their individual care. It is important to understand that age or date of birth has limited predictive value in terms of functionality or scope of dental treatment when dealing with our aging population. Likewise, policy makers should be aware of positive and negative stereotypes about older people as they work to set state or national health agendas to care for older adults at the societal level (Hooyman & Kiyak, 2010).

Health and social policies for older adults

The Social Security Act of 1935 established the first significant national public benefits program and consequently the federal government's role in protecting the social welfare of older adults (Bryce & Friedland, 1997). The act provided an implicit guarantee that the succeeding generations would provide for its older members through employees' Social Security contributions. Some policymakers at the time intended to expand the plan to include other public benefits including a nationwide health program. However, after the passage of the Social Security Act, national interest in policies to further support older adults diminished until the 1960s. Subsequent landmark legislation passed in 1965 included establishing Medicare and Medicaid (Hooyman & Kiyak, 2010). These public policies were critical in keeping many older adults out of poverty, and ensuring payment for most medical and hospital services.

Congress passed the Older Americans Act (OAA) in 1965 in response to concern by policymakers about a lack of community social services for older persons. The original legislation established authority for grants to states for community planning and social services, research and development projects, and personnel training in the field of aging. The law also established the Administration on Aging to administer the newly created grant programs and to serve as the federal focal point on matters concerning older persons (AoA, 2012).

While this federal legislation provides support for most medical services for older adults, public funding for adult dental services is much more limited. Consequently, the lack of public funding for dental care often results in older adults not receiving routine preventive and restorative dental services. As a consequence, many older patients only seek dental care when they have an emergency or a dental problem. About 70% of older adult patients do not have third party payment coverage for their care (McGinn-Shapiro, 2008). Funding for Medicaid is targeted at low-income people and is shared approximately equally between the state and the federal governments. Although Medicaid requires that coverage of certain dental benefits be provided for children, states can opt out of providing dental benefits for adults and seniors, and most have done so. Only about 2% of the total Medicaid budget is currently allocated to oral health care (CDC, 2003).

Funding for Medicare is fully supported by the federal government, and the primary beneficiaries are adults over age 65, although there are limited provisions for coverage of certain serious illnesses for all age groups. As further described in the next paragraph, Medicare provides no dental coverage for elders except in extraordinary circumstances. Sometimes dental services are covered through employer-provided healthcare plans. This coverage does not usually extend into retirement years. Even if privately or publicly funded plans provide some basic coverage beyond the work years, inadequate reimbursement can emphasize triage and symptomatic care only. Fear or anxiety may also limit dental care usage in older adults. Visual or hearing-impaired elderly can become frustrated trying to communicate with dental staff. As a result, dental care may not be pursued. Because such a small proportion of US elders have private dental insurance and Medicare and Medicaid's coverage of oral health care is minimal, the dental care needs of underserved older Americans will not be met without significant changes in health policy related to dental care for older adults.

"Medically necessary" oral health care

The US Surgeon General's report has declared that oral health problems represent the "silent X-factor promoting the onset of life-threatening diseases which are responsible for the deaths of millions of Americans each year" (NIDCR, 2000). Increasingly, studies find that oral disease can significantly affect systemic health. For example, bacteremia or cytokinemia from diseased periodontal tissues may trigger inflammatory and/or immunologic responses contributing to tissue or organ damage (see Chapter 11, Periodontal Disease). Compelling associations exist between oral disease and cardiovascular and respiratory diseases, but oral disease can also exacerbate the effect of diseases such as diabetes. Data-driven conclusions about a potential direct cause-and-effect relationship for many oral–systemic linkages remain lacking, but ongoing research continues to suggest strong inter-relationships. Medical and oral health research collaborations to study these relationships are urgently needed to improve the delivery of oral health care and to set public policy and direct public resources to the most effective therapies, including oral health care.

In establishing the Medicare legislation, Congress included a blanket exclusion of dental services. The enabling legislation specifically omitted payments "for services in connection with the care, treatment, filling, removal, or replacement of teeth or structures directly supporting the teeth" (Section 1862(a)(12) of the Social Security Act). The exclusion was later amended in 1980 when Congress made an exception for inpatient hospital services when the dental procedure itself made hospitalization necessary (CMS, 2013). The exception allowed payment "in the case of inpatient hospital services in connection with the provision of dental services if the individual, because of his/her underlying medical condition and clinical status, or because of the severity of the dental procedure, requires hospitalization in connection with the provision of such services." Currently, Medicare will pay for dental services that are an integral part either of a covered procedure such as reconstruction of the jaw following accidental injury, or for extractions done in preparation for radiation treatment for cancer involving the jaw (Committee on Medicare Coverage Extensions, 2000). Medicare will also make payment for oral examinations, but not treatment, preceding kidney transplantation or heart valve replacement, under certain circumstances. The Medicare coverage as specified in statue is summarized in Table 21.2.

In 2011, Congress considered but ultimately disapproved funding medically necessary dental procedures associated with prosthetic heart valve

Table 21.2 Medicare coverage of dental services as specified in statute or by the Health Care Financing Administration*

Clinical condition	Medicare-covered service
Underlying medical condition and clinical status requires hospitalization for dental care	Inpatient hospital services only (Medicare Part A)
Severity of dental procedure requires hospitalization for dental care	Inpatient hospital services only (Medicare Part A)
Any oral condition for which nondental services are covered	All dental services if incident to and an integral part of a covered procedure or service performed by the same person (Medicare Part B)
Neoplastic jaw disease	Extractions prior to radiation and prior to oral examination if extractions occur (Medicare Part B)
Renal transplant surgery	Oral or dental examination on an inpatient basis (Medicare Part A if performed by hospital-based dentist; Part B if performed by a physician)

*Adapted from Field *et al.* (2000).

replacement, organ transplantation, head and neck cancer, lymphoma, and leukemia. Medically necessary dental procedures were defined as those that diagnose, prevent, or treat a condition; prevent the condition from progressing or becoming more painful or severe; or help improve a condition and/or provide rehabilitative effects. Given the growing scientific evidence that preventing oral infection significantly benefits health, Congress should revisit the need to revise the statutory Medicare language to include more oral health care that prevents or reduces complications of medical conditions or their treatment. In addition to the proposed 2011 Medicare inclusions, special considerations are warranted for several chronic conditions.

Expanding the evidence base

Diabetes mellitus is a chronic metabolic disorder that affects an estimated 26 million people in the USA, 11 million of whom are adults age 65 years or older (NIDDK, 2011). It will likely become the leading cause of overall disease burden by 2023. Complications associated with diabetes include increased risks for heart disease and stroke, hypertension, blindness and eye disorders, kidney disease, neuropathies, amputations, dental disease, and problematic pregnancies. Persons with diabetes have a risk for death about twice that of nondiabetic people the same age. Even prediabetes, a condition involving blood glucose levels higher than normal

but not high enough to be classified as diabetes, increases the risk of heart disease and stroke. The Scottsdale Project assembled medical and dental experts to assess the quality of evidence linking periodontal disease and diabetes. They concluded there is support for a bidirectional relationship between the two conditions (Li *et al.*, 2011). Diabetes mellitus modifies the risk for periodontal disease and can increase its prevalence, progression, and severity. Poorly controlled diabetes increases the risk of developing periodontal disease three fold. In addition, diabetes and severe periodontal disease increases mortality from ischemic heart disease and the risk of developing end-stage renal disease. Treating periodontitis may improve metabolic control in diabetic patients, reduce the risk of complications, and improve a person's quality of life.

Aspiration pneumonia is perhaps the most common infectious result of poor oral health in elderly patients, especially those in nursing homes. Medical risk factors for aspiration pneumonia include swallowing and feeding problems, less effective lung defense mechanisms, diabetes, impaired immune status, positioning influences, neurologic issues, and functional status. Dental risk factors include dental decay, periodontal disease, high salivary levels of *Staphylococcus aureus*, diminished salivary flow, infrequent visits to the dental hygienist, and generally poor oral hygiene. Pneumonia can be life-threatening and very expensive for older institutionalized patients, yet routine daily oral care can reduce these healthcare costs (Tarpenning, 2005).

Focus on the future: innovation to improve the oral health of vulnerable elders

Innovative models of care delivery

The delivery of dental care to older persons must address problems specific to this population. The 2008 Institute of Medicine (IOM) *"Retooling for an Aging America"* report found older adults are often poorly served by the current healthcare system (IOM, 2008). Quality of care may be compromised when services are provided by various practitioners in an uncoordinated, inefficient, and overly expensive way. Additionally, seniors are often passive partners in their own care. The vulnerable elderly health needs must be addressed comprehensively and efficiently, and in a way that equips them to be active partners in their care. This report specifically recommended that models of care with the best outcomes should be identified and disseminated. In 2011, another IOM report (IOM & NRC, 2011) underscored the need for quality-based dental care in traditional and nontraditional settings. The report recommended more use of nondental healthcare providers to deliver preventive oral health services, expansion of the service capabilities of allied dental staff, and consideration of innovative dental provider personnel roles. (See Chapter 19 for discussion of the role of allied dental providers in long-term care facilities.)

Current dental care delivery models that perform well for older adults must be publicized and replicated where possible. Most older adults receive their dental care in traditional private practice dental offices, representing more than 90% of practicing dentists. Community dwelling older adults may have difficulty accessing care in general practices due to their need for longer appointments and the limited amount of training in geriatrics received by the typical general practitioner. A comprehensive, coordinated approach focused on prevention and health promotion is essential. Office settings should also be more "senior friendly" (see Chapter 5, The Senior Friendly Office.) This includes good lighting; supportive and stationary chairs; efforts to minimize falling risks; handicap-accessible entrances, restrooms, and dental operatories; and effective wheelchair transfer assistance. Positive attitudes toward the elderly should be promoted, with extra time and attention directed toward effective communication strategies and flexible financing options for low-income elderly. Cost-effective clinical approaches that promote good oral health outcomes must be more broadly shared among private practitioners.

"Safety net" healthcare systems may help reduce disparities in dental care access for lower income elderly (ADA, 2011). Included are Federally Qualified Health Centers (FQHCs), hospital emergency departments, free clinics, local health departments, long-term care and special needs services, and charity and volunteer programs. FQHCs are the most common safety net clinic approach, with about 1000 centers providing dental care services across the USA. In 2009, 8.4 million dental visits were recorded and about 3.5 million people received care (McGinn-Shapiro, 2008). However, limited public funding for dental care has resulted in many of these clinics focusing on children, particularly those with insurance through Medicaid and other federally funded programs that aim to expand access to healthcare services for children. Their facility planning and professional development strategies are more likely to be focused on pediatric than geriatric healthcare delivery. To improve dental care access for the vulnerable elderly, all safety net systems should promote quality geriatric dental care, leverage their resources, reduce redundancy, coordinate care more effectively, and work collaboratively with private practices for better integration. To attract dentists into these systems, publicly supported programs including local, state, and/or federal incentives such as loan forgiveness programs for dentists should be expanded.

Integrated models of care

Interdisciplinary team approaches are essential for new healthcare models for older adults. Particularly because of the growing recognition of the importance of good oral health to overall health and well-being, interdisciplinary approaches are needed to provide oral health services in the context of an integrated healthcare home. Managing one's own health care in a fragmented marketplace can limit the accessibility of oral health care for elders and their families. Resources are scattered among multiple providers and locations; communication among providers, caregivers, and patients is often poor; and patient health suffers. In contrast, care management systems using a central point of contact and coordinator allow integration and collaboration of efforts. In addition, patients must be empowered to take a more active role in managing chronic diseases. If this is to be accomplished, they must be educated and equipped with the knowledge and tools to maintain their health and well-being. However, frail elders should not be expected to be successful at creating interprofessional communication where the channels do not yet exist. Caregivers must be better educated about care for elder patients and given the communication channels needed for rational care management.

Integrating oral health into health professionals' educational curricula would provide important foundational knowledge to facilitate preliminary screenings and appropriate referrals. The national efforts to enhance interprofessional education are an important step to improve communication and provide more patient-centered and integrated health care (Interprofessional Educational Collaborative, 2013). In 2009 six national education associations of health professions schools formed a collaborative to promote and encourage efforts that would advance interprofessional learning experiences to help prepare future clinicians for team-based care of patients. These organizations representing the disciplines of allopathic and osteopathic medicine, dentistry, nursing, pharmacy, and public health came together to create core competencies for interprofessional collaborative practice that can guide curricula development at all health professions schools (IPEC Expert Panel, 2011).

Redefining roles

State practice acts for healthcare providers often do not consider problems that accompany shortages in the healthcare workforce and are not adaptable to disparities in workforce distribution. With updated scope of practice acts, roles for dental practitioners and their staffs can be expanded through job delegation. Using such approaches to manage elder patients increases their access to care. Training in geriatric dentistry ensures quality care provision and it is possible that dental hygienists with advanced training in geriatrics might also enhance access and coordination.

An evidence-base and a way to measure additional competence would be required for such an effort to succeed. Care providers, whether they are dentists, dental hygienists, or other dental providers who choose this path, should receive greater professional recognition with a well-defined and appropriate scope of practice and a commensurate salary.

Use of new technology

Health information technologies are starting to help providers better meet the oral health needs of frail and functionally dependent elderly. For example, digital technology now allows dental hygienists or other oral healthcare workers to collaborate with dentists in remote locations, employing "telehealth." Using a properly configured laptop computer, digital portable X-ray unit, and USB intraoral camera, older patients can be assessed, digital radiographs and/or photographs taken, electronic records created, and prevention education provided/transmitted to and from remote, dentally underserved sites. This information is shared with the dentist – who can then diagnose problems, develop a clinical care plan, and task onsite care providers to perform needed preventive and limited restorative services before referring the patient for comprehensive care. Examples of programs effectively utilizing dental telehealth technologies include the Dental Health Aide Therapist (DHAT) program in Alaska, Apple Tree Dental based in Minnesota, and those at the University of the Pacific School of Dentistry.

PACE program: interdisciplinary geriatric care in action

An effective comprehensive healthcare model identified and praised by the 2008 IOM report is the Program of All-Inclusive Care for the Elderly (PACE) (IOM, 2008). This national system of more than 80 managed long-term care programs in nearly 30 states supports low-income frail elderly and their families. Conceived by a dentist in the early 1970s, the PACE model helps seniors while respecting their desire to remain autonomous and at home with maximum physical, social, and cognitive function. PACE supports adults age 55 years and older through a comprehensive care package of integrated acute and long-term care and all Medicare and Medicaid services, plus community long-term care (Fig. 21.2). No benefit limitations,

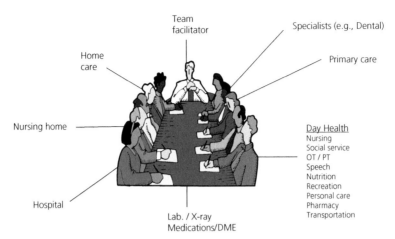

Figure 21.2 The PACE model of integrated and team-managed care for older patients. DME, durable medical equipment; OT/PT, occupational therapy/physical therapy.

copayments, or deductibles, even for dental care services, are imposed (Hirth *et al.*, 2009).

Among the advantages of PACE are centralized resources, home-based care, proactive approaches, and improved patient, provider, and payer experiences. The integrated, community-based collaborative teams provide comprehensive opportunities for seniors to access care and support for basic daily living. Primary care providers; home care and nursing home providers; hospital staff; laboratory, X-ray, and medications experts; day health providers such as occupational therapists, physical therapists, speech therapists, and nutritionists; and specialists such as geriatric dentists or vision care providers participate on interdisciplinary teams. PACE offers nursing home and hospital care, but focuses on outpatient care and home care. Providers are drawn to PACE because there are fewer regulatory restrictions and improved ability to focus on elderly patients' needs. Cost savings for payers such as Medicare and Medicaid are realized because patients are served in home situations for longer periods rather than higher-cost nursing homes and assisted living facilities. Older adults often prefer aging-in-place at home to living in a long-term care facility.

The PACE program supports everything from primary, specialty, and home medical and dental care to social services, transportation, meals, and support resources. Programs range from PACE vans that transport elders from home to a day center for services or social support to home care visit providers who administer medications and make home-cooked meals. Innovative care is encouraged because there is no constraint to a fee-for-service payment model. Services are provided as needed, supported by federal grants plus Medicare and Medicaid. Some services not covered by Medicare or Medicaid are built into the PACE model to improve overall health, including dental care, optometry, hearing aids, podiatry, prosthetics, and medical supplies. The system is capitated with a per-member, per-month payment structure. Barriers to access are overcome by supporting patients with lifetime enrollment, without limits on the amount or duration of care, and without co-payments, and deductibles.

The Denver-based InnovAge Greater Colorado PACE (IGCP) program is the largest PACE provider in the USA, and serves as a national model. It provides a rich setting to teach, treat, and implement progressive, cost-effective services for seniors with challenging care needs. IGCP includes a teaching component in which dental practitioners mentor and help advance the clinical skills of dental assistants, hygienists, and senior dental students. The IGCP dental staff teams with primary care providers so that patients receive all needed medical screenings and referrals as well as physical functioning assessments related to oral health, such as chewing and swallowing.

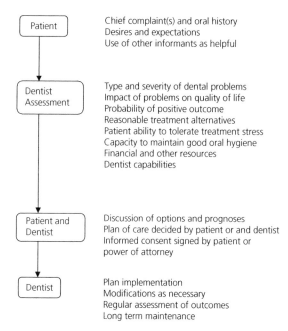

Patient	Chief complaint(s) and oral history Desires and expectations Use of other informants as helpful
Dentist Assessment	Type and severity of dental problems Impact of problems on quality of life Probability of positive outcome Reasonable treatment alternatives Patient ability to tolerate treatment stress Capacity to maintain good oral hygiene Financial and other resources Dentist capabilities
Patient and Dentist	Discussion of options and prognoses Plan of care decided by patient or and dentist Informed consent signed by patient or power of attorney
Dentist	Plan implementation Modifications as necessary Regular assessment of outcomes Long term maintenance

Figure 21.3 Steps in clinical decision making for geriatric dental patients.

IGCP delivers quality geriatric dental care while honoring aging adults using innovative delivery, interdisciplinary planning, and clinical care that regularly monitors outcomes and informs quality assessments. A key element is the use of the electronic health record to note relevant findings from multidisciplinary assessments in order to make effective clinical decisions based on factors pertinent to older patients. This includes considering the patient's ability to tolerate the stress of treatment, whether or not the patient can reasonably give informed consent, whether they can self-administer pain medications, and what staffing resources are available for patients with special needs. Students are especially encouraged to consider the steps outlined in Fig. 21.3 pertaining to appropriate treatment planning approaches.

IGCP also partners with other caregivers and social workers to provide comprehensive care for seniors. Overall this system helps improve and integrate oral health within a health home, especially for underserved populations. The needs of vulnerable populations are the top priority, with the focus on prevention as foundational for good health and an emphasis on quality care rather than administrative costs.

Advancing a policy agenda to improve the oral health of vulnerable elders

The National Elder Care Advisory Committee (NECAC) of the American Dental Association organized the National Coalition Consensus Conference on the Oral Health of Vulnerable Older Adults and Persons with Disabilities (ADA, 2010). The participants at this working conference generated recommendations that were refined and disseminated through a national webcast. Recommendations related to oral health delivery systems included the further establishment of delivery systems that meet the needs of vulnerable adults. They also recognized the value of replicating existing models of care that bring services to places where vulnerable adults live and receive general health services, social services and education services such as the PACE programs. The group acknowledged that as more clinicians, practices, and health systems use electronic health records, it will be important to ensure the inter-operability of the electronic records and telehealth technology. (In practical application, this would ensure that disparate systems can "talk" to each other.) This would ensure effective communication, collaboration, and referrals within and among dental professionals and other health professionals serving the elderly. Similarly, in the spirit of interdisciplinary education and collaboration, the group recommended the development and dissemination of guidance for general health and social service professionals about oral health prevention and treatment in order to function and make appropriate referrals within a comprehensive health home.

Conference participants recognized the importance of advocacy and efforts underway to expand Medicaid covered services for aged, blind, and disabled adults. This expanded coverage could include comprehensive preventive and restorative dental care in outpatient and inpatient settings, application of preventive medications such as fluoride varnish by nondentists, and reimbursement for behavioral management and home-based care, which is often necessary when caring for vulnerable elders. Funding is also needed to promote continued research on the general health implication of oral diseases in order to expand the evidence base and prepare advocacy positions to support payment for dental care that supports treatment of general health conditions. The complete

Case study 1

Heart transplantation for 77-year-old man

A 77-year-old man has a new heart, and his operation has kindled a debate on transplant surgery ethics. Ray Nelson received the heart from a 55-year old donor whose organ normally would have been rejected because of its advanced age. "One has to wonder whether or not the process was being manipulated to provide some advantage to someone who otherwise might not be eligible," said Dr. Atwater, a lecturer on medical ethics at the University Hospital.

Complications after a bypass operation last year forced Nelson, an active man who used to swim at least 50 laps a day, to be hospitalized in September. Ten days after his transplant at the University Hospital, he was up and talking.

The regional director of the hospital's cardiac science program said the hospital's transplant committee asked the hospital's ethics board for guidance in Nelson's case. The ethics board said that while age alone should not be the determining factor, it also noted that patients needing hearts far exceed the number of donor organs available. After rigorous debate, the transplant committee voted in a secret ballot to permit a transplant, but only if Nelson received a heart that would otherwise go unused. When the heart of a 55-year-old brain dead patient became available, no emergency cases were pending and Mr. Nelson received the transplanted heart.

Case study questions

1 Do you consider Mr. Nelson a "vulnerable elderly" patient? Why, or why not?
2 What is the average life expectancy for a white male born in 1920? Is Mr. Nelson "typical" in terms of the quantity and quality of life thus far as compared to other adults in his age cohort?
3 As a member of the transplant committee or the hospital's ethics board, would you approve Mr. Nelson's transplant? Why or why not?
4 Did "ageism" factor into the decision making of any of the individuals or groups in the news story? If so, how? And was it justified?
5 If Mr. Nelson lived in your state, would he be eligible for any publicly funded medical, dental and/or social service benefits?

Case study 2

Mrs. Ellie King's dentures

Mrs. Ellie King is a 77-year-old white female who lives in a federally subsidized senior apartment complex. She presents to a new dentist with a chief complaint that her "dentures don't fit. I feel like my jaws are melting away. I think it has something to do with my pyorrhea I had when I was young and my osteoporosis."

Past medical history

Mrs. King has been diagnosed with hypertension, poor circulation, occasional angina (chest pain), shortness of breath and ankle edema. She also complains of poor vision, even when she is wearing her glasses. She experiences occasional incontinence, and she was diagnosed with adult onset diabetes and osteoporosis about five years ago

Dental history

Mrs. King's teeth were extracted at age 27 due to "pyorrhea" (periodontal disease). At that time, her family dentist fabricated maxillary and mandibular dentures. She has been wearing the original dentures comfortably until about 2 years ago when the dentures became loose and began irritating her gums. She also commented that her mouth feels dry, especially with the new hypertension medicine that her doctor prescribed.

Health behaviors

For the previous 3 years Mrs. King has been taking nutritional supplements including a multivitamin, vitamin C, and vitamin E. She recently purchased additional supplements from a local health food store in order to prevent the aging process (superoxide dismutase and Coenzyme Q10). She thinks these supplements have been helpful to her, but they are very expensive and she sometimes has little money left to pay for groceries.

Mrs. King's doctor told her that exercise would be helpful in preventing her osteoporosis and heart disease from getting worse. She would like to exercise more, but she develops shortness of breath when she walks more than 50 yards, and she is afraid to walk in the downtown area because her neighbor recently had her purse stolen while walking in the neighborhood. So she spends most of her time in her apartment reading and watching television. Mrs. King recently read an article in *Reader's Digest* about the relationship between osteoporosis and tooth loss, as well as osteoporosis and "shrinking jaw bones" in people who wear dentures. She came to your office seeking advice and answers.

Case study questions

1 Do you consider Mrs. King a "vulnerable elderly" patient? Why, or why not?
2 What diseases or limitations is Mrs. King experiencing, are they common in her age cohort, and how are they impacting her oral health as well as her overall well-being?
3 If Mrs. King lived in your state, would she be eligible for any dental benefits under the Medicaid program?
4 What advice will you offer Mrs. King at her next dental appointment? Outline a specific set of recommendations and rationale.

Case study 3

Mr. Ellis's toothache

Mr. Ellis, an 82-year-old man, is very proud that he has retained almost all of his natural teeth with the exception of tooth no. 30, which was extracted when he was 17 years old. After enlisting in the Navy, he started to pay more attention to his daily mouth care, and became determined to retain all of his remaining "adult" teeth. After completing his tour of duty and returning home, he married his wife, June, and had three children. Mr. Ellis visited the family dentist at least once a year throughout his adult life until his dentist retired about 5 years ago. He and June recently enrolled in the Denver-based InnovAge Greater Colorado PACE (IGCP) program, and were happy to receive a comprehensive dental examination as a service provided by the program. He has found it increasingly difficult to maintain good oral hygiene because of his diabetes and related vision problems, as well as his Parkinson's disease. One of his upper molars has been causing him some discomfort while eating. He was discouraged to learn that four of his teeth have active root decay.

Case study questions

1 What are the key goals and characteristics of PACE programs? Who is eligible to participate in these programs? How are PACE programs funded, and what dental services could Mr. Ellis receive as a member of IGCP?
2 What are the advantages of utilizing an interdisciplinary team approach to address Mr. Ellis's oral health needs?
3 Explain the challenges associated with treatment planning for Mr. Ellis. Identify and discuss the key assessment and diagnostic information needed to develop an appropriately sequenced treatment plan for Mr. Ellis.

DISCUSSION QUESTIONS

1 What is meant by the "demographic imperative," and why is this important from political, social, financial, and healthcare perspectives?
2 What is a chronological definition of aging, and is this the most appropriate way to assess the healthcare needs of older adults?
3 Define the term "vulnerable elders."
4 What are "activities of daily living" and why are they important to the oral health assessment and treatment planning for vulnerable older dental patients?
5 Explain the concept of "ageism" and how it could potentially affect public policy or the health care of an older patient.
6 List and describe the most important health and social policies for older adults enacted in the USA during the 20th century. Explain the public funding currently available to fund dental services for low income and vulnerable elders.
7 What is meant by the term "medically necessary dental care?"

8 Provide examples of the growing evidence base suggesting a bidirectional relationship between oral health and overall health and well-being.
9 What is a "safety net" healthcare delivery system?
10 Provide an example of the use of technology in practice to better meet the needs of older patients.
11 Describe the key features of a PACE program, and compare and contrast this model of care to the more traditional model of health service delivery in the USA.
12 Select a strategy from the policy agenda to improve the oral health of vulnerable elders recently developed at an American Dental Association (ADA) -sponsored consensus conference, and describe how you would work to advocate, implement, and evaluate this strategy.

list of recommendation from the conference can be found in the published proceedings (ADA, 2010).

Summary

The aging of America is often referred to as the demographic imperative or "Age Wave." This dramatic growth in the number and proportion of older adults in the USA has important policy implications. This chapter explored the impact of our aging population on health policies, the preparation of health professionals, and the delivery of oral health services. In looking to the future, this chapter also explored innovative models of care delivery to better meet the health needs of older patients. Case studies are included to illustrate some key concepts in geriatric dentistry and to help the reader integrate their understanding of demographic and sociological shifts in the USA and their relationship to the delivery of dental care for older adults.

References

ADA (American Dental Association) (2009) *2007 Oral Health Care of Vulnerable Elderly Patients Survey.* From http://www.ada.org/sections/publicResources/pdfs/oral_elderly_survey.pdf. Accessed April 18, 2014.

ADA (American Dental Association) (2010) *Proceedings: National Consensus Conference on Oral Health of Vulnerable Older Adults and Persons with Disabilities.* From http://www.ada.org/sections/newsAndEvents/pdfs/2010_nccc_proceedings.pdf. Accessed April 18, 2014.

ADA (American Dental Association) (2011) *Breaking Down Barriers to Oral Health for All Americans: Repairing the Tattered Safety Net. A Statement from the American Dental Association.* American Dental Association, Chicago.

AoA (Administration on Aging) (2012) *Older Americans Act.* From http://www.aoa.gov/AoA_programs/OAA/index.aspx. Accessed April 18, 2014.

Bryce, D.V. & Friedland, R.B. (1997) *Economic and Health Security: an Overview of the Origins of Federal Legislation.* The National Academy on Aging, Washington, DC

Bureau of Health Professions (1993) *Grants for Faculty Training Projects in Geriatric Medicine and Dentistry, Program Guide.* Health Resources and Services Administration, Washington, DC.

CDC (Centers for Disease Control and Prevention) (2003) *Health, United States, 2003.* DHHS Pub No. 2003-1232. National Center for Health Statistics, Hyattsville, MD.

CMS (Centers for Medicare and Medicaid Services) (2013) *Medicare Dental Coverage.* From http://www.cms.gov/Medicare/Coverage/MedicareDentalCoverage/index.html?redirect=/MedicareDentalCoverage/. Accessed April 18, 2014.

Committee on Medicare Coverage Extensions (2000) *Carriers Manual, Section 2136 [HCFA, 1999b].* Centers for Medicare and Medicaid Services, Baltimore.

Dolan, T.A. & Atchison, K.A. (1993) Implications of access, utilization, and need for oral health care by the noninstitutionalized and institutionalized elderly on the dental delivery system. *Journal of Dental Education,* **57**(12), 876–87.

Dolan, T.A., Atchison K.A. & Huynh, T.N. (2005) Access to dental care among older adults in the United States. *Journal of Dental Education,* **69**(9), 961–74.

Dolan, T.A., Peek, C.W., Stuck, A.E., *et al.* (1998) Functional health and dental service use among older adults. *Journal of Gerontology: Medical Science,* **53**(6), M413–18.

Dychtwald, K. & Flower, J. (1989) *The Age Wave: How The Most Important Trend Of Our Time Can Change Your Future.* Bantam Books, New York.

Ettinger, R.L. & Beck, J.D. (1984) Geriatric dental curriculum and the needs of the elderly. *Special Care in Dentistry* **5**, 207–13.

Field, M.J., Lawrence, R.L. & Zwanziger, L., eds. (2000) *Extending Medicare Coverage for Preventive and Other Services.* The National Academies Press, Washington, DC.

Hirth, V., Baskins, J. & Dever-Bumba, M. (2009) Program of All-Inclusive Care (PACE): past, present, and future. *Journal of the American Medical Directors Association,* **10**, 155–60.

Hooyman, N. & Kiyak, H.A. (2010) *Social Gerontology: A Multidisciplinary Perspective,* 9th edition. Allyn and Bacon, Boston.

IOM (Institute of Medicine) (2008) *Retooling for an Aging America. Building the Health Care Workforce.* The National Academies Press, Washington, DC.

IOM (Institute of Medicine) & NRC (National Research Council) (2011) *Improving Access to Oral Health Care for Vulnerable and Underserved Populations.* The National Academies Press, Washington, DC.

IPEC Expert Panel (2011) *Core Competencies for Interprofessional Collaborative Practice: Report of an Expert Panel.* Interprofessional Education Collaborative, Washington, DC. From http://www.aacn.nche.edu/education-resources/ipecreport.pdf. Accessed April 18, 2014.

IPEC (2013) Interprofessional Education Collaborative website. From https://ipecollaborative.org/. Accessed April 18, 2014.

Katz, D.L. (1997) *Epidemiology, Biostatistics and Preventive Medicine Review.* W. B. Saunders Co., Philadelphia.

Katz, S., Ford, A.B., Moskowitz R.W., *et al.* (1963) Studies of illness in the aged. *Journal of the American Medical Association,* **185**, 94–9.

Li, S., Williams, P.L. & Douglass, C.W. (2011) Development of a clinical guideline to predict undiagnosed diabetes in dental patients. *Journal of the American Dental Association,* **142**, 28–37.

McGinn-Shapiro, M. (2008) *Medicaid Coverage of Adult Dental Services.* National Academy for State Health Policy. From http://nashp.org/publication/medicaid-coverage-adult-dental-services. Accessed April 18, 2014.

NIDCR (National Institute of Dental and Craniofacial Research) (2000) *Oral Health in America: a Report of the Surgeon General.* US Department of Health and Human Services, National Institutes of Health, Rockville, MD.

NIDDK (National Institute of Diabetes and Digestive and Kidney Diseases) (2011) *National Diabetes Statistics, 2011.* NIH Publication No. 11-3892. US Department of Health and Human Services, Bethesda, MD.

Tarpenning, M. (2005) Geriatric oral health and pneumonia risk. *Clinical and Infectious Diseases,* **40**, 1807–10.

US Census Bureau (2002) Population by Age and Sex for the United States: 1900 to 2000, Part A. Census 2000 Special Reports, Series CENSR-4, Demographic Trends in the 20th Century, 2002.

US Census Bureau (2006) *Facts for Features.* From http://www.census.gov/newsroom/releases/pdf/cb06-ffse01-2.pdf. Accessed April, 18, 2014.

US Census Bureau (2008) *Projections of the Population by Age and Sex for the United States: 2010 to 2050 (NP2008-T12),* Population Division, US Census Bureau; Release Date: August 14, 2008.

Answer Section

Chapter 14: Multiple choice questions

Question 1 Correct answer is B
Question 2 Correct answer is D
Question 3 Correct answer is D
Question 4 Correct answer is C
Question 5 Correct answer is B
Question 6 Correct answer is A
Question 7 Correct answer is A
Question 8 Correct answer is C
Question 9 Correct answer is B
Question 10 Correct answer is E
Question 11 Correct answer is D

Chapter 17: Multiple choice questions

Question 1 Correct answer is B
Question 2 Correct answer is D
Question 3 Correct answer is A
Question 4 Correct answer is C
Question 5 Correct answer is E
Question 6 Correct answer is E
Question 7 Correct answer is B

Chapter 18: Discussion questions

Question 1 Benzodiazepines Valium®, Halcion®, and Ativan®, plus nitrous oxide
Question 2 Aribex's NOMAD® or NOMAD-Pro® portable handheld unit, plus DEXIS® instant imaging systems with a laptop, or Ergonom-X® self-developing dental film
Question 3 Rainbow® Stabilizing System with Velcro® hand, knee and head gentle restraints
Question 4 Open Wide® mouth rest, Molt mouth gag, Jennings bilateral mouth prop, Logibloc®, McKesson, and Isolite® systems
Question 5 Mobile units are readily wheeled from room to room within a facility, whereas portable dentistry units are assembled, disassembled and transported off-site.
Question 6 If a piece of equipment fails or if a supply is exhausted, the procedure may need to be aborted and completed at a later date.

Chapter 20: Discussion questions

Question 1 Correct answer is Case 1
Question 2 Correct answer is Physician and Nursing Staff
Question 3 Correct answer is Bisphosphonates and Denosumab
Question 4 Correct answer is B
Question 5 Correct answer is C
Question 6 Correct answer is A
Question 7 Correct answer is B
Question 8 Correct answer is D
Question 9 Correct answer is B
Question 10 Correct answer is C

Geriatric Dentistry: Caring for Our Aging Population, First Edition. Edited by Paula K. Friedman.
© 2014 John Wiley & Sons, Inc. Published 2014 by John Wiley & Sons, Inc.
Companion website: www.wiley.com/go/friedman/geriatricdentistry

Index

Note: page numbers in *italics* refer to figures, those in **bold** refer to tables, case studies and boxes

---

Geriatric Dentistry: Caring for Our Aging Population, First Edition. Edited by Paula K. Friedman.
© 2014 John Wiley & Sons, Inc. Published 2014 by John Wiley & Sons, Inc.
Companion website: www.wiley.com/go/friedman/geriatricdentistry

Printed and bound by CPI Group (UK) Ltd, Croydon, CR0 4YY

27/10/2024

14580246-0004